D1552326

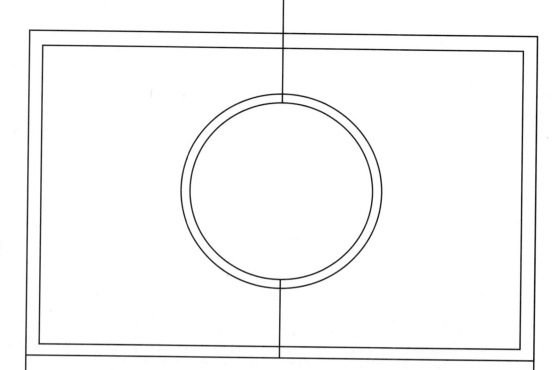

Understanding
Medicare
Managed Care
Meeting Economic, Strategic, and Policy Challenges

Louis F. Rossiter

Health Administration Press, Chicago, Illinois

Copyright © 2001 by the Foundation of the American College of Healthcare
Executives. Printed in the United States of America. All rights reserved. This book
or parts thereof may not be reproduced in any form without written permission of
the publisher. Opinions and views expressed in this book are those of the author
and do not necessarily reflect those of the Foundation of the American College of
Healthcare Executives.

05   04   03   02   01   5   4   3   2   1

Library of Congress Cataloging-in-Publication Data

Rossiter, Louis F.
    Understanding medicare managed care : how competing choices meet the
economic, strategic, and policy challenges facing our health care system /
Louis F. Rossiter.
        p.   cm.
    ISBN 1-56793-143-X (softcover : alk. paper)
    1. Medicare.   2. Managed care plans (Medical care). I. Title.
RA412.3 .R675   2000
368.4'26'00973—dc21   00-058207
                                                                    CIP

The paper used in this publication meets the minimum requirements of American
National Standards for Information Sciences—Permanence of Paper for Printed
Library Materials, ANSI Z39.48–1984. ⊚ ™

Health Administration Press
A division of the Foundation
    of the American College of
    Healthcare Executives
One North Franklin Street
Suite 1700
Chicago, IL 60606
(312) 424-2800

CONTENTS

Dedicated to Diana, Emily, Mary, and Pearl

ACKNOWLEDGMENTS

This book began to take shape around the time enrollment in Medicare managed care reached five million beneficiaries and the program turned 15 years old. Fifteen years and five million beneficiaries were proof that the program had matured into a permanent feature of Medicare, despite the ebb and flow of new enrollees. The time had come to document the development of this program in a book. So much had changed since the start of the program, and so much more is likely to change. As a result, someone needed to take a strategic, rather than a strictly operational, view of crucial events.

Having served on the initial selection panel for the very early Medicare managed care demonstration programs, I thought I had a unique sense of what Medicare was like before managed care. I remember well the initial excitement of seeing an entirely new alternative take seed. From 1983 to 1989, I was one of the principal investigators of the Health Care Financing Administration's (HCFA) national evaluations of what was then known as the "Medicare Risk-Contract" program. I am extremely grateful for the years of challenging health services research of a huge social experiment with my good friends Kathy Langwell and Randall Brown, who were both of Mathematica Policy Research at the time. Mathematica Policy Research and the Medical College of Virginia held the two evaluation contracts of the Medicare managed care program for nearly ten years. I am also extremely grateful for the wonderful friends and colleagues from the Medical College of Virginia who participated and led the research, especially Sheldon Retchin, M.D., and Barbara Brown. Later, Sheldon Retchin and Dolores Gurnick Clement did an outstanding job of taking over the leadership of the evaluation for HCFA when I joined the Office of the Administrator at HCFA.

There are many people at HCFA I must thank for contributing to the perspective I have of Medicare managed care. First, Gail Wilensky, former Administrator of HCFA and good friend, colleague, and coauthor on numerous publications, deserves special acknowledgment for trusting in my advice and offering so much of her own all along the way. Mike Hudson, former Deputy Administrator of HCFA, provided insightful views of the political economy of this program and its major players. All of the many folks who helped to manage the program in the past and in the present deserve special thanks. I am indebted to Ed Moy, Elizabeth Handley, Carlos Garaborzo, Gary Bailey, and especially Jean LeMaseurier for their experience and expertise. The researcher learned much from the people who really made the program what it is today. A special word of thanks goes to Sol Mussey for his helpful comments on an early version of Chapter 5. I want to mention Peter Neumann, who was the first to show me, even after a brief life at HCFA, it was still possible to find a book inside oneself.

I am grateful to a number of people who assisted along the way in the time leading up to preparation of this book and during its writing. Over the years, I had many graduate students who participated in the research and evaluation of Medicare managed care. These graduate students, who helped either by direct involvement in the topic or by extending my time and energy, include Terri Pointer, Eric Bell, Pat Randall, Jin Chern, Dawn Parker, Margaret Smith, Charles Shasky, Amy Heberger, Brian Jenkins, Brian Searles, William Carpenter, Chi-wen Pai, Tripp Welch, Viktor Bovbjerg, Leslie Kress, Dana Taylor, Ahmad Okasha, Jennifer Green, David McMillen, Ibrahim Ibrahim, Scott Johnson, Imre Solti, Michael Jurgensen, Kathy Scott, Julie Sydnor, Ron Fisher, Lawrence Patrick, David Meyer, Jennifer Troublefield, Jennifer Jackson, Sinan Sanvar, Raleigh Heard, Dan Goodwin, Susan Roman, and Michael Morrical.

I am grateful for the help received from the primary editor of the earliest drafts of the manuscripts, Jeff Finn. Jeff Finn has a superb store of practical, common-sense understanding of Medicare; the culture of the Medicare beneficiary; and older Americans in general. He also brought to the assignment a wealth of experience in communicating with the main audience of this book, gained during his years with the communications arm of the American Hospital Association and his time at HCFA. I will always be grateful for his honest assessments and "big picture" view of each chapter. He is responsible, more than anyone, for the readable, take-away messages that are so easy to find in the template we developed together. A second gifted writer and editor, David Hogge, dealt with the final versions of the manuscript and made the words all come together, unlocking the academic prose and opening it to a level of clarity I did not think was possible. My thanks also go to Rob Fromberg, former Associate Director, Health Administration Press, for his excellent good nature and encouragement.

The responsibility for the research rests solely with me. But I want to acknowledge the help I received from Susan Roggenkamp, Karen Swisher, and Deborah Draper, who lent me some of their research into medical groups, medical liability, and demand management programs. My dear colleague Roice Luke deserves special recognition for lending me his data on local hospital markets. I also drew heavily from the work done by my colleagues in the national evaluations of the program, including that done by Randy Brown, Kathy Langwell, and Sheldon Retchin. Thank you for publishing and disseminating your excellent research so that I could provide an assimilation in this form.

All of my faculty colleagues in the Department of Health Administration, Medical College of Virginia, Virginia Commonwealth University deserve a big thank you for allowing me to use my research time to prepare this book. I hope I made up for missed administrative duties after the draft was completed. I appreciate each one of you.

My thanks also go to the many millions of Medicare beneficiaries who have chosen the competitive option to the traditional federal program. Their revealed preferences demonstrate their concern with the cost and quality of their personal healthcare. Their actions display for all of us how competing choices support them in meeting the challenges they face in the healthcare system.

Louis F. Rossiter, Ph.D.
November 2000

PREFACE

The Medicare program provides health coverage to 40 million older and disabled Americans at a cost that approaches one-quarter trillion dollars in public expenditures, about 2.5 percent of the gross domestic product. On the basis of the sheer magnitude of these figures, few people would consider Medicare a small government program. Fewer still would even entertain the thought that the program offers limited benefits.

But when one considers the facts, one realizes that these perceptions need to be challenged. In reality, Medicare pays only about half the cost of medical care for beneficiaries because of its cost sharing, coverage limits, and noncoverage for certain types of nursing home care, drugs, and other services. And as a result of these factors, 70 percent of Medicare beneficiaries purchase supplemental health coverage in the private market. These beneficiaries—millions of people in thousands of local healthcare markets—voluntarily pay premiums to hundreds of private insurance companies for supplemental coverage or, in some cases, entirely private coverage that is publicly financed.

This private version of coverage, called Medicare managed care, competes for beneficiaries with the federally provided version of Medicare, which comes with nationwide benefits and mandatory rules governing coverage decisions and payments to hospitals and physicians. In most parts of the country, beneficiaries have a competing choice. Approximately 15 percent of beneficiaries (and this number is growing) choose to have the government pay a private health plan on their behalf to deliver health services. The private health plan then pays hospitals and physicians under essentially private rules. Normally, beneficiaries have financial incentives to use a defined network of hospitals and physicians that relies on special administrative systems for managing utilization and assuring quality of care.

In this competitive choice arrangement, administrators and providers face a variety of challenges. For instance, how can health plans, hospitals, and physicians participate in this market with sometimes arcane and complicated government rules? What operating strategies should hospital and health plan administrators pursue if they intend to manage utilization and assure quality of care? How can physicians attract and retain patients from this growing segment of beneficiaries and then treat them cost effectively? What policy

xvii

issues do healthcare executives need to address as they come to terms with the special economics of Medicare managed care?

Understanding Medicare Managed Care addresses these challenges. The book serves as a vital reference resource for managers of Medicare managed care plans, healthcare executives, and physicians—people who are dealing with the economics of Medicare managed care and who are looking for proven methods of operating strategically and successfully in the private side of the market. This book provides fresh insights into the trends and policy issues that affect Medicare managed care, and it gives healthcare professionals a structure for thinking strategically as they plot a long-term plan for competing in this market.

Understanding Medicare Managed Care is divided into 12 chapters, and each one could serve as a one-hour program to educate boards of directors, healthcare executives, physicians, administrators, and staff about Medicare managed care. These chapters fall comfortably into three parts. The first part is a primer or overview of the economics of the way the current system works. In this part, you will read about the trends and major players in the market, the history of Medicare managed care, and the current ways you can decide to participate as a private health plan under the new Medicare+Choice provisions of participation. The second part deals with the strategic planning and strategic marketing of Medicare managed care. The chapters in this part cover a variety of topics: pricing and the capitation dollar; benefit design, marketing, and enrollment; quality and cost-control techniques; disease management and the three imperative diseases; basic primary care; demand management; and provider liability. The third part speculates about future changes in this system and the healthcare marketplace and their implications for health plan participation.

Ultimately, the private domain of Medicare managed care and its variations is as vital and influential as the public domain, traditional fee-for-service. This public–private structure creates a competitive healthcare system that gives beneficiaries an essential set of choices, and these choices help drive transactions and shape human behavior. Without choice, Medicare loses its capacity to continually evaluate what people want from the program and how much it costs to provide the care they want. With choice, beneficiaries are free to continually examine the benefits and costs of alternatives and select the one that meets their needs. So far, nearly seven million older and disabled Americans have opted out of traditional fee-for-service Medicare and into Medicare managed care. Whether this level of enrollment increases depends on several critical factors, some of which are beyond the direct control of managed care plans. But many factors are within control of managed care plans. To that end, success derives from how well the leaders of managed care plans, healthcare executives, physicians, and other clinicians understand the competitive system in which they acquire and then care for patients.

The Economics of Medicare Managed Care

The purpose of Part I is to provide the leaders of health plans—board members, physicians or other clinicians, and managers—with a concise, simple description of the private side of Medicare, which is better known as **Medicare managed care**, for those unfamiliar with the various elements of the program. Part I serves as a useful set of readings that define the institutional and marketplace characteristics of Medicare managed care. In the four chapters that make up Part I, readers will learn how the private Medicare managed care market evolved, what decisions led to its early development, and how the program is organized. At the end of each chapter is a table that summarizes strategic decisions, providing a quick checklist for managed care plans operating in the market.

Chapter 1 begins with a brief explanation of the key economic aspects of Medicare and managed care. The traditional fee-for-service Medicare program is compared with the new Medicare+Choice program in the context of private Medicare supplement policies sold in the market. With these supplemental policies, a beneficiary can select either traditional fee-for-service medicine or managed care. Each selection offers a range of choices in terms of benefits and plan features, which affect the cost beneficiaries pay for coverage.

The changing nature of the Medicare program, given the broad alternative offered by managed care, has implications for the future of the program. For example, new Medicare beneficiaries are increasingly familiar with managed care because they are more likely to have been in a managed care plan through their employers, and this exposure is likely to have an impact on plan selection and service use. Changes in the program, as well as the shift in beneficiaries, set in motion the elements required to convert Medicare from a defined-benefit program to a defined-contribution program. Chapter 1 explains this conversion.

Chapter 2 examines trends, especially those that have determined and will determine who seeks coverage under Medicare and how these beneficiaries are distributed across the country. This chapter describes who the major players

Medicare managed care is a method used to deliver health services and to pay hospitals and physicians caring for Medicare beneficiaries. This method attempts to control or coordinate the use of services to contain expenditures, improve quality, or both. It always involves beneficiaries making a choice to enroll in an alternative to traditional fee-for-service Medicare. The alternatives have (1) a defined network of hospitals and physicians, (2) administrative systems for utilization management and quality assessment and improvement, and (3) financial incentives for enrollees to use the network of hospitals and physicians.

are in today's managed care market and the reasons for their success. In addition, the chapter describes the active markets and how they are structured. This chapter also includes a discussion on consumer perception about various health plans and the aspect of protection that each plan offers.

Chapter 3 provides a history of the program, including the legislative rationale for some of the features seen today in the program.

Chapter 4 provides more detail on the types of managed care arrangements permitted in Medicare. This chapter takes a close look at Medicare SELECT, a form of managed care with perhaps both its feet still in traditional fee-for-service. Chapter 4 also examines the range of new Medicare+Choice plans: HMOs, PPOs, PSOs, private fee-for-service plans, and high-deductible medical savings accounts.

INTRODUCTION TO MEDICARE MANAGED CARE

The purpose of Chapter 1 is twofold. First, it introduces readers to the basics of Medicare managed care. Second, the chapter examines Medicare, a regulated federal program, in the context of the largely voluntary private insurance market that has grown up around it. The chapter begins with a summary of traditional economics regarding the supply and demand of health services, and this is followed by a discussion of the important role choice plays in competitive markets. Subsequent sections of the chapter highlight the basic features of Medicare and the contrast between traditional fee-for-service and managed care. The chapter ends with a discussion about the economics of consumer choice as related to Medicare and explains the implications that choice will have on the future funding of Medicare.

The Economics of Medicare Managed Care

Social programs are not often considered laboratories for market-driven reform. Yet one of the largest public sector programs in existence anywhere—the Medicare program—offers an ample number of features of a dynamic, competitive marketplace. In fact, these features account for the widespread acceptance of Medicare. The acceptability comes from not only the millions of Americans who are beneficiaries of Medicare, but also from the physicians, hospitals, and **health plans** that offer health services to these people. To understand how these competitive forces work in Medicare, it is important to examine the supply and demand sides of healthcare.

Health plans are organizations licensed by a government entity to act as insurer for an enrolled group of individuals or families.

Supply Side

First, consider that many of the 5,100 hospitals and 790,000 physicians participating as suppliers in the traditional Medicare **fee-for-service** program view the payments they receive for services as regulated pricing. Although these providers, or suppliers, are free to leave Medicare at any time and serve markets other than Medicare, few do. Instead, the vast majority of physicians and other providers take what the program will pay, no matter how much the hospital or physician chooses to provide in the way of services. In this fashion, then, Medicare competes with the rest of the healthcare economy. It does so with some level of success, given the participation levels of hospitals and

Fee-for-service is any method used to pay hospitals and physicians for individual medical services where the health plan pays more when more services are used.

physicians: 100 percent for hospitals and nearly 100 percent for physicians in the relevant Medicare medical specialties.

Demand Side

Now, consider that beneficiaries have the Medicare program and its contractors as broker, representative, and agent. As broker, the program helps beneficiaries purchase health services in the market. It standardizes information on the types of services purchased, and it organizes resources for answering questions about available hospitals, physicians, and managed care plans. Medicare also serves beneficiaries as a representative, taking steps to promote, if not influence, a more uniform quality of care. It even exacts legal sanctions against the few physicians, hospitals, nursing homes, laboratories, and health plans that repeatedly perform poorly. And, finally, Medicare strives to be a perfect agent for beneficiaries, improving their ability to be informed consumers of healthcare services and ensuring that they can compete in the private market for access to high-quality care. The demand for specific services and health plans varies widely by geographic area, health status, diseases, income, and other demographic factors. The variation in demand has little to do with what Medicare provides in the way of management or information. Rather, Medicare is a largely unmanaged, open-demand system on the public side.

Competitive Model and Economic Markets

Medicare promotes competition at a number of levels for beneficiaries who can make choices by voting "with their feet." On one level is the traditional program, in which beneficiaries are free to switch to any hospital or physician they please in any part of the country and still receive benefits under the program. This arrangement, which has been a feature of Medicare since its inception, sets up economic forces for physicians and hospitals to compete on perceived or real quality and amenities.

When there were no alternatives to the traditional fee-for-service sector, beneficiaries were largely shielded from the financial implications of their healthcare decisions. They had no choice but to accept a monolithic one-size-fits-all approach. This is not as true today; thanks to the competition taking place on a new level with Medicare managed care.

The Medicare managed care program allows beneficiaries to make choices "with their feet" regarding the entire financing and delivery system that will serve them. In the Medicare+Choice program, also known more generically as Medicare managed care, beneficiaries are free to change how their hospitals or physicians are paid and who pays them. They do so by choosing a particular Medicare+Choice health plan that gives them access to Medicare benefits. This aspect of beneficiary choice sets up a very strong economic force for managed care plans to compete on perceived or real quality and amenities and to adopt strategies for coordinating care.

At yet another level is the grand competition between the two sectors—traditional fee-for-service Medicare and Medicare managed care. An abundance of choice exists.

Medicare will soon limit the number of times a beneficiary can change between the traditional fee-for-service sector and a Medicare+Choice health plan to once every six months. This selection between plans will become more systematic with an annual government-organized open-enrollment period.

With such a formal enrollment process, and with better information for making decisions, the program is evolving toward a competitive model. The government's approach will encourage market behavior that will make it easier for beneficiaries to switch between sectors and among private health plans within sectors, and this will help the demand side of Medicare become more informed and deliberative. The regulated prices paid for covered services on the fee-for-service side of Medicare will remain. But managed care plans that can accept the equivalent of those regulated service prices and cover the same services (and more) while retaining satisfied beneficiaries will compete successfully in enrolling beneficiaries from the fee-for-service sector. The opportunity to make some reasonable financial return will provide health plans with the incentive to be successful.

As suppliers enjoy the freedom to enter private contracts with beneficiaries, they create new choices that are alternatives to the traditional fee-for-service Medicare program. With these choices, a more competitive market should evolve. This arrangement could also reveal ways of producing alternative services at a cost to beneficiaries that is just enough to keep them satisfied. Such levels of satisfaction distinguish the competitive model.

Money for Medical Care

At its inception in 1965, Medicare was hailed as representing a new dimension of Social Security and rights of citizenship for millions of Americans. "The main goals of the [Medicare] program were to decrease the financial burdens that the elderly incur in obtaining medical care services and to increase access to care" (Pauly, Kissick, and Roper 1988). By fiscal year 2002, under current law, Medicare is projected to grow to be the second largest category of federal spending (15 percent), exceeded only by Social Security (22 percent) (Congressional Budget Office 1997).

The United States currently devotes nearly 14 percent of all spending on goods and services in the economy on healthcare. Medicare pays 30 percent of that bill, which is the largest single source of payment for healthcare. At the same time, however, beneficiaries spend 30 percent of their largely fixed incomes on Medicare premiums and out-of-pocket costs (Kaiser Family Foundation 1998). Medicare costs working Americans, through payroll taxes,

Part A of Medicare (Hospital Insurance Program) pays providers directly and covers inpatient hospital care with a large deductible and further cost sharing over 60 days. Part A also covers skilled nursing facility care following a hospital stay, home health care, and hospice care.

Part B of Medicare (Supplemental Medical Insurance Program) has a monthly beneficiary premium and pays providers directly. Part B covers physician and other medical services, outpatient hospital care, ambulatory surgical services, laboratory services, outpatient mental health services, and some preventive services with a deductible and coinsurance of 20 percent for most services.

Part C of Medicare (Medicare+Choice) pays approved managed care plans to cover the services under Part A and Part B, usually combined with other supplemental services.

Defined-benefits coverage is an approach to providing medical benefits. With this coverage, Medicare

at least 1.45 percent of their working wage each and every labor hour, and that covers just the hospital portion of Medicare. The general tax funds of the U.S. Treasury have increasingly been used to pay for Medicare.

The money coming into the program is used to purchase much needed medical services in the open market, largely and traditionally on a fee-for-service basis. However, as described in Chapter 2, the creators saw a place for managed care plans even at the start of the program. Only now are such plans becoming major players in the program, and this is occurring in several parts of the country. Enrollment has been growing at a rate of about 100,000 new enrollees per month. Projections indicate enrollment in Medicare managed care plans will grow to 34 percent of enrollment in the year 2007 (Congressional Budget Office 1997).

This large, costly, essential program has always been big business to physicians and hospitals. Medicare pays more than $100 billion to hospitals and home health care agencies through **Part A of Medicare**. Through **Part B of Medicare**, nearly $50 billion is paid to physicians in private practice, and another nearly $20 billion is paid to the facility operators and physicians in the outpatient setting. The funds paid to Part B of Medicare are up for grabs, and current and still emerging varieties of managed care plans view it as big business, as Chapter 3 describes.

Managed care plans have an unprecedented opportunity to compete with the traditional fee-for-service program, still nearly in its original form, and offer better price and quality of care to Medicare beneficiaries. Health plans that successfully provide care at a better price will be rewarded with enrollment in their plans and premium payments per member per month from Medicare. They will also be rewarded with beneficiaries who will greatly add to overall health plan revenues and possible operating margin, although the profit made under Medicare is capped.

When managed care plans receive premium payments from Medicare, they have an obligation to pay for covered services for each enrolled beneficiary. These plans know that the predetermined per-member-per-month premium payments are all they will receive. This arrangement is known as **Part C of Medicare**.

Successfully operating in Part C of Medicare takes careful strategic efforts on the part of health plans. It can mean a major shift in the way dollars are used to deliver medical care. This book aims to help health plans make more effective strategic decisions concerning their participation in Part C of Medicare.

Traditional fee-for-service coverage (Part A and Part B) is known as **defined-benefits coverage**, and managed care coverage (Part C) is **defined-contribution coverage**. Defined-benefits coverage establishes a package of services that will be paid regardless of cost. The responsibility to pay for the services rests with the sponsor of the package, not the beneficiary. From the federal government's viewpoint, traditional fee-for-service is an open-ended fiscal arrangement because it is defined-benefits coverage. Managed care is a closed-ended fiscal arrangement because it is defined-contribution coverage. Defined-contribution coverage establishes an amount paid toward a service benefit. Thus, the contribution from the sponsor is capped, but the beneficiary can augment that amount. The next sections explain why this distinction is of utmost importance in the long run for physicians, hospitals, and managed care plans, and whether those entities view Medicare managed care as an opportunity or a threat.

Regulated Economics

The money for medical care flows out of the trust funds from Medicare in two highly regulated mechanisms, and Figure 1.1 illustrates this process. Each dollar sign represents a key payment to a supplier in the Medicare program. The program has two mechanisms for paying suppliers: the traditional fee-for-service system and the managed care system.

The traditional fee-for-service system, indicated on the left side of the diagram, pays hospitals and physicians through two mechanisms.

The first mechanism is the Hospital Insurance Trust Fund (labeled "A" in the diagram), which pays hospitals directly through private bill-paying contractors (intermediaries) using federal government rules. Under the current rules for hospitals, known as the prospective payment system, each hospital is paid a predetermined dollar amount for each hospital discharge. Known as **diagnosis-related groups (DRGs)**, the payments to hospitals are adjusted up and down for the various diagnoses assigned to the patient and several other factors. Hospitals receive more revenue from Medicare if they log more hospital discharges or discharges of a higher case mix.

or another sponsor provides funding for a specific package of medical services and is responsible for paying for that package.

Defined-contribution coverage *is another approach to providing medical benefits. With this coverage, the sponsor provides funding for a specific dollar contribution toward the cost of coverage and is responsible only for paying that contribution.*

Diagnosis-related groups *(DRGs) are classifications of patients by case mix, used for payment to hospitals. Patients are classified into groups with different levels of payment per inpatient hospital*

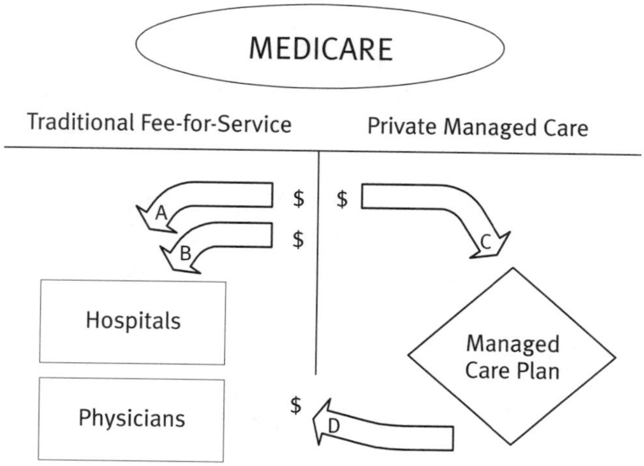

FIGURE 1.1
Traditional Fee-for-Service Medicare Versus Private Managed Care

Two choices: The regulated economics of Medicare managed care

The second mechanism for paying hospitals and physicians is the Supplemental Medical Insurance portion of Medicare (labeled "B" in the diagram). This mechanism primarily pays physicians directly through private bill-paying contractors (carriers) using federal government rules. Under the current rules, each physician is paid a predetermined dollar amount for each type of visit, service, or procedure. Based on a **resource-based relative-value scale** (RBRVS), payments to physicians are adjusted up and down for differences among visits, services, and procedures, as well as for the medical knowledge expected and for the time normally required to provide these services. These payments are also adjusted for office expenses, including malpractice costs. Physicians receive more revenue from Medicare if they provide more visits, services, or procedures, or if they serve a broader case mix.

The significant factors about A and B in Figure 1.1 are that they are fee-for-service and are directed almost entirely by the U.S. federal government through complex, uniform rules that are used throughout the country. Prices are given to the hospitals and physicians on a take-it-or-leave-it basis by the federal government. A physician has two choices for serving Medicare beneficiaries. The first option is to become a participating physician. To become participating, the physician agrees to receive the regulated payment as the only payment allowed, plus an allowed amount in cost sharing paid by beneficiaries, for all Medicare patients seen. The second option is to serve Medicare beneficiaries without becoming a participating physician. To become nonparticipating means the physician agrees to charge beneficiaries somewhat more than the allowed fee (up to a limit). However, Medicare pays the physician less. Nearly all physicians are participating physicians.

The managed care side of Figure 1.1 reflects an entirely different economic arrangement. To begin with, the dollars flow from Medicare to the managed care plan. The Medicare+Choice program (labeled "C" in Fig. 1.1) pays managed care plans directly from Medicare, and Chapter 4 describes this process in more detail. The payment, known as a Medicare+Choice payment, is an all-inclusive monthly premium payment for each person enrolled, and the amount is based on federal rates published once per year for the coming year. The current pricing rules allow each managed care plan a capitation payment, per member enrolled per month. These payments to managed care plans are adjusted up and down for differences in expected costs depending on the gender and age of the enrollee, as well as his or her institutional and Medicaid status. The system is described more fully in Chapter 5. Managed care plans receive more revenue if they enroll more beneficiaries. They receive no additional revenue for a beneficiary if he or she uses more services or costs the plan more than expected.

Competitive Economics

There are two profoundly different implications stemming from the regulated traditional fee-for-service (left) side versus the private managed care (right) side of Figure 1.1.

First, there are lofty implications for the strategic behavior of health plans. The managed health plan must know how to design benefits to supplement the Medicare-covered services, market to elderly and disabled individuals rather than employer groups, and retain its enrollment. After all, beneficiaries are allowed to switch health plans or return to the traditional fee-for-service program with only six months notice. The care must also be managed in a cost-effective, high-quality manner if the plan is to remain competitive in the market and maintain its financial health. In most major urban areas of the country, different managed care plans are designed to accomplish the same things, often to the detriment of other managed care plans in the local market. Thus, strategy is played out in a significantly more complex and competitive market than traditional fee-for-service Medicare.

Second, and perhaps the most significant aspect of Figure 1.1, is the change represented by the arrow labeled "D." The managed care plan, *not Medicare*, sets the rules for payment to hospitals and physicians, as well as to other providers. All dollars flow through private hands on the managed care side of Medicare, and the rules for paying each hospital and each physician are negotiated among the hospitals, physicians, and the managed care plan. These rules can take almost any form the health plan wishes to strike with the hospitals and physicians, subject to certain tests of substantial financial risk. As a result, hospitals and physicians compete with each other to be awarded the contracts, setting in motion unforgiving competitive pressures to maintain low costs for the health plan by minding prices and the use of services.

Consumer Choice Economics

Consumer choice enters the economic picture of Medicare managed care as illustrated in Figure 1.2. This figure presents Medicare from the standpoint of

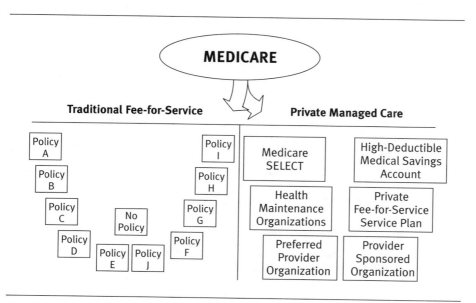

FIGURE 1.2

Ten Standard Medicare Supplemental Plans Versus Six Managed Care Plans

Consumer choice: The economics of Medicare managed care

Medicare supplemental policies fill Medicare coverage gaps in the market. Gaps in coverage that are paid by beneficiaries without supplemental policies include:

Inpatient hospital: Deductible $764. Copayments for days 61–90 are $190 per day. Copayments for lifetime reserve days 91–150 are $380 per day. Beyond day 150: all costs.

Skilled nursing facility care days 21–100: $95 per

a beneficiary eligible for the program, for whom two choices exist. The first is whether to enroll in traditional fee-for-service care or managed care. The second is which type of health plan to choose under each sector.

If the first choice is traditional fee-for-service care, a beneficiary may choose to have no supplemental Medicare policy. In that case, the beneficiary would face Medicare's substantial gaps in coverage. The most notable gaps include paying an inpatient deductible of more than $800 for each illness spell in the hospital, as well as 20 percent of approved charges for coinsurance for physician expenses.

Most beneficiaries, however, select from among ten standard so-called **Medicare supplemental (Medigap)** policies offered by private health insurance companies. These policies are not meant to organize the delivery of care. Rather, they are strictly a means for beneficiaries to prepay the likely costs of the gaps in Medicare coverage. These policies must be certified by the state in which the policy is sold as a Medicare supplemental policy, according to regulations passed by the Congress in 1990 (Omnibus Budget Reconciliation Act of 1990). Table 1.1 summarizes the ten traditional fee-for-service policies approved for marketing to Medicare beneficiaries as Medicare supplements. The premiums are generally progressively higher from Policy A through Policy I.

According to one study, three policy types dominate the market, accounting for about 60 percent of the premium sales of all policy types (Rice,

TABLE 1.1
Ten Standard Policies and Benefits

The federal way or the highway: Traditional fee-for-service supplemental policies approved for marketing to Medicare beneficiaries under OBRA, 1990

	Policies									
	A	B	C	D	E	F	G	H	I	J
Core Benefits[a]	√	√	√	√	√	√	√	√	√	√
SNF Coinsurance[b]			√	√	√	√	√	√	√	√
Part A Deductible		√	√	√	√	√	√	√	√	√
Part B Deductible			√			√				
Part B Excess Charges						Hi[c]	Lo[c]		Hi[c]	Hi[c]
Foreign Travel			√	√	√	√	√	√	√	√
At-Home Recovery				√			√		√	√
Prescription Drugs								Lo[d]	Lo[d]	Hi[d]
Preventive Medical Care					√					√

Source: NAIC. Medicare Supplemental Insurance Minimum Standards Model Act 6. July 30, 1991.
[a] Core benefits include coverage of all part A (hospital) coinsurance for stays longer than 60 days, the 20% Part B coinsurance, and the Parts A and B blood deductible.
[b] SNF is skilled nursing facility.
[c] Low excess charge coverage pays 80 percent of the difference between the physician's charge and the Medicare-allowable rate; high coverage pays 100 percent of the difference.
[d] Low prescription drug coverage has a $250 annual deductible, 50 percent coinsurance, and a maximum annual benefit of $1,250; high coverage is similar, but it has a $3,000 annual benefit.

Graham, and Fox 1997). Policy F is by far the most demanded type. Its core benefits include coverage of inpatient hospital copayments for stays longer than 60 days, the 20 percent physician services coinsurance, and the blood deductibles. In addition, Policy F covers skilled nursing facility coinsurance, the inpatient hospital deductible, the physician deductible, 100 percent of the excess charges of physicians above the approved amount, and foreign travel.

The next most demanded type is Policy C. In addition to core benefits, this policy covers skilled nursing home facility coinsurance, the inpatient deductible, the physician deductible, and foreign travel.

The third most demanded type is Policy B. This policy covers core benefits along with the inpatient hospital deductible. The remaining seven policies account for 2 percent to 8 percent of the market demand.

The private market is dominated by individual beneficiaries who decide which policy to purchase. These beneficiaries then pay the premium entirely out of pocket based on their understanding and their family's understanding of their needs. Approximately 70 percent of the market is individual coverage, and this is marketed either directly by the supplemental insurer through print and electronic media or through independent brokers who receive a commission.

In 1995, 352 insurance companies sold Medicare supplemental policies and collected premiums totaling $12.5 billion. Of those companies, 33 dominate the market, reporting premiums of more than $100 million and accounting for almost 75 percent of the total (GAO 1998). The most notable of these companies are United HealthCare, Bankers Life & Casualty Company, Empire Blue Cross & Blue Shield, and many other local and regional Blue Cross and Blue Shield health plans.

Approximately 30 percent of the market with insurance is provided by group policies paid for in full or in part by the current employer or previous employer of someone on Medicare. In this case, the benefits manager makes the purchase decision as part of an overall package of retiree benefits. Depending on how much of the premium is paid for by the employer, the choice of policy type will be made by the employer. Group policies in the Medicare supplement market tend to be found in the Northeast and the Midwest in connection with large manufacturing employers with a history of unions and large retiree populations.

An emerging issue is to what extent group policies, which are primarily traditional fee-for-service policies, can be converted to managed care policies. There are associated issues regarding mandatory enrollment in a managed care plan that might restrict choice of physician or hospital to receive the premium payment from the employer.

Approximately 25 percent of beneficiaries have no private supplemental policy (Fig. 1.3). Many are eligible for state Medicaid programs and are considered dually eligible for Medicare and Medicaid. Others are eligible

day. Home health and durable medical equipment: 20% of approved amounts.

Physician: Annual deductible: $100, 20% of approved charges. Physicians not accepting assignment 100% of limited excess charges.

Outpatient drugs: all costs. Routine exam: all costs. Podiatry care: all costs. Care outside the US: all costs. Dental, hearing, and vision care: all costs.

for the benefits of coverage from the Department of Veterans Affairs. Many, however, face Medicare coverage gaps with no assistance, paying out of pocket for the cost-sharing provisions of Medicare.

Those dually eligible for Medicare and Medicaid and the dually eligible for Medicare and Veterans coverage are extremely specialized population groups, with very high expenses, and very low likelihood of enrollment in private Medicare managed care. They are unlikely to be in Medicare managed care because coordinating benefits from two government payers for very high cost groups is complex. Experiments are under way to demonstrate how coordinated premiums and benefits can be administered to enroll in Medicare+Choice plans, but dually eligible beneficiaries rarely select the Medicare managed care option. As a result, they will not be discussed in this book.

On the managed care side of the market in Figure 1.3, Medicare managed care accounts for less than 20 percent of the market nationwide. Enrollment in Medicare+Choice HMOs has about 13 percent market share, Medicare SELECT has less than 3 percent of the market, and other Medicare+Choice managed care plans have less than 1 percent of the market. But all that could change.

As Figure 1.2 demonstrates, beneficiaries have two broad choices with Medicare: traditional fee-for-service and Medicare managed care. Under managed care, a beneficiary may choose from among six basic types of managed care plans. Unlike the traditional supplemental policy, these also arrange for the delivery of care. Yet they all offer beneficiaries the economic protection from Medicare cost-sharing provisions equal to or exceeding those offered by the traditional supplemental policies. That is one of the principal drawing cards for Medicare managed care. There are no rules or regulations regarding the mix of supplemental benefits as long as Medicare coverage is included, but coverage generally tends to be richer compared with the fee-for-service

FIGURE 1.3

Traditional Fee-for-Service and Private Managed Care Market Share, 1998

Private coverage rules: Most beneficiaries have some or all private insurance

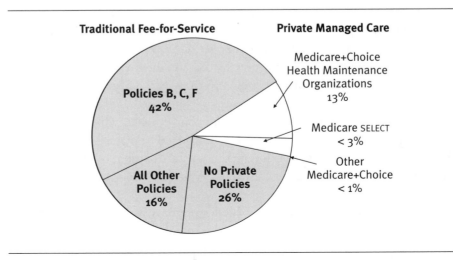

Traditional Fee-for-Service

Policies B, C, F
42%

All Other Policies
16%

No Private Policies
26%

Private Managed Care

Medicare+Choice Health Maintenance Organizations
13%

Medicare SELECT
< 3%

Other Medicare+Choice
< 1%

supplements. Those in Medicare managed care do not need any other supplemental coverage. Some beneficiaries retain their supplemental coverage as
further assurance that if they drop out of a Medicare+Choice plan they will
still have traditional supplemental coverage.

The dominant type of managed care coverage selected by beneficiaries
today is the **Medicare+Choice HMO**. This type of coverage must be licensed
by the state insurance commissioner or federally qualified under the HMO
Act of 1973. The benefit package for HMOs is flexible in terms of how
it supplements and coordinates with Medicare coverage, and it normally
has minimal cost-sharing arrangements, including no deductibles. In other
words, Medicare+Choice plans are under no obligation to adhere to ten
standard policies. They are free to experiment with benefits and respond to
the local market.

Most managed care plans request that new enrollees select a primary
care doctor from those who are part of the plan. If a selection is not made, one
will be assigned to the enrollee. Normally a primary care doctor is responsible
for managing the patient's medical care, admitting to a hospital, and referring
to specialists. To that end, the primary care doctor serves as a type of case
manager for the beneficiary who gains access to services through the managed
care system.

HMOs have lock-in requirements. That means the enrollee generally
is locked into receiving all covered care from the doctors, hospitals, and other
medical care providers who are affiliated with the HMO. In most cases, if
the enrollee goes outside the plan for services, neither the plan nor Medicare
will pay. The enrollee will be responsible for the entire bill. Medicare+Choice
plans recognize two exceptions to this lock-in policy. The first is emergency
services, which may be received anywhere in the United States, and the second
is urgently needed care, which may be received while temporarily away from
the plan's service area. Some plans offer coverage while traveling overseas
or out of the country for an extra fee as well. Medicare does not provide
this coverage.

A variation on the HMO option is the **point-of-service option**. Under the point-of-service option, the plan permits enrollees to receive certain
services outside the plan's established hospital and physician network, and the
plan will pay a percentage of the charges. In return for this flexibility, enrollees
must pay a portion of the cost, usually at least 20 percent of the bill.

To end enrollment in a managed care plan and return to the traditional
fee-for-service sector, Medicare beneficiaries send a signed request form to
the plan or to their local Social Security Administration office. Beneficiaries
return to traditional fee-for-service Medicare the first day of the next month.
To change from one managed care plan to another, beneficiaries simply enroll
in the other plan through the new plan. Disenrollment from the first plan
is automatic. Coverage under the new plan begins on the first day of the
following month.

Medicare+Choice HMO is a type of managed care plan that acts as both insurer and provider of a comprehensive set of healthcare benefits to an enrolled population. Benefits are paid for through a predetermined premium that does not change with service use of the enrollee. Services are furnished through a network of affiliated hospitals and physicians that must be used or no coverage is provided.

Point-of-service option lets HMO enrollees decide whether they will use network or non-network hospitals and physicians when they need care. Patients are usually charged sizable copayments for selecting hospitals and physicians not in the health plan's network.

Medicare SELECT plans are traditional Medicare supplement insurers that provide supplemental benefits through a defined network of hospitals and physicians. Coverage of supplemental benefits is limited to those services furnished by participating network hospitals and physicians, plus emergency and out-of-service-area care. Enrollees can use the hospitals and physicians outside the network and receive Medicare coverage, but they face the gaps in Medicare coverage in doing so.

Medicare SELECT **plans** are currently the second largest form of Medicare managed care and must adhere to the ten standard policies. They are a hybrid policy, falling somewhere between traditional fee-for-service policies because they are marketed like the regular supplements, and they do not change the fee-for-service relationship between Medicare and hospitals or physicians. Medicare continues to pay on a fee-for-service basis as usual. On the other hand, they act as managed care plans because they provide strong incentives for beneficiaries to use a defined network of hospitals and physicians. Beneficiaries enrolled in Medicare SELECT plans use the network of hospitals and physicians or pay the gaps in Medicare coverage for each service they access outside the network. The requirement to use the network of hospitals and physicians or face Medicare cost sharing is offered by Medicare SELECT plans in return for a lower monthly premium for the beneficiary. The policies are viewed as a modest adoption of managed care to permit beneficiaries to try a limited network with minimal consequences.

The government authorizes several other types of Medicare+Choice managed care plans. They possess virtually no market share (Fig. 1.3) and are still evolving as known players in the market. They were added to the mix by the Balanced Budget Act of 1997 for two reasons: to expand beneficiary choice and to capture innovations for Medicare in the private sector that are so apparent in the non-Medicare commercial market.

These innovations have been widely adopted in the commercial market because employers are being pressured to lower their premium costs for the employment-based private coverage they provide employees. The share of workers in firms with ten or more employees in traditional service benefits plans has plummeted from 65 percent in 1986 to less than 33 percent in 1996 (Gabel et al. 1997). In addition to the growing enrollment in HMOs, the innovations have encompassed preferred provider organizations (PPOs) and provider sponsored organizations (PSOs).

Medicare+Choice Preferred Provider Organizations (PPOs) offer benefits through a defined network of hospitals and physicians for all benefits. Coverage for Medicare and supplemental benefits is limited to those services furnished by participating network hospitals and physicians, plus emergency and out-of-service-area

The new provisions for Medicare are designed as a possible vehicle for the same sort of choice and innovation in the commercial market to come to Medicare. Briefly, these innovations include **Medicare+Choice PPOs** and **Medicare+Choice PSOs.** When compared with HMOs, both these forms of Medicare managed care may have weaker incentives for cost control when it comes to paying hospitals and physicians and for encouraging beneficiaries to use their network of hospitals and physicians. From a beneficiary's point of view, they look like any HMO in terms of benefits and requirements to use hospitals and physicians within the network. In practice, they are more likely to have different ownership than HMOs, and they are much more closely aligned with hospitals and physicians. Both types of plans, nevertheless, receive a predetermined monthly premium payment from Medicare to cover all Medicare services. Thus, these plans assume a large risk when compared with the risk assumed by any HMO.

The same is true for **Medicare+Choice private fee-for-service plans** and **high-deductible medical savings accounts (MSAs).** Private fee-for-service plans must rely on high premium payments to remain financially healthy. The Medicare+Choice payment is all they will receive from Medicare, and they must provide all Medicare covered services with little in the way of cost controls. However, such plans face no limits on the premiums they charge, so they can raise sufficient premium revenue to cover all their costs as long as beneficiaries are willing to enroll in the plan. Physicians in private fee-for-service plans may also charge beneficiaries up to 15 percent above the health plan fee schedule (which may be higher or lower than Medicare's). Private fee-for-service plans offer significant flexibility in premiums, payments to physicians and hospitals, and the delivery system, but their costs could be high when compared with alternatives.

High-deductible MSAs should be very attractive to beneficiaries who wish to arrange for their own care and have maximum flexibility over the funds they use to pay hospitals and physicians. Beneficiaries can use the MSA account to pay for services not normally covered by Medicare. Medicare's contributions and interest or gains on the account are exempt from taxes. Withdrawals are not taxed or subject to penalties if used for qualified medical expenses, such as hospital and physician fees. Other withdrawals will be included in beneficiary gross-income calculation for tax purposes to discourage the use of MSA accounts for purposes not related to healthcare.

High-deductible MSAs are only experimental at the time of this writing. Up to 390,000 Medicare beneficiaries may enroll between 1999 and 2002. The Health Insurance Portability and Accountability Act of 1995 (P.L.104-191) authorized an MSA demonstration for employed individuals who are not yet eligible for Medicare, but high-deductible MSAs are unprecedented in Medicare. They are likely to be most attractive to beneficiaries with very low expected spending for Medicare-covered services and high disposable income to pay for services as they require them.

Enough Money for Medical Care

At one level, the economics of the program are quite clear and very simple. Funds flow in to the Medicare program from beneficiary contributions, payroll tax revenues, and general fund tax revenues. Funds flow out of Medicare to hospitals, physicians, home health agencies, nursing homes, and device manufacturers to pay for medical services eventually required by nearly every person in this country before they die.

One side of Medicare achieves the flow of funds via a traditional fee-for-service system that has been at work for nearly 35 years. The other, newer, private side of Medicare achieves the flow of funds by means of large, well-established managed care plans under a system that has been at work for about 15 years.

care. Enrollees can use the hospitals and physicians outside the network, but they are usually charged sizable copayments for doing so.

Medicare+Choice Provider Sponsored Organizations *(PSOs) are like HMOs or PPOs, except in ownership and organization, rather than the product they offer. They are managed care plans formed by hospitals or physicians (or both), with a requirement that the hospitals and physicians be affiliated with each other and that PSOs in urban areas deliver at least 70 percent of Medicare services themselves.*

Medicare+Choice private fee-for-service plans *cover Medicare benefits and supplemental benefits. However, they must pay all hospitals and physicians on a fee-for-service basis at rates determined by the plan without placing the hospital or physician at financial risk. They may not vary payment rates on the basis of utilization, and they may not restrict hospital or physician participation.*

Apart from this picture of the economics of Medicare managed care is the looming economic issue of whether there is sufficient public and private money to sustain both sides of the system. Medicare expenditures account for roughly 2.5 percent of all the goods and services produced in the U.S. economy. Is this level of spending sustainable? Will it be cut? Or will it be augmented with funds for other types of spending, such as prescription drugs for the elderly?

Where the Money Comes From

Part A of Medicare, the Hospital Insurance Trust Fund, is funded primarily by a payroll tax on current workers. This trust fund earmarks money for primarily paying Medicare Part A hospital expenses. The Part A Trust Fund receives revenues equal to 2.9 percent of worker-earned income, half paid by the employer and half paid by the employee. Expenses have exceeded trust fund revenues since 1995, forcing money to be spent from Part A Trust Fund reserves. Without legislative action, the Part A Trust Fund will be exhausted by 2008 (Board of Trustees 1998).

The Part B services are also paid by a trust fund that depends on beneficiary premium payments, but this fund has been primarily supported by general tax revenue for many years. Any reduction in the expenses covered by the Part B Trust Fund or an increase in premiums has the effect of reducing annual federal budget deficit or increasing the surplus.

Every day of the year, the funds flowing into the program from all sources must be balanced with the funds flowing out of the program. The Medicare budget can be balanced either by increasing the in-flow or decreasing the out-flow of dollars. If a balance is not achieved, public confidence in the program will be severely undermined, hospitals and physicians might not be paid, and beneficiaries might not receive services unless they pay for them out-of-pocket. It is difficult to imagine this could happen, of course, because the program is so large, and politically powerful forces would ensure a balanced budget. But thoughtful legislators know they must fashion a long-term solution to the looming Medicare Trust Fund deficits.

Where the Money Goes

Medicare managed care represents an approach to balancing the Medicare budget based on the outflow of funds. By offering an alternative to Medicare beneficiaries, it provides a competitive check on the fee-for-service sector. If Medicare fee-for-service payments are cut too far and hospitals and physicians provide poor-quality care or refuse to accept new Medicare patients, beneficiaries can join a health plan in the managed care sector. If managed care plans raise their supplemental premiums too high, skimp on necessary services, or provide poor care coordination, beneficiaries can join the fee-for-service sector.

In a sense, the private managed care portion of Medicare offers beneficiaries a clear option. They can take what Medicare would pay a managed care plan and supplement that payment with their own funds to purchase what they want and what they can find in the market. Managed care plans in the market can continually strive to design the benefit packages, network of hospitals and physicians, and plan administration features that are enough to make beneficiaries switch to managed care. The monolithic Medicare traditional fee-for-service sector is fundamentally the same today as it was at its inception. The newer Medicare managed care sector, on the other hand, is still evolving. And it is precisely that feature, the plan's inclination to innovate, that makes it ultimately alluring through its advertising and drive for attractive benefits beyond the standard Medicare package.

Strategic Implications: Will the Balance Tip?

As Medicare managed care reaches about half the life span (15 years) of traditional fee-for-service (35 years) and approaches one-fifth its size, it seems clear that a number of forces are fostering managed care's progressive gain in strategic importance for hospitals, physicians, and traditional and managed care health plans.

Forces Driving Change

Current legislative forces and long-term demographic forces are driving change in Medicare managed care. The legislative forces today are new provisions in the types of managed care plans that can participate. They give nearly every type of private market player an opportunity to compete for market share. Legislative forces are also pressuring Medicare to set adequate payments that respond to the requirements of Medicare managed care plans and their enrollees. In the longer term, however, demographic forces will provide the most persuasive rationale for Medicare managed care. A growing share of beneficiaries will be coming into the program as they age. They will already be familiar with managed care because they are likely to have belonged to well-known health plans during their working careers.

Nevertheless, the competitive nature of the traditional fee-for-service market and the private managed care market allows the scales to tip toward private managed care as illustrated in Figure 1.4.

Medicare continues to see increases in the volume and intensity of services that push up expenditures. Inpatient hospital length of stay has fallen, and spending for inpatient hospital services has slowed to 6.7 percent per enrollee between 1990 and 1996. But spending per beneficiary in the same period for outpatient services grew 10 percent per year, skilled nursing facilities 25.1 percent per year, home health 28.7 percent per year, and hospice 34.3 percent year. The growing share of federal and national health expenditures and the historical contribution of healthcare spending to the federal budget deficit make Medicare a primary focus when attempting to constrain federal spending. The Congress has dealt with this problem by cutting payments

FIGURE 1.4

The Forces
Driving Change
in Medicare

*The strategic
implications:
Could the
balance tip
toward private
managed care?*

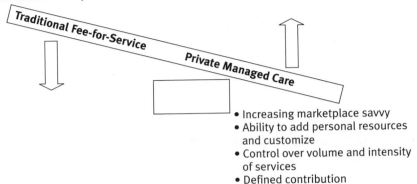

- Increasing volume and intensity of services
- Regulated payments to providers
- Fraud and abuse
- Defined benefit plan

Traditional Fee-for-Service

Private Managed Care

- Increasing marketplace savvy
- Ability to add personal resources and customize
- Control over volume and intensity of services
- Defined contribution

to hospitals and physicians under traditional fee-for-service Medicare. But such regulations on payments to hospitals and physicians are unlikely to keep pace with private offers from Medicare managed care plans to reconfigure the payments to serve their enrollees. New regulations attempting to slow the spending on skilled nursing facilities, hospital outpatient services, inpatient rehabilitation facilities, and home health agencies will have a similar effect.

Growth of fraud and abuse will make the traditional fee-for-service program increasingly costly to operate. In the end, however, the open nature of traditional fee-for-service Medicare as a defined-benefit plan make it economically untenable without significant increases in the public revenues that support it. Conversion to a defined-contribution plan gives the medical marketplace, rather than the government, the hard task of saying: "There is only so much money to go around for healthcare."

As long as payments to managed care plans are even partially pegged to fee-for-service costs, as they are today, managed care plans should be successful. These plans should be able to take the Medicare payment, combine it with what beneficiaries are willing to pay, improve on the efficiency of the fee-for-service sector, and continue to gain enrollment by offering enhanced benefits. The relative balance of the Medicare system should not be affected by payments that are adjusted to account for the health risk of enrollees. Nor should the Medicare system be affected by overall payment limits for balanced federal budgets that equally affect both sides of the system. The flexibility offered on the private side of the Medicare system should help managed care plans emerge as the dominant force in the future.

Private-sector managed care addresses each of the economic forces imposed on traditional fee-for-service Medicare. Managed care plans specifically control the volume and intensity of services. They offer more flexibility to physicians and hospitals to receive higher payments for services, rather than regulated fees. They are free to adopt any private sector approaches to fight fraud and abuse. They are not defined-benefits coverage from the public standpoint.

Managed care plans are showing savvy approaches to benefit design, marketing, and network features. They offer beneficiaries the ability to add personal resources and to create a customized health plan that meets their needs better than traditional Medicare supplemental coverage that only wraps around the traditional fee-for-service Medicare program. With Medicare managed care, a beneficiary can take what would have otherwise been paid in the fee-for-service sector, combine it with the beneficiary's own premium, and find a benefit package that best suits the beneficiary's own needs. Managed care plans lower costs through various cost-control techniques that involve physician payment incentive systems, hospital and physician selection, utilization management, case management, disease management, and demand management. All these issues are discussed further in Chapters 7 through 11.

Economic Outcome

For long-term policy reasons, however, there is every reason to think that managed care will continue to be on the ascendancy and traditional fee-for-service in continued decline in policy importance. The difference lies in the social contract represented by each.

Because traditional fee-for-service is defined-benefits coverage while managed care is defined-contribution coverage, policymakers will be attracted to defined-contribution coverage. The open-ended fiscal commitment posed by defined-contribution coverage is not sustainable unless elected officials are willing to ask the taxpayers for more tax revenues to maintain the status quo. Managed care represents a closed-ended commitment per beneficiary. The growth in Medicare spending can be better controlled by Medicare managed care. As long as the combined Medicare+Choice payment per member per month plus premium contributions from beneficiaries is sufficient to maintain enrollment in managed care plans, the Medicare program can experience gradual conversion from defined-benefits coverage to defined-contribution coverage for health services.

Will there be a sweeping conversion to Medicare managed care? That is the crucial strategic question. The inexorable application of the competitive model combined with little or inadequate response for marketplace change in the traditional fee-for-service sector could gradually continue the process of conversion. Eventually the time could come when enough Medicare beneficiaries have enrolled in Medicare managed care that financial disincentives are put in place to remain in a costly, open-ended fee-for-service program.

Strategic Decisions Checklist

Strategic Questions	Strategic Analyses
What are the economics of private Medicare managed care?	Suppliers (primarily physicians and hospitals) operate in a private marketplace in which Medicare must compete to provide access to care.
	Demanders (Medicare beneficiaries) make a two-stage choice concerning their Medicare coverage.
How is Medicare structured to handle the transaction of money for medical care?	The market is structured for consumers to make a two-stage choice.
	In stage one, consumers must decide whether to remain in the regulated traditional fee-for-service side or the private managed care side.
	In stage two, consumers choose either supplemental insurance, in the case of traditional fee-for-service, or Medicare+Choice plan, in the case of private managed care.
	This structure forces a constant reassessment on the part of suppliers and demanders regarding their participation on both sides of Medicare.
What trends affect whether there is enough money for medical care?	Traditional fee-for-service Medicare confronts increasing volume and intensity of services, regulated payments to providers, fraud and abuse, and the inherent open-ended nature of a defined-benefit plan.
What trends affect whether Medicare has enough money for medical care?	Private managed care represents increasing marketplace savvy, an ability to add personal resources and customize benefits, control over volume and intensity of services, and the inherent closed-ended nature of a defined-contribution.

THE CHANGING PRIVATE MEDICARE MANAGED CARE MARKET

Medicare managed care is connected to several types of markets. The most important is the market for the financing of private health plan coverage. The next most important is the market for the delivery of private health services. Understanding where a Medicare managed care plan fits and where it is going requires knowledge or assumptions about the overall and local markets for the financing of health plan coverage and the delivery of health services. You need a clear vision of how your health plan belongs in a larger context, including the people it serves, market rivals, beneficiary perceptions, and how all of these fit together.

The purpose of Chapter 2 is to present a national and regional strategic overview of the changing Medicare managed care market, the people covered, the major players in financing and delivery, some description of selected active regional markets, and beneficiary perceptions. Chapter 2 illustrates the types of data and analysis you as a health plan manager should develop for your own situation to answer important strategic questions: What determines Medicare managed care market share in your market? What determines delivery system market share in your market? What combination of price and quality features will your managed care plan adopt to achieve market share? What structure and process of care yield delivery system market share?

Let's begin by examining the national trends for Medicare managed care enrollment and delivery system process and structure features. The end of this chapter presents a framework any health plan can use for self-examination.

People Covered in Medicare Managed Care

Since the start of the program more than 15 years ago, and despite two periods of high disenrollment of plans and beneficiaries, millions of people have elected Medicare managed care. One reason for the solid place of managed care in the Medicare program is *choice*. Almost two-thirds of all beneficiaries now have the option of selecting private health plans instead of receiving medical services through traditional fee-for-service Medicare (Physician Payment Review Commission 1997). About one in seven beneficiaries obtain Medicare coverage through a managed care plan at the end of 1998. Figure 2.1 illustrates the trends since the beginning of Medicare and into the future. This chart shows only risk-contract enrollment, excluding Medicare SELECT, cost, and

FIGURE 2.1

People Covered
in Medicare
Managed Care
and Traditional
Fee-for-Service
Medicare,
1965–1998
(Actual) and
1999–2007
(Projection)

*Could it be
one-third of
enrollment?
Medicare
managed care
has grown
rapidly and
could be much
larger*

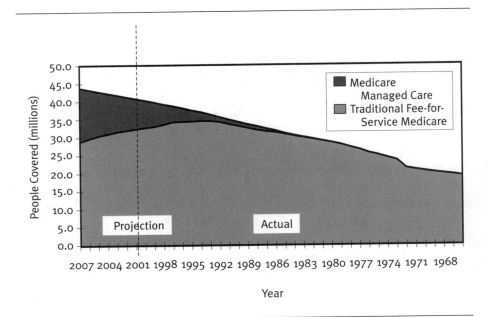

other types of contracts discussed further in Chapter 3. Despite transitory declines in the number of plans and enrollees in 1988 and 1998, the trend is that of gradual growth in the number of enrollees in Medicare managed care.

Defined as risk-contract enrollment, Medicare managed care enrollment was nonexistent in Medicare for the first 12 years of the program. By the beginning of the 1980s, several managed care plans had risk contracts with the program as demonstration projects, and growth was tentative for much of the decade even after Medicare managed care became official in January 1985. In the 1990s, the number of beneficiaries surpassed the double digits in percent of Medicare beneficiaries in Medicare managed care.

More typically today, compared with its beginnings, Medicare managed care is adding 500,000 to 700,000 net new beneficiaries every year. In some months, as many as 100,000 Medicare beneficiaries join managed care plans. As a result, Congressional Budget Office projections suggest the Medicare managed care portion of Medicare, not including Medicare SELECT but including all types of Medicare+Choice plans, will grow faster than overall program growth, shrinking further the traditional fee-for-service Medicare program into the year 2007. Medicare managed care in the form of Medicare+Choice could be more than 30 percent of the total Medicare enrollment in just a few years. Overall figures such as these mask the significant regional variation in Medicare managed care enrollment discussed below.

Table 2.1 provides a broad overview of several key characteristics of the people in traditional fee-for-service Medicare and in Medicare managed care for the latest year the data are available—1995. With nearly 10 percent of the population enrolled in Medicare managed care at the time shown, one of the most striking differences in the total versus managed care enrollment is the difference in age groupings. Those eligible for Medicare because of disability dominate the under age 65 group, and they are about 2.5 times *less* likely to join a managed care plan. The youngest beneficiaries account for 12 percent of the total Medicare program and less than 5 percent of the managed care enrollment. Those age 65–74 are *most* likely to be enrolled (57 percent), and they enroll disproportionately relative to their overall representation (47 percent). The 75–84 age group is nearly as equally represented in the total program as in the managed care program (30 percent). The oldest age category is less likely to join a managed care plan, accounting for 11 percent of total Medicare and 8 percent of managed care.

Figure 2.2 highlights the age distribution to illustrate the differences between the total Medicare program versus the Medicare managed care program. The bulk of enrollment, nearly 90 percent, is in the two middle age groupings. This phenomenon affects the flow of revenues to the health plans,

	TOTAL MEDICARE	MEDICARE MANAGED CARE
Total People	37.7 Million	3.1 Million
Age		Percent
<65	12	5
65–74	47	57
75–84	30	30
≥85	11	8
	100	100
Gender		
Male	43	44
Female	57	56
	100	100
Race or Ethnicity		
White	86	86
African American	9	7
Other/Unknown	5	7
	100	100
Medicaid-Eligible?		
Yes	16	4
No	84	96
	100	100

TABLE 2.1
Distribution of People in Medicare and Medicare Managed Care, 1995

Enrollees are different: Most enrollees are in the younger age groups

FIGURE 2.2

Distribution of People in Medicare and Medicare Managed Care by Age, 1995

Enrollees are younger: Age 65–74 most likely to enroll

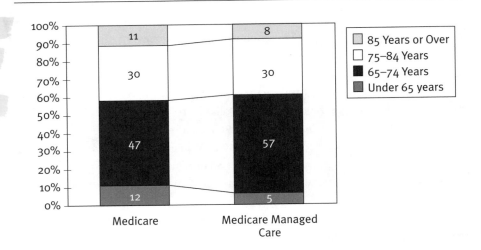

as explained in Chapter 5; strategic marketing issues for the plan, as explained in Chapter 6; and how patient care activities are carried out, as explained in Chapters 6 through 9.

Returning to Table 2.1, males and females are represented nearly exactly the same in the total Medicare program as in managed care. The same may be said about whites, but African Americans are somewhat less likely to join managed care plans.

Only 4 percent of managed care enrollment comes from those dually eligible for Medicare and Medicaid, yet the dually eligible account for 16 percent of total Medicare. Medicaid is a program jointly operated by the federal government and each state government. The reason those eligible for Medicaid do not enroll in Medicare managed care plans is that their home state often does not have separate coordinating contracts with the managed care plans. It is too complex to administer a joint Medicare–Medicaid contract with difficult payment issues to address. Thus, many people on Medicaid do not have the option to join a Medicare managed care plan because their Medicaid coverage is not set up to coordinate easily with such dual enrollment.

Major Players in Medicare Managed Care

Medicare+Choice contractors number nearly 300, with more expected in the future. HMOs dominate the Medicare managed care market today. Few PPOs, PSOs, or private fee-for-service plans have significant enrollment since their recently granted ability to enter the market.

The Medicare managed care program was purely experimental until the mid-1980s when only around 20 health plans participated. The number of plans grew sharply in the late 1980s and dipped in the early 1990s when the economy experienced a recession and many HMOs were busy growing their commercial enrollment.

By the mid-1990s, the trend was up again (Fig. 2.3), with the number of HMOs participating in Medicare managed care tripling from 1993 to 1998. In mid-1998 to early 1999, a number of plans sharply curtailed their enrollment in several counties, and several dropped out of the program because of lack of interest or merger or acquisition with another plan. Total enrollment continued to increase, but the number of plans declined by 12 percent. The direction of further growth is difficult to project because the future of model types such as PPOs, PSOs, or private fee-for-service plans is not known at this time.

One recent study (Pai and Clement 1999) suggested that more HMOs may participate in the Medicare program as a strategy to diversify revenues— especially if premium payments for other private commercial enrollment are curtailed—or face declining relative profit margins. In other words, the number of plans participating in Medicare does not depend on the Medicare payment rates alone, but the Medicare payments compared with other payments to HMOs. Larger for-profit HMOs are more likely to serve the Medicare market than smaller not-for-profit HMOs. Thus, further merger and acquisition activity by for-profit HMOs is likely to be associated with HMO interest in this market.

Active Markets in Medicare Managed Care

Enrollment is disproportionately concentrated today in key states in different parts of the country, as illustrated in Figure 2.4. Table 2.2 shows the number

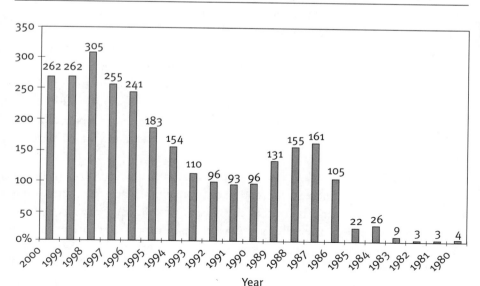

FIGURE 2.3

Number of HMOs in Medicare Managed Care, 2000

Many players: The number of plans has doubled in the 1990s

FIGURE 2.4

Distribution of People in Medicare and Medicare Managed Care by Top Four States in Managed Care Enrollment, 2000

Lopsided: Four large states have one-half the enrollment

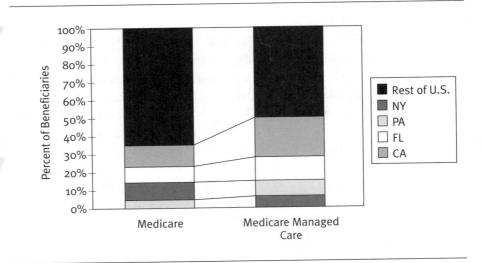

of beneficiaries enrolled in Medicare+Choice HMOs. California, Oregon, Arizona, Colorado, Rhode Island, Hawaii, Nevada, Pennsylvania, Florida, and Washington have the largest percent market share within the state of Medicare beneficiaries enrolled in Medicare+Choice. Of these, California, Florida, Pennsylvania, and New York have large absolute enrollment—around a half million in each state. Figure 2.4 shows that although the big four account for 29 percent of beneficiary enrollment in Medicare, they account for 50 percent of Medicare managed care enrollment. Below we will examine these major markets in terms of Medicare managed care enrollment and delivery system market share dominated by major players for possible clues about the way Medicare managed care could develop in other areas of the country. Round out the top four with four more (Massachusetts, Arizona, Ohio, and Texas), and two-thirds of Medicare+Choice enrollment is in the top eight states.

Fifteen states have more than 100,000 enrolled beneficiaries. California has more than 1.5 million; Florida has more than 750,000; Pennsylvania has 586,000; New York has nearly 500,000; and Texas has nearly 400,000 each, followed by Massachusetts, Ohio, Arizona, Washington, New Jersey, Illinois, and Colorado. The top 12 states in total enrollment account for 77 percent of enrollment.

Table 2.2 does not list the 13 states with fewer than 5,000 enrollment in Medicare+Choice. These states tend to have smaller urban areas, suggesting the involvement of nonurban areas is an issue that must be addressed by Medicare+Choice. But after this low market share group, the lowest market share states are (from highest to lowest percent market share) Wisconsin, Tennessee, Nebraska, North Carolina, Arkansas, Indiana, Virginia, Iowa, and Utah. This list contains a slight bias toward states in the southeast, suggesting that this part of the country has a potential for change and growth.

State	Total Beneficiaries	Medicare+Choice Health Maintenance Organization Enrollees			
		Enrollees	Percent Market Share Within State	Rank	Cumulative Percent Across States
US	40,101,432	6,849,918	17.08%		100%
CA	3,984,611	1,573,805	39.5%	1	23.0%
OR	499,981	181,161	36.2%	2	25.6%
AZ	685,924	247,294	36.1%	3	29.2%
CO	475,546	161,850	34.0%	4	31.6%
RI	174,636	57,347	32.8%	5	32.4%
HI	168,248	53,967	32.1%	6	33.2%
NV	240,269	76,441	31.8%	7	34.3%
PA	2,139,493	586,548	27.4%	8	42.9%
FL	2,857,971	769,992	26.9%	9	54.1%
WA	750,054	182,092	24.3%	10	56.8%
MA	982,934	236,205	24.0%	11	60.2%
CT	524,866	105,432	20.1%	12	61.8%
NM	238,607	45,977	19.3%	13	62.5%
NY	2,770,312	495,449	17.9%	14	69.7%
OH	1,742,591	293,884	16.9%	15	74.0%
TX	2,307,039	387,598	16.8%	16	79.6%
LA	622,038	99,797	16.0%	17	81.1%
NJ	1,225,768	184,729	15.1%	18	83.8%
MO	881,610	130,050	14.8%	19	85.7%
MN	667,443	88,728	13.3%	20	87.0%
MD	654,432	78,169	11.9%	21	88.1%
IL	1,677,573	189,247	11.3%	22	90.9%
OK	519,558	52,181	10.0%	23	91.6%
DC	78,569	7,750	9.9%	24	91.8%
ID	167,760	15,783	9.4%	25	92.0%
AL	701,293	58,060	8.3%	26	92.8%
WV	346,574	25,320	7.3%	27	93.2%
KS	399,306	28,762	7.2%	28	93.6%
GA	936,379	55,715	6.0%	29	94.4%
KY	638,998	34,780	5.4%	30	95.0%
WI	801,870	42,117	5.3%	31	95.6%
TN	849,286	44,017	5.2%	32	96.2%
NE	259,134	10,605	4.1%	33	96.4%
NC	1,155,005	46,271	4.0%	34	97.0%
AR	450,359	17,993	4.0%	35	97.3%
IN	872,195	34,329	3.9%	36	97.8%
VA	898,615	34,038	3.8%	37	98.3%
IA	487,748	16,752	3.4%	38	98.5%
UT	208,887	6,635	3.2%	39	98.6%

TABLE 2.2
Medicare+
Choice Health
Maintenance
Organization
Enrollment by
State, January
2000

*Market share is
concentrated:
Market share
and market size
are related*

Note: AK, DE, ME, MI, MS, MT, ND, NH, PR, SC, SD, VT, and WY each have fewer than 5,000 Medicare+Choice HMO enrollees.

Managed care is newest in these states in comparison to other states with large general enrollments for decades. There might be a competitive strategy that is in operation in these states that is not present in other states.

We have taken the top four states—California, Florida, Arizona, and Pennsylvania—with both large enrollment and market share, and examined several of the major cities in these states. The following section describes their Medicare managed care market share and their delivery system market share. By examining the major players on the financing and delivery sides of the market in these states, we hope to provide a framework for thinking about market dynamics and identify the determinants of market share. The results will also reveal a statewide strategy in several cases on either the financing or the delivery system sides of the market. By looking at these examples and visualizing the role of the major players in the market we can gain an understanding of what advanced markets look like. These should suggest how other markets might progress if Medicare managed care enrollment grows elsewhere in the country. The final section in this chapter poses a model for viewing financing and delivery in any market and for understanding how the major players are operating in the market.

Strategy and Market Share in California

No other state compares with California because of the size of Medicare managed care and its unique delivery system characteristics. Nearly 40 percent of beneficiaries in California are in Medicare managed care. Of the state's 3.9 million total Medicare beneficiaries, 1.5 million are in Medicare+Choice HMOs. Most of these are in four major urban areas, all in southern California.

Los Angeles County has 1 million beneficiaries, and 386,107 are enrolled in Medicare+Choice HMOs. The number of beneficiaries in this one urban area is more than those in all but four other states in terms of total Medicare enrollment. The number in Medicare managed care exceeds all but four states, rivaling only Pennsylvania, Florida, New York, and Texas. Nearby

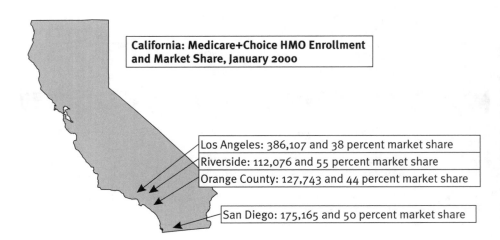

California: Medicare+Choice HMO Enrollment and Market Share, January 2000

Los Angeles: 386,107 and 38 percent market share

Riverside: 112,076 and 55 percent market share

Orange County: 127,743 and 44 percent market share

San Diego: 175,165 and 50 percent market share

Riverside boasts the largest percent Medicare managed care market share with more than half (55 percent) of all beneficiaries in Medicare managed care. San Diego comes in at 50 percent Medicare managed care. Orange County is the fourth largest in the state with 44 percent Medicare managed care. In each local area, the managed care plans and the delivery system major players are slightly different.

Three major players account for the managed care plan enrollment in Riverside: PacifiCare, Aetna, and Kaiser. PacifiCare is the dominant player with 44 percent of the Medicare managed care enrollment. Aetna and Kaiser account for roughly 20 percent each, with the remainder taken by much smaller health plans. In Riverside, Kaiser offers its own hospitals as a platform for the delivery system, whereas Adventist Health, Valley Health System, and Columbia/HCA finish the bulk of the delivery system measured in hospital beds for the Medicare population. Riverside represents a market of dominance on the Medicare managed care enrollment and delivery system side, with overwhelming control over hospital beds in strategic alliances, primarily involving four major players. The physician practice side is in constant flux and is difficult to quantify with any degree of stability.

Orange County, California is the major urban section of the Los Angeles area with 288,961 total Medicare beneficiaries. Medicare managed care plays a huge role with 40 percent of the beneficiaries enrolled. Again, most of them are enrolled in one of two plans: PacifiCare or Kaiser. PacifiCare, a large network-model HMO, uses strong physician incentives for cost control, maintains a high provider-to-member ratio, and commands discount prices compared with the market from hospitals and physicians because of its huge market share. PacifiCare has capitation payments extensively for its delivery systems, paying global rates to many of its affiliated physician group practices, and it negotiates vigorously with the hospitals. Kaiser is a distant second with less than one-fourth of PacifiCare's enrollment amount at 19 percent market share. Health Net has half that amount at 6 percent.

The distinguishing characteristic of Orange County is the concentration on the delivery system side. Four major hospitals and health systems dominate the delivery system, holding nearly 60 percent of the hospital beds: Tenet,

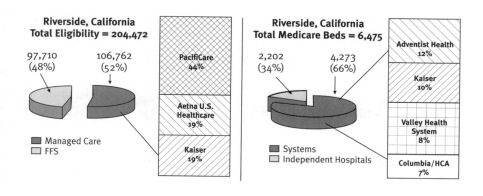

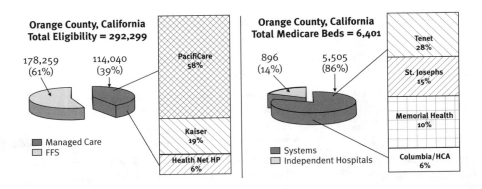

Orange County, California
Total Eligibility = 292,299

178,259 (61%)   114,040 (39%)

PacifiCare 58%

Kaiser 19%

Health Net HP 6%

■ Managed Care
□ FFS

Orange County, California
Total Medicare Beds = 6,401

896 (14%)   5,505 (86%)

Tenet 28%

St. Josephs 15%

Memorial Health 10%

Columbia/HCA 6%

■ Systems
□ Independent Hospitals

St. Joseph's, Memorial Health, and Columbia/HCA. Each participates with PacifiCare because it must or be excluded from almost 60 percent of the market. Medicare managed care has been a familiar fixture of this healthcare landscape since the start of the HMO program in the mid-1980s. The market would seem to have evolved into two major players on the Medicare managed care side and four major players on the hospital delivery system side, with a hospital delivery system almost completely controlled (86 percent) by major hospital alliances.

Although Riverside clearly beats its neighbors in the Los Angeles metropolitan area for market share in Medicare managed care, nothing compares with the size of Los Angeles for the number of enrollees in Medicare managed care. At 386,107 Medicare+Choice HMO enrollees, it represents the largest single market. Yet nearly two-thirds of the market in Los Angeles remains in fee-for-service. Meanwhile, on the delivery system side, four hospital systems dominate: Tenet, Los Angeles County Health Department, Kaiser, and UniHealth. Yet these have less of the delivery system, measured in hospital beds, than the previous locales. The four hospital systems control 42 percent of the delivery system, and 76 percent is in strategic hospital alliances.

Although smaller in total enrollment, San Diego's Medicare managed care market share is larger than Los Angeles's. San Diego market share is nearly one-half Medicare managed care. The huge population of 337,639 Medicare beneficiaries are enrolled largely in PacifiCare, which plainly dominates with 63

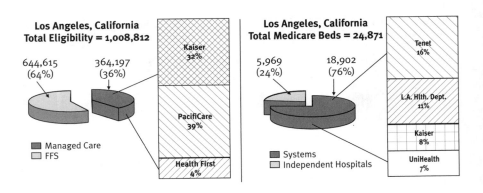

Los Angeles, California
Total Eligibility = 1,008,812

644,615 (64%)   364,197 (36%)

Kaiser 32%

PacifiCare 39%

Health First 4%

■ Managed Care
□ FFS

Los Angeles, California
Total Medicare Beds = 24,871

5,969 (24%)   18,902 (76%)

Tenet 16%

L.A. Hlth. Dept. 11%

Kaiser 8%

UniHealth 7%

■ Systems
□ Independent Hospitals

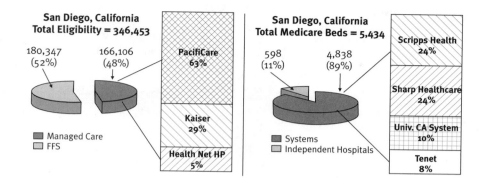

percent of the market. Kaiser has about 29 percent of the market and Health Net Health Plan has a small but respectable share of 5 percent. More than 5,000 hospital beds are available to this population, and four major players control them: Scripps Health, Sharp Healthcare, University of California–San Diego, and Tenet. These four have an overwhelming 66 percent control of the delivery system, represented by hospital beds, and 89 percent dominated by strategic hospital alliances.

What we learn from California is that the future of Medicare could be something that already exists in most major cities of southern California: a Medicare program that is already operated largely privately through big corporations on the financing and delivery systems sides. We see large Medicare+Choice health plans that have large networks, strong physician incentives for cost control, and a reputation for very low payments to physicians and hospitals. This is a highly price-conscious and price-driven market. The delivery system, at least among the hospitals, is consolidated, with few hospitals freestanding. However, the major players in each city are not the same. The hospital systems in each city are not always the same names, suggesting that although the financing side has developed a statewide strategy, the delivery system side has not.

Summary of California Market

Strategy and Market Share in Florida

Florida comes in second to California in number of Medicare beneficiaries in states with high market share in Medicare managed care. With more than 2.8 million Medicare beneficiaries and 27 percent in Medicare HMOs, four important metropolitan areas account for most of the enrollment. One managed care plan dominates the market in each local area, in this case Aetna U.S. Healthcare. But after that major player, the market is shared among a number of players, each different in each local market. Whereas southern California has two major players in each major market, Florida has one, with many different substantial but smaller HMOs in Medicare managed care.

South Florida has the largest market share in Medicare managed care. Ft. Lauderdale has a 48 percent market share, followed by Miami with a 45 percent market share. Tampa at 34 percent and West Palm Beach with 36

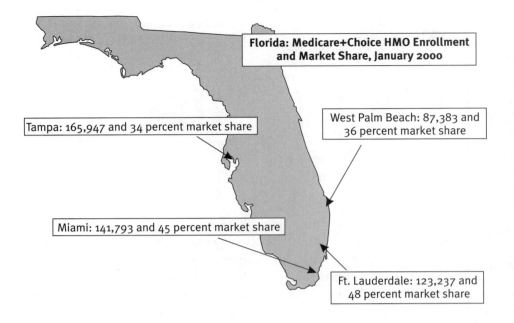

Florida: Medicare+Choice HMO Enrollment and Market Share, January 2000

Tampa: 165,947 and 34 percent market share

West Palm Beach: 87,383 and 36 percent market share

Miami: 141,793 and 45 percent market share

Ft. Lauderdale: 123,237 and 48 percent market share

percent are not far behind in market share. Aetna U.S. Healthcare dominates the market in Ft. Lauderdale and West Palm Beach, and United holds the largest market share in Miami. A number of plans have respectable numbers of enrollment and market share, but there is no pattern in terms of hierarchy across the different areas.

In Miami and Tampa, on the delivery system side, the major player is Columbia/HCA in hospital capital measured in beds. Columbia/HCA falls to second in West Palm Beach and third in Ft. Lauderdale. Tenet is the major player in Ft. Lauderdale, and Allegheny Health System is the largest in West Palm Beach. Yet market shares for the largest system in each metropolitan area is around 24 percent to 33 percent. The Florida delivery system is less consolidated than the California market and may have a ways to go. The current makeup of major players allows the managed care plans to have a large number of providers and to emphasize price negotiation, rather than quantity or quality interventions, to keep costs down.

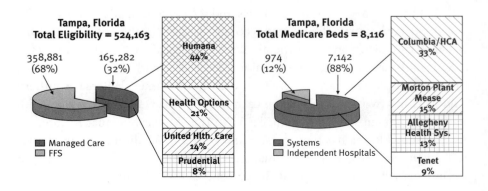

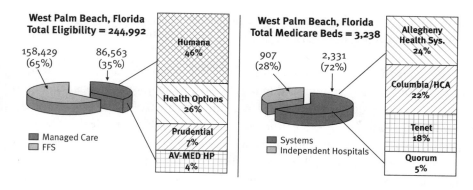

In West Palm Beach there is a healthy enrollment of 35 percent Medicare market share, and again Humana comes out as the leader in enrollment. The delivery system players are somewhat different, with Columbia/HCA having less than one-fourth of the market share and Allegheny Health System playing a role here it does not play elsewhere. Tenet hospitals are a major force, as are Quorum hospitals. The top four hospital systems make up 72 percent of the delivery system in terms of hospital beds.

Down in Ft. Lauderdale, the financing side of the market is very similar to West Palm Beach, with Humana, Health Options, and AV-MED Health Plan playing similar roles in both cities. On the delivery system side, however, Tenet comes to the forefront in Ft. Lauderdale and competes with Columbia/HCA and two other not-for-profit hospital systems. The

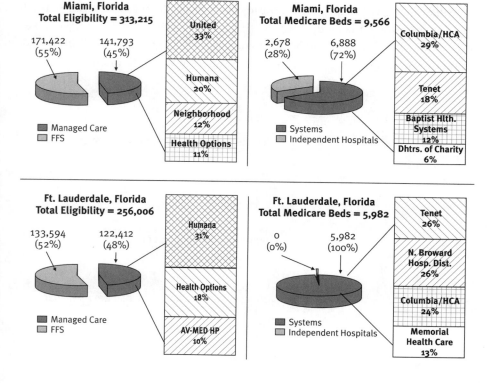

Ft. Lauderdale market has only four hospital systems to serve the Medicare market, and each system is of similar size in terms of beds.

Summary of Florida Market

Medicare managed care is a dominant force in Florida with about one-third to one-half of the market in several major cities. One major player has the largest market share in terms of Medicare managed care enrollment in each of the major cities—Aetna U.S. Healthcare. Another health plan, Health Options, consistently comes in second, along with two other health plans, consistently having a major presence but with a much smaller market share. A single statewide consolidator on the delivery system side, Columbia/HCA is a force to be dealt with by the health plans, especially in Ft Lauderdale where there are only three other choices for delivery system. Florida may be closer to the managed competition notions of selective groups of hospitals and physicians aligned with certain health plans. Because quality of care has been a visible issue over the years in south Florida and its Medicare managed care plans thanks to newspaper coverage, Medicare beneficiaries in that region are more attuned to concerns about quality of care and look for activities and signals of good quality from their financing and delivery system participants. The Medicare+Choice payments to health plans are still among the highest in the nation, allowing the managed care plans to pay rates closer to fee-for-service Medicare rates. But this situation could change if enrollment continues to grow and the zero-premium option is no longer sustainable in much of the Florida market.

Strategy and Market Share in Arizona

Arizona ranks near the 40th percentile, next to California, in overall market share in Medicare managed care. With 685,000 total beneficiaries, it ranks at the top of states with Medicare managed care in numbers, 247,000, and market share, 36 percent. Two Arizona cities have the bulk of enrollment.

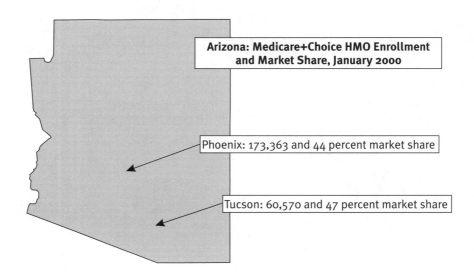

Arizona: Medicare+Choice HMO Enrollment and Market Share, January 2000

Phoenix: 173,363 and 44 percent market share

Tucson: 60,570 and 47 percent market share

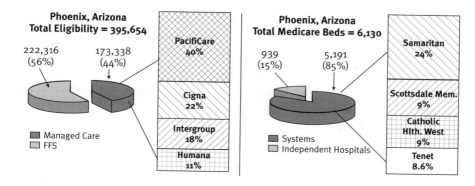

Phoenix, Arizona
Total Eligibility = 395,654

222,316 (56%)   173,338 (44%)

■ Managed Care
☐ FFS

PacifiCare 40%
Cigna 22%
Intergroup 18%
Humana 11%

Phoenix, Arizona
Total Medicare Beds = 6,130

939 (15%)   5,191 (85%)

■ Systems
☐ Independent Hospitals

Samaritan 24%
Scottsdale Mem. 9%
Catholic Hlth. West 9%
Tenet 8.6%

Phoenix has nearly 60 percent of all Medicare beneficiaries in the state, and 44 percent of them are enrolled in Medicare+Choice plans. Most of that enrollment is in PacifiCare, but Cigna also has significant enrollment. The rest of the enrollment is split with several smaller plans including Intergroup and Humana. These are names that appear in other states and other cities; thus, Phoenix is an amalgam of Medicare+Choice plans that have their base of enrollment elsewhere. Some of this may stem from beneficiaries who reside elsewhere most of the year and spend the winter months at their second home in Arizona—the so-called "snow birds." These non-Arizona-based health plans beat the local competition in terms of enrollment. Maricopa Senior Select, Blue Cross and Blue Shield of Arizona, and Premier Healthcare operated by Samaritan all have less than double-digit market share. This is despite the fact that Samaritan, for example, has a huge market share on the delivery system side of the market, with nearly 25 percent of the beds in Phoenix. Because of the large market share in beds enjoyed by the major players, 85 percent of the beds are controlled by only four or five of the top local hospital systems. These are all well-organized, well-respected organizations, and the fact that they have not been able to develop their own dominant financing system in the form of a retail Medicare+Choice health plan is a message for others.

The story is similar in Tucson, with PacifiCare again playing a dominant role on the health plan side of the market, and two large not-for-profit systems, Carondelet and Samaritan, owning most of the hospital beds. All the managed

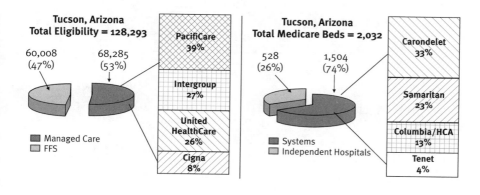

Tucson, Arizona
Total Eligibility = 128,293

60,008 (47%)   68,285 (53%)

■ Managed Care
☐ FFS

PacifiCare 39%
Intergroup 27%
United HealthCare 26%
Cigna 8%

Tucson, Arizona
Total Medicare Beds = 2,032

528 (26%)   1,504 (74%)

■ Systems
☐ Independent Hospitals

Carondelet 33%
Samaritan 23%
Columbia/HCA 13%
Tenet 4%

care plans include all of the local hospital systems in their networks and offer a zero-premium product. Most plans are committed to having a large network with a high provider-to-member ratio and to having tough negotiations on prices with the threat of being eliminated from the network. But thus far, each local system has been able to maintain its position as a provider to everyone.

Summary of Arizona Market

Arizona seems to be at a transitional phase between having some of the highest Medicare+Choice enrollment in the country and having a super concentration of Medicare+Choice enrollment exceeding 50 percent market share. Nearly half of the dollars for Medicare flow through the accounts of four national HMOs, and 75 percent of the beds are with four local hospital systems. The current major health plans will need to continue to grow enrollment from their already lofty levels, and the smaller local health plans will need to either expand or quit the market. The current large-network approach to contracting with the delivery system may shift toward more selective contracting as the realities of a lower Medicare+Choice payment level come to pass. The zero-premium product could be threatened, or it might be retained through a successful strategic alliance between a health plan and a delivery system that together can implement strong quality assessment and improvement, disease management, and product positioning around quality.

Strategy and Market Share in Pennsylvania

The state with the third largest total enrollment and seventh largest market share compared with other states has four cities that stand out in terms of Medicare managed care market share: Philadelphia, Allentown, Pittsburgh, and Scranton. Philadelphia is the city with the largest enrollment at 37 percent, followed by Pittsburgh at 32 percent, with Allentown barely breaking into double digits and Scranton at 28 percent.

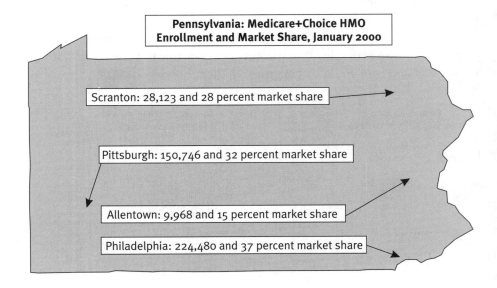

Pennsylvania: Medicare+Choice HMO Enrollment and Market Share, January 2000

Scranton: 28,123 and 28 percent market share

Pittsburgh: 150,746 and 32 percent market share

Allentown: 9,968 and 15 percent market share

Philadelphia: 224,480 and 37 percent market share

The Medicare managed care market in Philadelphia and Pittsburgh is dominated by the Blue Cross and Blue Shield HMO, Keystone, with 60 percent of the market in Philadelphia and a remarkable 72 percent of the market in Pittsburgh. The plan uses a large network of physicians and hospitals with strong physician incentives for cost control. The plan is large enough in Pennsylvania to demand below-market prices from its network for participation.

The second major player is Aetna U.S. Healthcare with a 35 percent market share in Philadelphia and a 16 percent share in Pittsburgh. It has a more select market with strong incentives to physicians for quality improvement as well as cost control. It also uses global capitation to pay groups of physicians or physician-hospital organizations to receive full risk for all Medicare-covered services after taking a portion of the Medicare+Choice payment for itself. In terms of market share, Keystone seems to be ahead in these markets and holding its own against the large, national chain HMOs.

On the delivery system side, the two cities are quite different. The market is highly fragmented in Philadelphia, with the top four hospital systems each accounting for less than 10 percent each of the beds, although 69 percent of beds are in local hospital systems. In Pittsburgh, the University of Pittsburgh system dominates the delivery system with 29 percent of the beds, and the other systems accounting for much less. Thus, Pennsylvania's two largest cities are a story of consolidation on the side of Medicare market share and fragmentation on the delivery system market share.

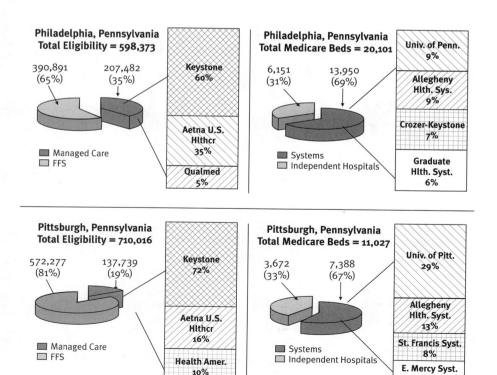

Two other cities are worth mentioning because, unlike our other three states where statewide strategies seemed to be in play, the participants are different on both sides of the marketplace. In Allentown and Scranton, the percentage of Medicare managed care market share is still in the teens. The managed care plans are an entirely different set of major players. In Allentown, Aetna U.S. Healthcare is the dominant player, and in Scranton, Health Maintenance Organization of North East Pennsylvania is the dominant player. The academic medical centers are out of the picture in these two cities and are replaced by a collection of smaller not-for-profit local hospital systems. The markets are characterized by a large network, physician incentives for cost control, and a large number of providers for the number of enrollees in the managed care plans.

Summary of Pennsylvania Market

Pennsylvania has a large number of beneficiaries enrolled in Medicare managed care, but still modest market shares of 15 to 37 percent. The delivery system side is substantially consolidated,with the top four major players in each city taking 66 to 70 percent of the market share in terms of hospital beds. Measured this way, the universities dominate the delivery system market share. Most markets have a zero-premium plan available for beneficiaries, reflecting the relatively high Medicare+Choice payment rates available to the plans. As a result, the product pricing for the managed care plans, where managed care is still a relatively new concept to the beneficiaries, is around price and benefits.

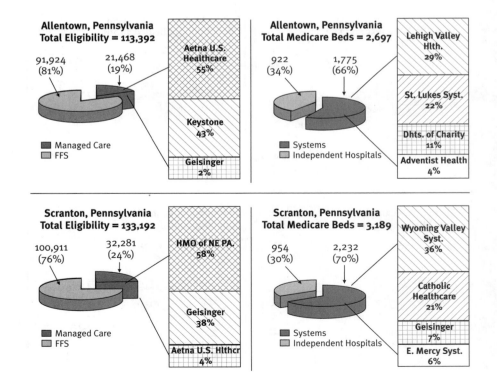

In the last section in this chapter we put these four prototype markets together, but first we examine the perceptions of beneficiaries regarding what the private financing and delivery system has to offer.

Consumer Perceptions About Private Medicare Managed Care

How do Medicare beneficiaries perceive the private Medicare managed care option? How do the members of Medicare+Choice managed care plans assess their experience?

On the first question, despite 17 years of operation as a full-fledged program, not many beneficiaries know about the option. This could change in 2000 when the Health Care Financing Administration (HCFA) attempts to conduct an open enrollment period for selecting the Medicare+Choice option. More than half the beneficiaries say they know little or nothing of what they need to know about the availability and benefits of Medicare HMOs (Murray 1988). This occurs despite the fact that more than two-thirds of beneficiaries have at least one Medicare+Choice plan in their area.

Among those who join a health plan, nearly half do so because of the lower cost and higher benefits of Medicare+Choice coordinated-care plans (Physician Payment Review Commission 1997). A relatively small number (8 percent) of beneficiaries left their plans. Among the disenrollees, 36 percent left because of perceived problems with the plan's physicians or concerns about access to care. Another 28 percent either moved out of the service area offered by the plan or left for some other involuntary reason. Thus, nearly 3 percent of *all* enrollees change plans because of problems with the plan's physicians or access, and nearly 2 percent of all enrollees change plans because they moved or for some other involuntary reason. The remaining disenrollees report a variety of reasons, including financial, for changing to another Medicare+Choice HMO. These reasons and rates of disenrollment are not unlike those reported for the alternative option, the traditional fee-for-service Medicare program.

Recent comparisons of satisfaction with comparable groups of managed care versus traditional fee-for-service enrollees are not available. But the best known results are from 1990 in a nationwide survey of nearly 12,000 beneficiaries (Clement et al. 1992). The findings mirror similar studies done in the 1980s (Rossiter et al. 1989B). Over 90 percent of beneficiaries covered by HMOs and traditional fee-for-service Medicare would recommend their health plan or physicians to others. The overwhelmingly consistent finding from the studies is that managed care enrollees tend to be more highly satisfied with the costs they incur, and are less likely to identify services that are not covered. Traditional fee-for-service Medicare enrollees are more likely to be very satisfied with access and quality measures. But the difference, while statistically significant, may not be substantial. Table 2.3 provides a full explanation.

TABLE 2.3

Percent Beneficiaries Rating Their Satisfaction Excellent, Adjusted for Differences in Beneficiary Characteristics, 1990

Trading off cost and quality: Beneficiaries rate satisfaction high for costs and low for quality

	Enrollees	Nonenrollees
Satisfaction with Overall Quality of Care	45.2	52.9
Safisfaction with Personal Attention		
Explanations	42.6	53.9
Attention to patient	42.5	56.0
Preventive advice	39.2	50.1
Personal interest	40.4	55.9
Respect and privacy	47.4	59.1
Satisfaction with Access to Care		
Ease of seeing MD of choice	42.9	61.3
Availability of emergency care	48.8	57.8
Ease of making telephone appointments	39.2	56.6
Convenience of office location	49.3	50.4
Convenience of office hours	40.7	48.3
Availability of specialty care	46.4	55.6
Availability of hospital care	51.0	56.2
Wait from appointment to visit	31.7	47.2
Wait at office	31.7	37.8
Ease of obtaining information by telephone	34.5	47.3
Ease of getting prescription filled	52.6	57.5
Satisfaction with Cost		
Amount of out-of-pocket costs	53.4	40.3
Satisfaction with Quality of Care		
Perceived quality of office/facilities	49.8	55.0
Thoroughness of exams	42.7	52.1
Perceived accuracy of diagnosis	40.5	50.8
Thoroughness of treatment	39.9	49.7
Perceived results of care	40.5	48.9
Recommend plan/provider to others	93.5	96.1

Source: Brown, R. S. et al. 1993. *The Medicare Risk Program for HMOs.* Princeton, NJ: Mathematica Policy Research. *Note:* Impact estimates were obtained with logit models that predicted the probability of receiving the services as a function of enrollment status, demographic variables, economic variables, attitudinal variables, and health and functioning variables. The estimated model was then used to predict probabilities for each individual as an enrollee and as a nonenrollee. The difference in the average of these two estimates across all sample members is the HMO impact.

Enrollees rated their overall satisfaction with care as excellent 45 percent of the time, compared with 52 percent of the traditional fee-for-service people. Certainly the managed care ratings are lower, but is 7 percent large or small? Put a different way, out of two hundred beneficiaries split between enrollment in HMOs or in traditional fee-for-service, a difference of seven beneficiaries will not rate the HMO as excellent. What may be more concerning is that nearly every dimension of care studied gives traditional fee-for-service the edge.

After differences in characteristics are controlled, Medicare beneficiaries who were enrolled at the time of this study were 11 to 15 percentage points less

likely than nonenrollees to give a rating of excellent to the following aspects
of the care process:

- explanations of the care received;
- attention received as a patient;
- advice on preventing health problems;
- personal interest taken in their care; and
- respect and privacy in regard to their care.

Enrollees were less likely to give an excellent rating to structural aspects of
care in the following areas:

- availability of different types of care (emergency, hospital, and specialty);
- ease of obtaining care (making telephone appointments, receiving
  information by phone, getting prescriptions filled, and the convenience of
  office hours);
- waiting times (from appointment to visit at the office); and
- ease of seeing the physician of their choice.

The ratings of perceived quality and overall outcomes receiving lower valua-
tions from enrollees were:

- quality of office/facilities;
- thoroughness of examinations;
- accuracy of the diagnosis;
- thoroughness of treatment; and
- overall results of care received.

The effect on satisfaction was similar among older and younger enrollees. Like
younger enrollees, older enrollees were generally satisfied with the care they
received but were less likely to give the highest marks to many dimensions
of quality. In addition, like their younger counterparts, older enrollees were
significantly more satisfied than traditional fee-for-service beneficiaries with
out-of-pocket costs.

There is little doubt that enrollees are satisfied, but not as much as traditional fee-for-service beneficiaries, except for the costs they incur. Medicare
managed care is a trade off for beneficiaries between quality to some extent
and cost.

The previous study is significant because it gives the comparison between enrollment in an HMO relative to the alternative, traditional fee-for-
service Medicare. Although that information dates back to 1990, it is the latest
source of comparative information. The most recent study of enrollees alone
was done in 1995 (Nelson et al. 1996). In that study, nearly all enrollees (96
percent) of Medicare HMO members were satisfied with their health plan in
1995–96. In fact, 91 percent would recommend their plan to a family member
or friend. Whereas HMO members were somewhat more likely to report access
problems than were traditional Medicare beneficiaries, less than 3 percent of

TABLE 2.4

Percent of
Beneficiaries
Reporting
Access to Care
Problems in
Traditional
Fee-for-Service
and Medicare
Managed Care,
1996

*Problems among
the vulnerable?
Access problems
are more likely
to be self-
reported by
enrollees*

Beneficiaries	All Beneficiaries	Nonelderly Disabled	Over Age 85	Low Income[a]	Fair or Poor Health
Traditional Fee-for-Service[b]	4.0	14.1	3.1	7.8	9.3
HMO[c]	12.0	21.3	23.1	16.5	26.1

Source: Survey sponsored by the Physician Payment Review Commission. 1996. Nelson, L. et al. *Access to Care in Medicare Managed Care.*
[a]Low income is defined as an annual household income of less than $10,000.
[b]For traditional fee-for-service beneficiaries, the access measure shown is the percentage who reported having trouble obtaining healthcare they wanted or needed within the past year.
[c]For HMO enrollees, the access measure shown is the percentage reporting one or more of the following problems since enrolling in the plan one year before or later: not being referred for specialist care wanted, not being admitted to a hospital when wanted, being discharged from a hospital before feeling ready, not receiving home health care wanted, experiencing delays obtaining care, and experiencing any other problems obtaining care.

HMO members disenrolled and returned to the traditional Medicare program. Most disenrollees merely switched to another HMO.

The Nelson study also found that, as in fee-for-service, certain subgroups of beneficiaries are vulnerable to access problems in HMOs. When asked about access to care problems experienced in the last year, the results were as indicated in Table 2.4.

The numbers in Table 2.4 come from two different surveys with different methodologies; thus, they are not strictly comparable. Nevertheless, the comparison reveals large differences in perceived access to care. The contrast seems to be too large to be entirely explained by the two different data sources. The most interesting aspect is that although a substantially higher percent of beneficiaries in HMOs appear to have had access problems, the differences between vulnerable beneficiaries in HMOs appear to be smaller in risk plans than they are in fee-for-service. In other words, disabled beneficiaries in fee-for-service were five times more likely than their nondisabled counterparts to have had any access problems. In managed care, it is only twice as likely. Each category follows this pattern.

As a final note on beneficiary perceptions of Medicare managed care, this information is now available on the Internet. Congress directed HCFA to collect data on beneficiary satisfaction with care, access, quality, and outcomes. Findings regarding member satisfaction are available on the Internet for each Medicare+Choice plan (http://www.medicare.gov/comparison/default.asp) and each market served.

Strategic Implications: Know the Financing and Delivery System

The importance of understanding your local market cannot be underestimated. You must know the financing system and the enrollment in health plans, the delivery system and the configuration of hospitals and physicians, and the beneficiaries and their perceptions. To assist with this understanding, a managed care plan should be able to place itself among the four boxes in Figure 2.5.

This framework for examining a local market and the place of the managed care plan in the market currently can be used by management to develop strategic assumptions and to help determine how the plan might want to change its place in the market. Answering the strategic questions at the end of this section should help to place your managed care plan in the matrix in Figure 2.5 along two dimensions.

The first dimension is Medicare managed care enrollment in Medicare+Choice plans, measured in market share. Medicare+Choice market share conveniently summarizes in one number the financing of health plan coverage. At a primary level, it can be viewed as the market share of Medicare managed care versus traditional fee-for-service. At a secondary level, it can be viewed as the market share of major players within the Medicare managed

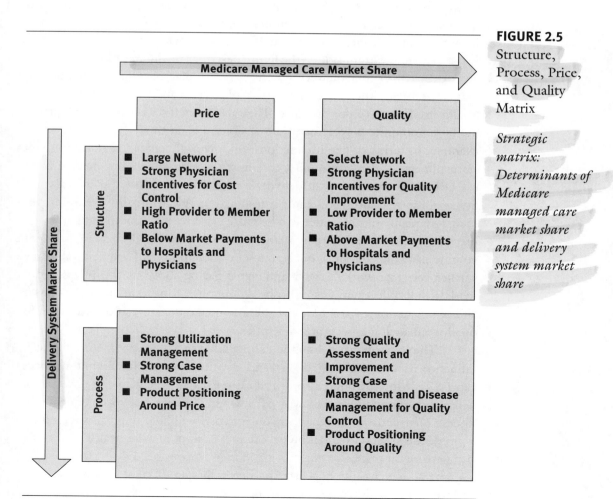

FIGURE 2.5
Structure, Process, Price, and Quality Matrix

Strategic matrix: Determinants of Medicare managed care market share and delivery system market share

care sector only. Price and quality in the market will largely drive health plan enrollment.

The second dimension is in terms of the delivery system, measured in market share among the hospitals and physicians. Delivery system market share will be driven largely by the way hospital and physician markets are structured and the various organizations and processes used to influence price and quality.

The upper-left side of the figure lists some of the major factors, which will be discussed in later chapters, at the intersection of PRICE and the STRUCTURE of the delivery system. A Medicare managed care plan using price to grow market share enrollment will rely on a large network of hospitals and physicians to play one group against another to receive price concessions. A large network (per the number of enrolled members) generally will ensure that no provider group is indispensable to the managed care plan; thus enabling the health plan to obtain price concessions and to lower health plan premiums. Yet price is only one determinant of health plan costs and premiums. Unnecessary service use increases costs and premiums. Thus, the plan should be structured to offer strong physician incentives for controlling costs. Because physician incentives for cost control can be diluted among a very large network of providers, the incentives must be clear and meaningful to the provider network.

The upper-right side of the figure describes the intersection of QUALITY and STRUCTURE of the delivery system. A health plan playing the quality card may do so by having a select network of physicians and hospitals with proven quality credentials or performance. They are selected for the perceived quality in the community across many dimensions. Quality may be perceived, for example, in terms of geographic location, medical center/teaching hospital status, image in the community, or a host of other issues. But market share can be built by structuring the delivery system around a select, quality network. Strong physician incentives can be designed to reward quality and improvements in quality of care. They can be more effective also among a small select provider network, rather than a large one. The promise of increased patient volume as quality and price goals are met is more powerful and believable in a smaller, select network. If the health plan is paying above-market prices, it can work with its select network of hospitals and physicians to retain the business, and it can to some extent expect them to make the time and effort to add quality-enhancing aspects and amenities.

The lower-left box lists the PRICE and PROCESS of care factors that can influence Medicare managed care and the delivery system. Premium prices can be kept low through strong utilization management in the network of hospitals and physicians. Likewise, strong and effective case management and disease management designed to control costs will help the plan succeed on a price basis. Marketing can be devoted to positioning the health plan to be competitive on price.

The lower-right box lists the determinants of QUALITY and PROCESS of care in the delivery system. Strong quality assessment and improvement efforts should reward the health plan with quality care. Case management and disease management efforts can also be geared toward improving quality under the notion that higher quality means lower costs. Finally, marketing can be devoted to positioning the health plan to be competitive on quality.

Use this matrix to score your health plan on each item in each quadrant relative to your rivals. On a scale of 1 to 10 assign numbers on the strength of agreement. Assign a 1 if you disagree that it describes your plan, and assign a 10 if it strongly describes your plan in the managed care market. You may wish to score the matrix yourself or use a group process to reach a consensus score for each item. Then, add the scores for the items and see first which quadrant on the upper half of the matrix (STRUCTURE) best describes your health plan and then which one in the lower half of the matrix (PROCESS) best describes your health plan relative to your rivals. Make the determination based on the quadrant with the highest score summed across items. In assigning the scores using the matrix, you should be answering the questions in the accompanying strategic questions table.

Based on the previous discussion, California represents the upper left of the matrix, Florida the upper right, Pennsylvania the lower left, and Arizona the lower right. In summary, California has a consolidated managed care health plan side, large networks with strong physician incentives for cost control, and low payments. Florida has more selective networks, incentives for quality improvement, and high payments. Pennsylvania has a consolidated delivery system side, with strong utilization management and product positioning around price. Arizona has a consolidated delivery system, strong quality assessment and disease management, and product positioning around quality.

The take-away message from this discussion is that Medicare managed care market share does not just happen. There are factors that health plans and beneficiaries bring to the market that determine the market share. Try to understand the factors and how they might be unique or the same for your market in comparison with others.

Likewise, whether there are two, three, or four major players on the delivery system side is not determined purely by accident. Study the hospitals and physicians as major players to quantify their importance in the marketplace through either the patients they see, the assets they hold, or their wealth or reputation. What delivery system is your health plan using? Understand what determines the market share the delivery system holds.

Finally, examine the combination scores down the matrix on the left side and then the right side. Which scores are higher for your health plan— the price features that drive Medicare managed care market share and delivery system market share or the quality features?

Strategic Decisions Checklist

Strategic Questions	Strategic Analyses
How many beneficiaries are in your market?	Obtain detailed data on the number of total beneficiaries and enrollment in Medicare managed care now and projected into the future.
	Create maps with indicators of the number of beneficiaries in your market and their location by zip code. Identify the pockets of Medicare managed care enrollment and understand why they exist.
What is the age and gender distribution of beneficiaries in your market?	Obtain detailed data on enrollment by personal characteristics such as age, gender, and race.
	Other characteristics are income or residence by income of the county or zip code, employment status, union status.
	Determine whether these features of the beneficiary population are similar or dissimilar from national figures.
Is enrollment in Medicare managed care proportional to the market by age, gender, ethnicity, or geographic location?	Determine whether enrollment in Medicare managed care is occurring disproportionately in certain age, gender, ethnicity, or geographic categories.
What determines financing and delivery system market share in your market?	Study your market compared with those with higher and lower financing and delivery system market share, and determine what makes your market unique or the same.
What are the determinants for your financing and delivery system?	Describe your financing and delivery system in the market and its positioning in terms of structure and process.
What are the determinants for rivals?	Describe rival delivery systems in the market and their positioning in terms of structure and process.

continued

Strategic Questions	Strategic Analyses
What combination of price and quality features will your managed care plan adopt to achieve market share?	List the changes in Medicare managed care product price, quality, structure of the delivery system, and process of care features that will enhance your position in the market.
What combination of delivery systems structure and process of care features will be used to achieve delivery system market share?	List the recent changes in delivery system structure and process of care and how they are likely to affect your position in the market.

EARLY DEVELOPMENT OF MEDICARE MANAGED CARE

The connection between Medicare and managed care is not a new phenomenon. Rather, it is a relationship that has evolved over many years. From the start of the original Medicare program in 1966 through the present, Medicare has offered a number of different contracting options to managed care plans. What is relatively new in the relationship is the large and growing *enrollment* in Medicare managed care.

Table 3.1 summarizes the significant events that occurred in the development of Medicare managed care, showing the highlights of the development between Medicare and managed care as four distinct phases:

Phase 1. Cost-reimbursement (1966–1979)
Phase 2. Experimentation (1980–1985)
Phase 3. Risk-contract program (1985–2001)
Phase 4. Structured choice (2002–)

Briefly, here is how the relationship has evolved. During the cost-reimbursement phase, Medicare attempted to treat payments for healthcare prepayment plans and group medical practices like cost payments to hospitals. For more than ten years, the concept of reasonable cost reimbursement was applied and worked reasonably well for the managed care companies that were emerging in the market. Then, during phase 2 large-scale social experiments ensued and Congress enacted new program legislation even before the first research results were reported. For nearly 15 years, during the risk-contract program phase, the program has remained much the same from the initial legislation and regulations. By 2002, a new period of multiple health plans will begin, with a structured process for choosing a plan and implications for being locked into a plan option.

Cost-Reimbursement Phase

Medicare's initial involvement with managed care entailed payment provisions that were based on the conventional benefit and cost-reimbursement philosophy of the original Medicare program. Those original provisions were the traditional service benefits of the predominant form of insurance at the start of Medicare: Blue Cross plans for hospital services and Blue Shield plans for physician services. The traditional program attempted to ensure that all

49

TABLE 3.1
Significant
Events in the
Development
of Medicare
Managed Care,
1965–2002

*Evolution of a
program: Four
distinct phases*

Year	Public Law or Code of Federal Regulations	Event
		Cost-Reimbursement Phase, 1966–1979
1965	89-97	Medicare enacted and signed into law by President Johnson.
		Group practice prepayment plans authorized to contract with Medicare for the prospective payment of Part B services.
1972	92-603	HMOs authorized to receive Medicare payments on a reasonable cost basis.
		Medicare eligibility expanded to disabled beneficiaries after being eligible for cash benefits for 24 months and to patients with end-stage renal disease (ESRD).
1973	93-222	HMO Act signed into law by President Nixon.
1977		Authorization of Health Care Financing Administration by President Carter.
		Experimentation Phase, 1980–1985
1980		Medicare capitation demonstrations begin.
1982		Medicare competition demonstrations begin.
1980	96-265	Reports of marketing abuses in traditional fee-for-service sector brings Medicare supplemental insurance under federal oversight.
1982	97-248[a]	HMOs and a new form of managed care, competitive medical plans, authorized to receive prospectively determined Medicare payments with a risk-based contract.
		Risk-Contract Program Phase, 1985–2001
1985	42 CFR Parts 405 and 417[b]	Rules established for managed care plans to receive a fixed payment from Medicare and enrollees, regardless of the volume of service provided.
1985	OBRA-1985	Stiffened requirements regarding maximum enrollment of 50 percent Medicare or Medicaid and 50 percent all other enrollment. Expanded role of peer review organizations and quality review organizations to handle beneficiary complaints and review Medicare managed care quality.

continued

TABLE 3.1
Continued

Year	Public Law or Code of Federal Regulations	Event
		Risk-Contract Program Phase, 1985–2001 (continued)
1986	COBRA-1986	Required Medicare to review and approve marketing material.
1987		Medicare ends contract with largest Medicare managed care plan, IMC in south Florida, because of widely publicized violations of enrollment rules and financial reporting. IMC purchased by Humana.
1987	COBRA-1987	Required managed care plans to arrange for the continuation of traditional Medicare supplemental coverage when not renewing a contract or changing service area.
1990	P.L. 101-508	Medicare supplemental insurance policies subjected to new standards regarding permitted policy types and allowable medical loss ratios.
1990	OBRA-1990	Permitted insurers in some states to offer a preferred provider organization product (Medicare SELECT) as a managed care modification of traditional Medicare supplemental insurance coverage.
1995		Guidelines were issued on Medicare point-of-service benefit offering available for HMOs.
1997	BBA-1997	Medicare+Choice program enacted, which broadened the array of health plans that may participate in Medicare and modified the calculation of the Medicare payment to managed care plans. Created the Medicare+Choice payment.
		Structured-Choice Phase, 2002–
2002		Start of open enrollment period with lock in. Beneficiaries can change health plan choice one time during the first six months of the year, in addition to changes that can be made during the annual coordinated election period.

[a] Section 1876 of the Social Security Act as amended by Section 226 of the Social Security Amendments of 1972 (P.L. 92–603), enacted October 30, 1972.

[b] *Federal Register*. Vol. 50, No. 7, Part IV: Department of Health and Human Services—42 CFR Parts 405 and 417—Medicare Program; Payments to HMOs and Competitive Medical Plans: Final Rules. January 10, 1985.

beneficiaries had access to virtually all hospitals and physicians. The benefits were defined in terms of hospital and physician services, and payments were made on a fee-for-service basis. The level of payments were determined by hospital costs and physician fees. Nearly every hospital and physician in the country was counted on to participate in Medicare. Prepaid group practice plans existed in certain parts of the country at the time and were already serving patients who would become beneficiaries of the new program. They wanted to participate in Medicare along with everyone else. Rather than an entirely different prepaid payment system, something akin to the hospital cost-based system was created for prepaid group practices.

Health Care Prepayment Plans

Group Practice Prepayment Plans (now called Health Care Prepayment Plans, or HCPPs) were one type of cost-based payment plan created during this early phase. HCPPs were authorized under the initial legislation to contract with the Medicare program for the prospective payment of Part B services (medical and other professional services). However, these prospective payments were based on the projected costs of the plans. Payments were adjusted at the end of the year to equal 80 percent of reasonable costs, with beneficiary copayments making up the additional 20 percent.

Section 1876 Plans

The Social Security Amendments of 1972 expanded the cost-based payment options for prepaid plans. These amendments allowed HMOs to provide both Part A and Part B benefits by entering into either cost-based or risk-based contracts with Medicare. Before the 1972 changes, only Part B cost reimbursement was permitted. A participating plan was required to be federally qualified as a HMO and to have at least 5,000 enrollees. As with the HCPPs, reimbursement was provided through interim monthly capitation payments, which were based on Medicare's estimate of how much it cost the plan to serve Medicare enrollees.

Both managed care contracts that were authorized in 1972 set cost limits. These limits circumscribed the risk to the plan, and they provided little financial incentive for the health plan to be concerned with the volume of services it provided. In fact, enrollees could seek care outside of the network of hospitals and physicians in the health plan, and the provider would still receive payment from fee-for-service Medicare. An adjustment at the end of the year would be made for out-of-plan service use.

If a managed care plan selected the cost-based contract, actual costs would be calculated at the end of the contract period on the basis of cost reports submitted by the health plan. The previous month's capitation payments would then be adjusted to reflect allowable and reasonable costs. This arrangement resembled the cost-based reimbursement contracts that hospitals entered at the time.

If a managed care plan selected the risk-based contract, actual costs would be calculated at the end of the contract period. These costs would then be compared with an adjusted-average per-capita cost that was determined retrospectively. This adjusted-average per-capita cost would be estimated for the geographic areas served by the health plan and represented what Medicare costs would have been for the enrollees in the health plan if they had remained in the fee-for-service sector. Costs were determined retrospectively only for the areas of the country with such contracts, but the early experiences with the Section 1876 payment provisions laid the groundwork for the prospectively determined adjusted-average per-capita costs used in the experimental phase and the risk-contract program phase.

The risk-based payment was lopsided, however. Under that arrangement, health plans could share in savings if the health plan's actual costs were less than the retrospective per-capita rate; but these shared savings could not exceed 10 percent of the adjusted-average per-capita cost. Meanwhile, these plans had to absorb all losses when their costs exceeded the adjusted-average per-capita cost. Thus, under Section 1876, Medicare managed care plans were fully at risk but limited in the amount of savings they could retain.

At the end of the cost-reimbursement phase, 13 years after the inception of the Medicare program, only 64 managed care plans had Medicare contracts. These included several with contracts going back to group practice prepayment plans (32 prepaid group practices or other organizations), HCPPs (31 HMOs), and Section 1876 risk contracts (1 HMO). Enrollment was significant, however. In 1979, more than 527,000 beneficiaries were enrolled in managed care plans (Langwell and Hadley 1986).

Start of Healthcare Reform: The Health Maintenance Organization and Resources Act of 1973

In 1970, there were only 33 HMOs in the United States and about 3 million members. Healthcare reform, in terms of dramatic change in the coverage of people with and without insurance, started from a base of largely fee-for-service or no coverage. The beginning of reform was the passage of the Health Maintenance Organization and Resources Act of 1973 (HMO Act of 1973). The effects of changes created by this act are still being felt nearly 30 years later as managed care, the current predominant form of health insurance, is increasingly providing new coverage for people without any health coverage. A recent example of this trend is the State Children's Health Insurance Program, which was passed in the Balanced Budget Act of 1997.

The HMO Act of 1973 offered grants and guaranteed loans of more than $350 million over ten years for new HMOs. With amendments to the original act, federal qualifications were established. These qualifications allowed health plans to obtain a permit to enroll members from the federal government. Previously, only state insurance commissioners were involved in licensing and regulating HMOs. The essentials of Federal qualification are shown in Table 3.2.

Initially, the HMO Act of 1973 only provided the development funding for not-for-profit community HMOs, and that seemed to be successful. By the early 1980s, there were nearly 300 HMOs. In fact, 92 new plans entered the market in 1984 alone.

But by the early 1980s, the method of development funding had changed. Many new plans were for-profit plans, and existing plans were converting to for-profit status. One prominent example was U.S. Health Care Systems, Inc., an early Medicare participant under a demonstration waiver. U.S. Health Care converted to for-profit status in 1981 and obtained venture capital. Within two years, the company went public, becoming the first HMO to sell stock to the public. Many other federally qualified plans followed suit.

The HMO Act of 1973 was one factor that led to the ability of U.S. Health Care and other federally qualified plans to expand quickly and seek capital successfully from private sources. The act and its amendments enabled HMOs to expand quickly in other states without having to grapple with the special demands of insurance commissioners from each state. The federal qualification provided some semblance of uniform regulation for quick expansion. It also proved to be the major criterion for determining a plan's acceptability as a Medicare managed care contractor.

TABLE 3.2
Health Maintenance Organization Act of 1973 and Its Amendments

Tough federal requirements: Essential provisions for federally qualified HMOs

Provide or Arrange for Basic Services	Physician services Outpatient and inpatient services, including short-term rehabilitation services and physical therapy Emergency services in and out of service area Mental health services Certain substance abuse services Diagnostic laboratory and radiology services Home health services Preventive services including voluntary family-planning services, infertility services, well-child care, adult periodic health exams, eye and ear exams for children, and immunizations
Community Rating	Premiums set on a per-person or per-family basis, with community rating by class by one of two methods, and with some exceptions
Quality Assurance Program	Stresses health outcomes, reviews providers, systematically collects data, and has remedial action procedures
Fiscally Sound Operation	Requirements on total assets, insolvency protection, minimum administration and management arrangements
Record Keeping and Reporting	Requirements regarding annual reporting and information needed by ERISA plans

Experimentation Phase

Medicare Capitation Demonstrations

In 1978, seven HMOs in five markets were solicited to participate in initial demonstration projects with prospectively determined payments for all Medicare-covered services. All but one are still enrolling today, albeit under different affiliation. In 1980, when these demonstration health plans began operating, each one received 95 percent of the adjusted-average per-capita cost in the local geographic area. They were permitted to retain and use at their discretion any savings between their actual costs and the prospective per-capita payment.

The seven plans, listed in Table 3.3, offered beneficiaries an alternative to the traditional fee-for-service approach, and they became the biggest market leaders in the history of Medicare managed care. Fallon Community Health Plan has the distinction of being the first HMO to receive risk-contract payments. Enrollment in Fallon and the others marked the first time that a comprehensive substitute for standard Medicare Part A and Part B benefits was offered by a private health plan, one that was not merely a supplement to Medicare.

In those days (and generally also today), the premiums for managed care plans were significantly below standard Medicare supplemental policies, both high and low options. With virtually no cost sharing, benefits often included physician exams, immunizations, prescribed medicines, eyeglasses, and skilled nursing services without prior hospitalization.

The seven demonstration plans represented a mix of model types: three plans were group models, one was a staff model, and three were network models (see Common Medicare Managed Care Terms for definitions.) Three of the initial plans that became market leaders were affiliates with Blue Cross and Blue Shield. It was notable that Blue Cross and Blue Shield plans in three states were among the leaders in testing models that had the potential to replace the traditional system. After all, the traditional fee-for-service Medicare program was modeled on the service-benefits insurance firmly associated with Blue Cross and Blue Shield plans around the country.

Even as the experimentation phase of Medicare managed care was coming to a close in 1985, enrollments remained relatively low for the leadership plans, with one exception. Share Health Plan in Minneapolis had enrolled more than 30,000 beneficiaries. Market share as a percent of all Medicare beneficiaries in the local market was also low during this phase. Most of the early leaders obviously were testing and sampling this new form of risk contracting with a very high risk population.

When the Medicare Capitation Demonstrations began, HMOs were still a relatively new approach to managed care in most parts of the country. These plans offered financing and delivery that were unfamiliar to Medicare beneficiaries, most of whom had never encountered a managed care option

TABLE 3.3
Medicare
HMO and City,
Form, and
Demonstration
Statistics,
1980–1981

Market leaders:
Early risk-based
experiments

HMO and City	Organizational Form	Demonstration Start Date	Affiliation	Medicare Enrollment, 1985	Medicare Market Share, 1985 (%)
Fallon Community Health Plan *Worcester, MA*	Group	April 1980	Blue Cross of Massachusetts	9,887	10.4
Greater Marshfield Community Health Plan *Marshfield, WI*	Group	June 1980	Marshfield Medical Foundation	—	—
Kaiser Health Plan *Portland, OR*	Group	August 1980	Kaiser-Permanente Medical Plan of Oregon, Inc.	7,640	4.0
Health Central *Lansing, MI*	Staff	September 1981	Blue Cross and Blue Shield of Michigan	1,717	4.5
HMO Minnesota *Minneapolis, MN*	Network IPA	May 1981	Blue Cross and Blue Shield of Minnesota	6,471	3.1
SHARE Health Plan *Minneapolis, MN*	Network Group	January 1981	None	31,695	15.0
MedCenters Health Plan *Minneapolis, MN*	Network Group	May 1981	St. Louis Park Medical Center and Methodist Hospital	8,626	4.1

during the years they were employed. Elderly and disabled beneficiaries were the chief prospects of these new plans and were more likely to have chronic conditions, which meant they were more likely to have a regular source of care by a physician. The likelihood of those beneficiaries switching to a new provider, which sometimes is required when enrolling in a managed care plan, was remote.

Who were the early converts to Medicare managed care? Rossiter, Fiedlob, and Langwell (1985) analyzed the demonstrations in the Minneapolis–

St. Paul metropolitan area. They discovered that beneficiaries enrolling in the demonstrations were less likely to have had a Medicare supplemental policy than beneficiaries who remained in the fee-for-service sector. Those enrollees were also less satisfied than nonenrollees with their usual fee-for-service source of care, and they described themselves as being healthier than nonenrollees.

Very soon after the initial Medicare Capitation Demonstrations, the effort to expand Medicare managed care intensified.

National Medicare Competition Demonstrations

The Carter administration initiated the Medicare Competition Demonstrations and started developing the terms for previously untried risk contracts. The Reagan administration expanded the demonstrations. By 1980, the new administration was very eager to interject more market competition into the Medicare program. The effort to expand the program began with a nationwide call for proposals to see what ideas and arrangements were available. More than 50 managed care plans of different types applied. Of those, 21 were selected to move forward and join the original seven starting as early as August 1982. Most were already federally qualified HMOs that represented all four regions of the country. To demonstrate competitive aspects of the program, five health plans were approved to enter the beneficiary-rich south Florida market and compete head to head for enrollment.

The years 1982 to 1985 marked the start of Medicare Competition Demonstrations and the establishment of a full risk-contract program with the publication of regulations. During these years, 27 HMOs entered the Medicare market as demonstration projects sponsored by HCFA. The 27 early entrants represented locations in all four census regions of the country, included all model types of HMOs, and were almost all not-for-profit organizations with federal qualification. Enrollment ranged from a high of 43,000 beneficiaries to a low of 130, and the average enrollment per plan was 5,300 beneficiaries. The disenrollment rate across all the demonstration plans was 13.2 percent.

The Medicare Competition Demonstrations were examined extensively from the time they began until the participating plans were converted to the national program that was to come in 1985. Until that time, no one had tested the financial risk associated with providing Medicare benefits to any Medicare beneficiary who applied (excluding end-state renal disease beneficiaries). The initial implementation and operational experience of these plans provided useful information and guidance for many new health plans that were interested in entering the market (Langwell and Hadley 1989; Brown and Retchin 1990).

These demonstrations revealed crucial information. For instance, whereas the rate of physician office visits was similar, hospital service use in the Medicare Competition Demonstration plans was 17 percent lower than under traditional fee-for-service Medicare. Approximately one-third of all plans experienced hospital days per thousand of 1,800 to 2,200 days. Five plans had rates of less than 1,800 days per thousand. The national average in traditional fee-for-service Medicare in 1984 was 3,174 days per thousand. Most of the plans experienced positive financial performance in 1984.

Even though the demonstrations used fewer hospital resources to treat beneficiaries, the quality of inpatient and ambulatory care was similar to traditional fee-for-service Medicare. These results came from intensive, detailed studies of patients with colorectal cancer, heart failure, and stroke in the inpatient setting and diabetes, hypertension, and other basic needs in the ambulatory setting. Overall satisfaction rates were similar for Medicare managed care enrollees compared with fee-for-service beneficiaries. These Medicare managed care enrollees were less satisfied with the information they received from physicians about their treatment, as well as with the ease of seeing the physician of their choice. Yet they were substantially more satisfied with the cost of their coverage.

South Florida Investigations

Negative reports surfaced in the south Florida press about enrollment in HMOs almost from the start of the Medicare Competition Demonstrations. Frequent accounts detailed cases of questionable marketing practices. Other anecdotes described confused beneficiaries who did not understand that their choice of physician or hospital became limited when they enrolled in a Medicare HMO. Most of these stories seemed to involve IMC, an HMO with more than 100,000 enrollees.

What was the truth behind the stories? Was the press reporting the sort of mistakes one would expect with a health plan that has such a large enrollment? Or did the reports offer an early indication that more widespread problems were taking place in south Florida?

Two Government Accounting Office investigations focused on problems with enrollment and disenrollment procedures (GAO/HRD-85-48 1985), financial solvency and grievance procedures, and appeal rights (GAO/HRD-86-97 1986). When released, these reports drew widespread national press attention, with south Florida and IMC prominently featured.

In early 1987, another report was released that used anecdotal information obtained by several staff members of the Senate Special Committee on Aging. The report reached several conclusions. HMOs abused risk contracts, reducing the ability of beneficiaries to access care. Marketing practices were inadequately monitored. The quality of care was inadequate. Medicare oversight of the program was insufficient.

But major changes began to occur in the south Florida market in April 1987 when the founder and president of IMC was indicted by a federal grand jury on charges of conspiracy. By May 1987, Medicare canceled its contract with IMC, and beneficiaries were allowed to disenroll. Nearly five years of scandal ended when Humana purchased the troubled plan.

Risk-Based Payment Phase

Tax Equity and Fiscal Responsibility Act (TEFRA) of 1982

TEFRA officially authorized the new risk-based payment system, largely still in place today, and ended the period of experimentation. The 1982 act established the requirements for organizational participation and the rights of beneficiaries to enroll, and it set the payment at 95 percent of the adjusted-average per-capita cost. Moreover, an adjusted community rate became a required calculation for the participating health plans. To guard against excessive profits, health plans were required to estimate the premium the plan would have charged its Medicare members on the basis of the premium-setting approach used for its non-Medicare members. At the beginning of the contract year, health plans were required to return any difference between the capitation payments and the adjusted community rate. The difference was to be returned either to Medicare or to the health plan's Medicare members in the form of additional benefits or lower cost sharing.

Other provisions of TEFRA were spelled out in the final regulation that implemented the mandate for Medicare's second method of paying providers: capitation payments (Rossiter and Langwell 1988).

June 1985 Final Regulation

The June 1985 Final Regulation implementing the TEFRA mandate is the most comprehensive and important event in the history of Medicare managed care. It transformed the relationship between the largest single payer for healthcare in the country and the hospitals and physicians that provided that care. The regulation also permanently established alternative means for receiving payment from the Medicare trust funds.

Generally, HMOs were required to demonstrate the ability to enroll Medicare beneficiaries and to deliver the Medicare-covered services. Minimum requirements were put in place regarding operating experience, beginning enrollment levels for non-Medicare members (no more than 50 percent Medicare), range of services, network-furnishing services, and quality-assurance programs. Specific steps defined the process for transitioning the demonstration plans to full program contracts.

The June 1985 Final Regulation described how the open enrollment process worked. Medicare beneficiaries could freely choose to join the plan at any time and begin receiving services through the HMO within 15 to 45 days. There were two exceptions to this open-enrollment process. The first was Medicare beneficiaries who were ineligible for Part B services. Those beneficiaries presented a burden to the system because of the administrative hassle of adjusting Part B premiums payments. The second exception involved patients with end-stage renal disease or hospice patients.

During this time, marketing also became strictly regulated. HMOs were required to submit all marketing materials to HCFA for approval at least 45 days before distribution. Medicare barred participating plans from discriminatory or misleading marketing. For example, plans could not offer gifts or financial inducements to enroll, and they could not solicit door-to-door. Health plans were expected to offer lower premiums than found in the local market for traditional Medicare supplemental coverage or additional non-Medicare services. Disenrollment procedures were stipulated.

The methodology for establishing adjusted-average per-capita cost payments was similar to the approach used originally in the demonstration programs. The regulation did not say specifically how the actuary was to calculate the adjusted-average per-capita cost, and this later became an issue in terms of appropriate adjustment factors, including risk adjustment. However, the regulation generally provided for monthly predetermined payments. These payments had to reflect geographic costs, enrollment, and age, gender, and disability status. The actuary could also make adjustments for Medicaid status, institutional status, and other factors. Two additional factors influenced the capitation payment rate: the process for setting adjusted community rates and the implications for health plans that exceeded the adjusted community rate limits.

OBRA 1991 and Medicare SELECT

For nearly six years, the fully authorized yet budding HMO strategy became a permanent aspect of the Medicare program. As enrollment grew, the new Bush administration thought more could be done to provide beneficiaries with even greater choice. At the time, Medicare beneficiaries had a dual option: traditional fee-for-service Medicare or risk-based contract HMOs. The private sector, however, had evolved to a triple option: traditional fee-for-service, PPO, or HMO. Moreover, there were numerous variations on those options, including point-of-service plans (see Common Medicare Managed Care Terms).

There was no reason Medicare could not offer something in between entirely fee-for-service and entirely risk-based contract. Like many private insurers, Medicare had deductibles and coinsurance for hospital and physician services. Could the cost-sharing provisions of Medicare be leveraged to give beneficiaries a PPO?

OBRA 1991 created just such a program: Medicare SELECT. This program authorized new Medicare supplemental plans that were in all aspects like one of the ten standard policies (see Chapter 1). The one exception (other than for emergency care) was that full benefits were paid only when network providers were used.

States regulated Medicare SELECT plans to ensure that they offered sufficient access, had an ongoing quality-assurance program, and provided full and documented disclosure at the time of enrollment of the beneficiary. The disclosure encompassed restrictions on the network and provisions for out-of-area and emergency coverage. The disclosure also addressed the availability and cost of all other Medicare supplemental policies without the network restrictions.

At the time, the Medicare SELECT program was viewed as being both too much managed care and not enough. It was not enough managed care because Medicare worked as it always did, whereas only the private Medicare supplemental insurance changed. Medicare supplemental insurers applied network restrictions to only the cost-sharing provisions of Medicare, whereas the inner workings of Medicare remained the same. It was viewed as being too much managed care because beneficiaries had to give up some freedom of choice in the sense of having to face normal Medicare cost sharing if they went out of the network of providers. Some thought protections would not be available if a plan, regulated only by the state, became insolvent. As a result, the original law authorized demonstrations in just 15 states. HCFA approved demonstrations in the following states: Alabama, Arizona, California, Florida, Indiana, Kentucky, Michigan, Minnesota, Missouri, North Dakota, Ohio, Oregon, Texas, Washington, and Wisconsin. Medicare SELECT became available to all states in 1996, following the release of several HCFA reports that showed mixed results in terms of cost savings but also expanded choices for beneficiaries.

Further Regulatory Changes in the 1990s

By 1994, several unpublished studies had shown that the cost and HCPP plan contracts were not cost effective for Medicare. HCFA also found that they were complicated to administer alongside a rapidly growing risk-contract program. To address these issues, HCFA was successful at getting presumptive payment limits for cost-contract plans. The limit was set at 100 percent of the adjusted per-capita cost. After this regulation went into effect, several prominent health plans with much of the cost-contract enrollment switched to risk contracts.

Participating HMOs had long complained that when new benefits were added to the Medicare-covered services midyear, the monthly capitation payment was not immediately adjusted. Plans were required to provide new benefits immediately even though they did not receive payment for them until much later. A new regulation in 1994 known as "national coverage limits" addressed that problem.

By the mid-1990s, many private health plans were offering the point-of-service option. This option allowed members to use an out-of-network provider if they agreed to a higher copayment. New rules established when and how a plan could offer a point-of-service option to encourage enrollment. Point-of-service could be offered as a mandatory feature of enrollment or as an optional supplement for beneficiaries. It could also be an added benefit if the risk-based payment was enough to cover the benefit. The premiums from employer group enrollment could be used to pay for the point-of-service option. The regulation for national coverage limits described how the option could be marketed and how beneficiaries needed to be informed and educated about the option.

Press reports and lawsuits in the early 1990s raised concerns about financial arrangements between HMOs and physicians or physician groups.

These arrangements were thought to cause substantial financial risk. In some cases, individual physicians were being paid a capitation payment to provide certain services that they themselves did not provide. This put the individual physician in the position of acting like an insurance company in terms of risk bearing, so a new regulation was issued in 1997 to clearly define substantial financial risk and available remedies. These new regulations required health plans to arrange stop-loss protection for their physicians, conduct annual enrollee surveys, or change their financial arrangements to eliminate the excessive risk to physicians or groups of physicians.

Also in 1997, a new regulation required Medicare managed care plans to establish and maintain an expedited appeals process for reconsidering decisions about coverage. The expedited review process was to come into play when an adverse determination could seriously jeopardize the life or health of the enrollee. The regulation spelled out when Medicare managed care plans must use their expedited review process, the rights of beneficiaries to have a reconsideration, and the time limits for reconsideration.

Structured-Choice Phase
Medicare+Choice

The recent history of Medicare managed care ends with the Balanced Budget Act of 1997 and the Medicare+Choice regulations that took effect in 1999. Medicare+Choice is described more fully in Chapter 2 as the current Medicare managed care program. But placed in the context of the evolving story of Medicare managed care, Medicare+Choice is important for several reasons.

First, Medicare+Choice allowed organizations other than HMOs to enter the Medicare managed care market. The new options included coordinated-care plans, such as HMOs, point-of-service plans, PSO plans, PPO plans, high-deductible plans used in conjunction with a Medicare medical savings account, and private Medicare fee-for-service plans. Chapter 4 provides greater detail about each of these.

Second, the Medicare+Choice program eliminated the prior adjusted-average per-capita cost payment except as a beginning base for calculating payments. This action gradually moved Medicare managed care toward a national regulated rate. Chapter 5 discusses the new payment in more detail. Rather than tying payments to local market conditions, which the traditional Medicare fee-for-service costs reflected, Medicare+Choice established a payment formula. It retained adjustments for age, disability status, gender, institutional status, and other factors including a risk-adjustment mechanism. Beginning in 1999, Medicare+Choice plans were paid the greater of a $367 per-member-per-month floor, a 2 percent increase over 1997 rates, or a blended payment 90 percent based on local rates and 10 percent based on an input-adjusted national rate. A 50-50 payment rate will be phased in nationally by 2003.

Third, and most important, Medicare+Choice instituted an annual, coordinated, open-enrollment period (Table 3.4). This new open-enrollment period held considerably more promise for educating Medicare beneficiaries about their choices than any program before it. An annual open-enrollment period will also force the next generation of beneficiaries eligible for Medicare to consider their options. Some of these options will be very familiar, especially for those beneficiaries who have experienced managed care through the private coverage they will be leaving.

Information on coverage options will be broadly disseminated to beneficiaries. Beneficiaries will receive certain information through the mail, and a toll-free number and an Internet site (http://www.medicare.gov) will provide them with immediate access to information about plan options. Beginning in 2002, beneficiaries will be able to change a personal election one time during the first six months of the year. They will also have opportunities to make additional changes during the annual coordinated election period. This

TABLE 3.4 Rules for Enrollment in Medicare+Choice Plans Transition, 1999–2002

Enrollment means lock-in: The choice of private managed care plan is structured around periods of lock-in for enrollment

Enrollment Year	Information Availability	Timing of Enrollment in a Medicare+Choice Plan or Traditional Medicare	Ability to Disenroll from a Medicare+Choice Plan, Return to Traditional Medicare, or Switch
1999	Special information campaign in November 1998	Continuous open enrollment	Any time during year
2000	Health information fair in November 1999	Continuous open enrollment	Any time during year
2001	Health information fair in November 2000	Continuous open enrollment	Any time during year
2002	Health information fair in November 2001	Open season held in November 2001; enrollment effective January 1, 2002	One time during the first six months of the year
2003 and thereafter	Health information fair in November of each year	Open season held in November of preceding year; enrollment begins January 1	One time during the first three months of the year

Source: Medicare Payment Advisory Commission analysis of the Balanced Budget Act of 1997. 1998. *Report to Congress.* Washington, DC: MedPAC.

provision establishes an approximate six-month lock-in period to any Medicare managed care plan and marks the start of a new phase.

The new phase will have much more involvement from Medicare in forcing people to choose a plan rather than be assigned to traditional fee-for-service Medicare. Patients will also have more rights about appealing coverage decisions and seeking external review of the decisions on a timely basis. These and other changes will continue to influence the structure of choices and foster a properly functioning private market.

Strategic Decisions Checklist

Strategic Questions	Strategic Analyses
What is the historical context of managed care and Medicare managed care?	You need to determine the history of your local market in each phase of Medicare managed care. You should understand where your health plan and your market have been and where they are now in terms of regulations, willingness to experiment, and readiness to change.
What are the pros and cons of federal qualification for your plans?	Know the costs and benefits of federal qualification versus state-only qualification.
How will upcoming changes in the Medicare managed care program affect your plan?	You can begin by following the changes in structuring beneficiary choice and new lock-in provisions. Then, you must get involved in explaining to beneficiaries how the changes will work in the future.

4

THE PRIVATE SIDE OF MEDICARE TODAY

Previous chapters discussed the fundamentals of the Medicare managed care marketplace and the trends and major players that have been crucial to its development. They also provided a brief history of managed care. Chapter 4 reviews the wide array of options that health plans have to serve Medicare beneficiaries and then compares the features of each plan.

To offer the Medicare managed care option, a managed care plan must realize the relationship between enrollment and revenues. Figure 4.1 illustrates this relationship with the Medicare+Choice market, the highest risk market available for health plans. Simply expressing the risk of enrolling Medicare beneficiaries in terms of the number of people enrolled is misleading. Suppose the enrollment of the average Medicare managed care plan was proportional to the national population of beneficiaries from Medicare, private commercial plans, and Medicaid. If that were the case, an average of 12 percent of the members would be Medicare beneficiaries. But this 12 percent segment translates into an average of 40 percent of the revenues. Why is that? Elderly and disabled Medicare beneficiaries have higher levels of use and cost more to service than any other group.

It is crucial to keep the vital relationship between enrollment and revenue in mind as we sift through the methods available to serve the Medicare managed care market. This chapter covers the various contractual arrangements in terms of regulatory, quality of care, and financial issues. All the options carry substantial financial risk and significant regulatory oversight.

Public Law 105-33, The Balanced Budget Act of 1997, defines three broad types of managed care plans: coordinated care, private fee-for-service, and medical savings accounts (MSAs). Table 4.1 describes each of these plans in terms of licensure, solvency, quality, and beneficiary financial liability. Although Chapter 1 discusses each of these plans and the glossary gives a brief definition, a brief review might be helpful.

Coordinated-care plans include HMOs, PPOs, and PSOs. To receive benefits through HMOs, enrollees must use the provider network offered by the health plan. With PPOs, the plan pays higher benefits when enrollees use the approved provider network and lower benefits for using unapproved providers outside the network. A PSO can operate like either an HMO or a PPO. Its distinction is that it is established by healthcare providers themselves. Enrollees receive a substantial portion of healthcare directly from affiliated providers who share, directly or indirectly, substantial financial risk. These

FIGURE 4.1

Relationship
Between
Enrollment and
Revenues to a
Medicare+
Choice
Organization

*Membership in
proportion to
national share
in private
commercial,
Medicaid, and
Medicare?*

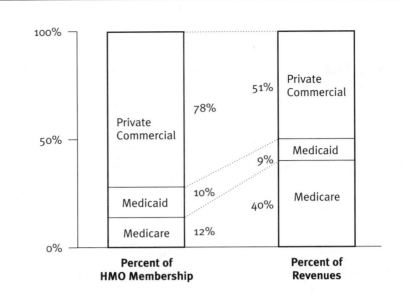

three types of health plans make up the first broad category of coordinated health plans.[1]

The next type of plan, fee-for-service, reimburses providers on a strictly fee-for-service basis. Such a plan is thought to have a broad, open network of providers and is authorized to charge enrolled beneficiaries up to 115 percent of the plan's payment schedule. As a result, these plans could be quite expensive. If beneficiaries are willing to pay to join, however, they can make up these costs. These plans offer a mechanism for unbridled fee-for-service arrangements to receive a Medicare+Choice payment and make up the higher costs out of beneficiary premiums and coinsurance.

The third broad option is an experimental MSA. Under this option, beneficiaries obtain high-deductible health policies that pay for all Medicare-covered services after they meet the annual deductible. Regulations cap this deductible at $6,000. The difference between the premiums for such high-deductible policies and the applicable amount of the Medicare+Choice payment is placed in a special account, which beneficiaries can use to meet their deductibles.

The following sections discuss these three broad types of plans and compare the provisions each one offers.

---

[1]A fourth plan is what the law calls a religious fraternal benefit society plan. These may restrict enrollment to members of the church, convention, or group with which the society is affiliated. Payments to such plans may be adjusted, as appropriate to take into account the actuarial characteristics and experience of plan enrollees. This health plan is highly specialized and is not included in this discussion.

Standard	Coordinated Care	Private Fee-for-Service	Medical Savings Account
Licensure	Must be licensed by the state as a risk-bearing entity, normally an HMO or PPO. Waivers are available to PSOs.	Must be licensed by the state as a risk-bearing entity, normally a service-benefits insurance company.	Must be licensed by the state as a risk-bearing entity, normally a high-deductible insurance company.
Solvency	Covered by state licensure requirement. Waivers are available to PSOs.	Covered by state licensure requirement.	Covered by state licensure requirement.
Quality	Must meet federal standards.	Must meet federal standards that are less restrictive than for coordinated-care plans.	Must meet federal standards that are less restrictive than for coordinated-care plans.
Beneficiary Financial Liability	Generally allows no balance billing.	Generally allows balance billing by any provider up to 15 percent above the private fee schedule amount.	Generally allows unlimited balance billing.

TABLE 4.1

Differences in Standards for Medicare+ Choice Plans by Type of Plan

Basic differences: Standards for plans vary

Source: Medicare Payment Advisory Commission analysis of the Balanced Budget Act of 1997. 1998. *Report to Congress.* Washington, DC: MedPAC.

Coordinated-Care Plans

For the most part, **coordinated-care plans** are HMOs. They resemble the type of health plan that has participated in Medicare managed care since the beginning of the program. Essentially, any managed care plan with a restrictive network that is not a private fee-for-service or MSA plan falls into this category.

Coordinated-care plans provide healthcare services, including but not limited to HMOs (with or without point-of-service options) PPOs, and plans offered by PSOs.

Medicare HMOs already dominate this category and are expected to continue to do so. PPOs, however, are less likely to participate in this category of plans. With their less restrictive provider networks, generally weaker financial incentives, and less rigorous utilization management systems, PPOs are less likely to do well financially.

In the future, PSOs will assume greater involvement in Medicare managed care. Those organizations can be not-for-profit or for-profit, but they must be controlled by the providers serving the enrollees. Moreover, providers in PSOs must offer a substantial share of services. PSOs in urban areas must have approximately 70 percent of Medicare expenditures provided by the controlling network. PSOs in rural areas must provide 60 percent.

Those providers must be affiliated with PSOs in one of two ways, either by contract or by ownership. If the affiliation is through ownership, then either one provider will control another or both providers will share control. Some sharing of substantial financial risk is required. Thus, the physicians and hospitals in a community can form a corporation with both having ownership or control. This entity can then obtain a contract with Medicare to become a coordinated-care plan if it meets all the requirements. The level of risk may vary by the type of provider, so physicians might have less risk than the hospital system. But providers must be at risk for more than their own services to meet the test of substantial financial risk.

PSOs that do not meet state licensure requirements as a state licensed HMO or PPO may apply to Medicare for approval as a coordinated-care plan. These organizations must have a net worth of $1.5 million at application. They must also have a written financial plan for projected losses and how they will maintain their net worth, including guarantees, letters of credit, or other transfers from the owners. After all, PSOs assume risks. And as any risk-bearing entity, these organizations must have an insolvency deposit and provisions for paying any bills incurred with creditors in case they have financial trouble or go out of business.

Generally speaking, PSOs must meet all the quality and reporting responsibilities of an HMO. As such, the PSO is a variation of the familiar HMO that currently dominates the program.

Private Fee-for-Service Plans

Private fee-for-service plans must pay all providers on a fee-for-service basis at rates determined by the plan without placing the provider at financial risk. At the same time, these plans may not vary payment rates based on the amount of services used, and they may not restrict provider participation.

Private fee-for-service plans are an entirely new and distinct option under Medicare managed care contracting. Any plan adopting this option must pay all providers on a fee-for-service basis at rates determined by the plan without placing the provider at financial risk. A private fee-for-service plan can set payment levels above or below Medicare payment rates. If the plan pays less, special checks are required to ensure that the provider network willing to contract with the plan is large and varied enough to serve the enrollees. Payment rates may not vary based on patient use of services.

The one feature that most distinguishes this type of plan from the coordinated-care plan has to do with providers. Any provider who can legally provide services and who agrees to the terms and conditions offered by the plan must be accepted into the plan to provide services.

Although coordinated-care plans are subject to the adjusted community rate limitations on beneficiary premiums and extra benefits, private fee-for-service plans may set beneficiary premiums at any level. Balanced billing, whereby physicians bill additional amounts beyond the Medicare payment, in addition to deductibles and coinsurance, are capped at 15 percent above the fee schedule used by the plan (which may be higher or lower than the Medicare fee schedule).

These plans are thought to cater to beneficiaries who would be willing to pay a higher premium in exchange for access to a wider range of providers, especially providers unwilling to accept Medicare patients at going Medicare rates. It is not obvious, however, why a health plan would not simply enter the Medicare market as a traditional Medicare supplemental insurer. One possibility is that a plan might decide it could offer a more desirable package with benefits beyond those included in the ten standard policies required by federal law. Taking the private fee-for-service plan option would offer the right organization the opportunity to receive the Medicare+Choice payment at risk, freely set payments to providers, and charge any profitable premium to beneficiaries. The real trick would be convincing beneficiaries to enroll in a high-premium plan, with few managed care provisions to hold down costs. Such a plan is likely to be prohibitively expensive. The extra benefits would have to be very attractive to beat other options that are likely to come at a lower cost.

One other major area of distinction between coordinated-care plans and private fee-for-service plans is in the quality assurance arena. Coordinated-care plans must meet all the requirements listed in Table 4.2, including specific ones to safeguard overzealous utilization management. Private fee-for-service plans are not required to meet these provisions because they pay fee for service and are not permitted to pay in a way that would be tied to service use for the patient. The payment system offers built-in incentives to encourage access to care. Nevertheless, unlike the traditional fee-for-service Medicare program, private fee-for-service plans are required to collect health outcomes data, monitor certain services, and evaluate the process of and the satisfaction with care.

High-Deductible Medical Savings Accounts

One other type of Medicare+Choice plan option is available for those willing to serve this market in pioneering fashion: the Medicare **high-deductible medical savings account** (MSA). This option is available on an experimental basis. Currently, up to 390,000 beneficiaries are authorized to enroll in a Medicare MSA before 2002.

There are two components to a MSA. The first is an interest-bearing account at a financial institution that can be used to pay for healthcare. The second is a high-deductible insurance plan to provide benefits for catastrophic healthcare expenses.

Funds in an interest-bearing account for a medical savings plan are intended to pay for medical services, but they can also be used for any sort of spending. In the case of Medicare MSAs, funds are normally restricted to Medicare-covered services plus other medical services as defined by the IRS. The IRS definition of medical services extends far beyond those covered by Medicare. Medicare's contributions and the interest earned by the account are

High-deductible MSA plans provide coverage only after an annual deductible of as much as $6,000 is met. Medicare deposits the difference between the Medicare+ Choice payment and the plan's premium into a medical savings account, which can be used by the beneficiary to pay expenses below the deductible.

TABLE 4.2
Quality
Requirements
for Medicare+
Choice Plans by
Type of Plan

*Quality is
regulated: Plan
quality
assurance
program*

Requirement	Coordinated Care	Private Fee-for-Service	Medical Savings Account
Stress health outcomes and provide for collection, analysis, and reporting of data that will permit measurement of outcomes and other indices of plan quality	√	√	√
Monitor and evaluate high-volume and high-risk services and the care of acute and chronic conditions	√	√	√
Evaluate the continuity and coordination of care that enrollees receive	√	√	√
Be evaluated on an ongoing basis as to its effectiveness	√	√	√
Include measures of consumer satisfaction	√	√	√
Provide Medicare with access to information appropriate to monitor and ensure the quality of care provided	√	√	√
Provide review by physicians and other healthcare professionals of the process followed in the provision of healthcare services	√	√	√
Provide for the establishment of written protocols for utilization review based on current standards of medical practice	√	A	A
Have mechanisms to detect both underutilization and overutilization of services	√	B	B
Establish or alter practice parameters after identifying areas for improvement	√		
Take action to improve quality and assess the effectiveness of such action through systematic follow-up	√		
Make available information on quality and outcomes measures to facilitate beneficiary comparison and choice of health coverage options	√	B	

Source: Medicare Payment Advisory Commission analysis of the Balanced Budget Act of 1997. 1998. *Report to Congress.* Washington, DC: MedPAC.
A: If the plan chooses to establish written protocols for utilization review, they must be based on current standards of medical practice.
B: Must have mechanisms to evaluate utilization of services and inform providers and enrollees of the results of such evaluation.

exempt from taxes. Withdrawals from the plan are neither taxed nor subject to penalties if they were used to pay for medical expenses. Certain withdrawals, however, are included in a beneficiary's gross income for tax purposes. And if beneficiaries spend all the funds in their account on nonmedical items, leaving them short on funds to pay for medical services, they have to pay a penalty. This penalty is significant. Nonmedical withdrawals during a year are subject to a 50 percent penalty to the extent they reduce the account balance to less than 60 percent of the deductible. The current rules ban additional supplemental Medicare policies for beneficiaries electing to have a medical savings account.

Several companies have expressed interest in the medical savings account concept, including Lincoln National and Golden Rule Health Insurance. But no one has entered the market, and beneficiaries do not seem to be demanding the option in great numbers at this writing.

A MSA works in the following manner. If Medicare's monthly payment rate is $450 and the high-deductible medical savings account premium is $150, $300 is placed in the MSA. A beneficiary may access the account to pay Medicare-covered benefits below the annual deductible amount. In 1999, the annual deductible was limited to $6,000. The amount of the deductible is updated for each subsequent year by the percentage growth of the national per capital Medicare+Choice. Noncovered Medicare expenses may be paid from the account also, and these are tax free if they are for medical services. As mentioned above, other withdrawals are taxable and may carry a penalty if they reduce the medical savings account balance too much.

Table 4.3 highlights the differences among the various Medicare+ Choice plans in terms of financial liability. Given their restrictive provider network and utilization management provisions, coordinated-care plans are likely to offer the lowest out-of-pocket cost to beneficiaries. Private fee-for-service plans are likely to require more expensive premiums to pay for unlimited provider network choice. Medical savings accounts present the greatest incentives for beneficiaries with some private plan coverage to control their use of services themselves. Table 4.3 shows why.

All beneficiaries are assumed to pay the Part B monthly premium. The traditional Medicare hospital deductible of over $800 in 2000 is a major reason beneficiaries opt for additional coverage. Those in medical savings accounts subject themselves to an even larger deductible across all services, but they have the medical savings account to help meet those expenses.

Traditional Medicare and private fee-for-service plans have similar balanced-billing provisions. The concept of balanced billing does not apply in coordinated-care plans. And with MSAs, balanced billing is allowed and unrestricted.

Only in traditional Medicare does Medicare pay providers directly and beneficiaries are responsible for their own cost-sharing amounts. In the other three plan types, the money is turned over to the Medicare+Choice plan, which must negotiate payments to providers.

There are several reasons why beneficiaries in the Medicare managed care program have the potential to be dissatisfied: provisions for sharing costs, the chance of denied benefits, and payment for out-of-service area and emergency care for enrollees in coordinated-care plans. When grievances occur, any Medicare+Choice plan must have meaningful procedures for resolving them, and this includes making coverage determinations, reconsidering decisions about coverage, expediting reviews about decisions by an outside source, and initiating appeals.

TABLE 4.3

Rules Affecting Beneficiary Financial Liability and Provider Reimbursement for Enrollees in Medicare+ Choice Plans by Type of Plan

Economic rules: Traditional Medicare compared to managed care

Item	Traditional Medicare	Coordinated Care	Private Fee-for-Service	MSA
Beneficiary liability for premiums, deductibles, copayments, and coinsurance	In 2000, beneficiaries pay a $44 monthly premium for Part B.	In 2000, beneficiaries pay a $44 monthly premium for Part B.	In 2000, beneficiaries pay a $44 monthly premium for Part B.	In 2000, beneficiaries pay a $44 monthly premium for Part B.
	Part A deductible for hospital care is $764 for each benefit period. The annual deductible for Part B services is $100. Beneficiaries with hospital stays of more than 60 days pay $191 per day. Beneficiaries with skilled nursing facility stays of more than 20 days pay $96 per day. Beneficiaries also have 20 percent coinsurance for most Part B services.	The actuarial value of cost sharing (not including the premium) on average cannot exceed the average actuarial value of cost sharing under traditional Medicare.	The actuarial value of cost sharing (not including the premium) on average cannot exceed the average actuarial value of cost sharing under traditional Medicare.	A deductible of no more than $6,000 (indexed for inflation after 1999). Amounts above traditional Medicare payments (including coinsurance) do not have to be counted toward satisfying the deductible. Above the deductible, MSA plan must pay all Medicare-covered expenses including cost sharing (but not balance billing).
Beneficiary liability for balance billing	Physicians who do not participate in Medicare may bill beneficiaries up to 15 percent above the allowed Medicare charge for nonparticipating physicians. Other providers may not balance bill.	Beneficiaries are not liable for any balance-billing amounts.	Contract providers can bill up to 15 percent above the private fee schedule (which can be higher or lower than Medicare rates). Noncontract providers cannot balance bill beneficiaries.	Balance billing is allowed and not subject to any limits regardless of whether the deductible has been met.

continued

TABLE 4.3
Continued

Item	Traditional Medicare	Coordinated Care	Private Fee-for-Service	MSA
Plan payment obligation to physicians, hospitals, and other providers	Medicare pays providers using a number of different methods, including prospectively set payment rates and retrospective cost-based reimbursement.	Plans pay contract providers based on privately negotiated fees or rates, minus beneficiary cost-sharing amounts. Plans pay noncontract providers at fees or rates based on traditional Medicare payment systems, including allowable balance billing.	Plans pay contract providers based on privately negotiated fees or rates, minus beneficiary cost-sharing amounts. Fees or rates must be as high as Medicare unless the plan has a sufficient number and range of provider contracts. Noncontract providers: same as in coordinated-care plans.	Above the deductible, the plan reimburses the provider for at least traditional Medicare payment amounts including coinsurance.
Sources of payments to physicians, hospitals, and other providers	All providers receive payments from Medicare and cost-sharing payments from beneficiaries (or their secondary insurers).	Contract and noncontract providers receive payments from plans and cost-sharing payments from beneficiaries.	Contract providers receive payment from plans and may collect cost sharing and balance bill (up to 15 percent) from the beneficiary. Noncontract providers receive payments from plans and cost-sharing payments (but no balance bills) from beneficiaries.	Below the deductible, providers receive payments from beneficiaries based on their charges. After the deductible is met, providers receive the plan's payment (based on traditional Medicare payment systems), but may collect unlimited balance bills from the beneficiary.

Source: Medicare Payment Advisory Commission and Congressional Research Service analysis of the Balanced Budget Act of 1997. 1998. *Report to Congress.* Washington, DC: MedPAC.

Reconsideration must be made within 60 days after receiving a request for the plan to reconsider a denied claim. A doctor with appropriate expertise who was not involved with the initial determination must make the reconsideration. Beneficiaries and providers can request expedited determinations and reconsideration if any delay would seriously jeopardize the life, health, or ability of the beneficiary to regain maximum function. Once the doctor receives the request or receives all the information needed to make a decision, the beneficiary must be notified of the decision within 72 hours.

Medicare Cost Contracts

The cost-contract option is all but eliminated. Since the Balanced Budget Act, Medicare may no longer enter into any section 1876 cost contracts, except with entities that had Health Care Prepayment Plan (HCPP) agreements immediately prior to entering a section 1876 cost contract. No section 1876 cost contracts can be entered into or renewed after December 31, 2002. A report is due by January 1, 2001, on the potential impact of eliminating the reasonable cost-contracting option on beneficiaries enrolled in any remaining plans at that time. A new or renewal HCPP agreement is permitted only with entities sponsored by a union or employer or with entities that do not provide or arrange for inpatient hospital services.

Medicare SELECT

Medicare SELECT offers insurers and provider organizations a mechanism to enter the Medicare managed care market with substantially lower risk than the Medicare+Choice option. Any state-licensed entity that meets the requirements of a Medicare supplemental insurer could market Medicare SELECT policies (Table 4.4). These would be in all respects like one of the ten standard policies in Chapter 1 (Table 1.1), except that full benefits are paid only when beneficiaries use providers in the network. As with Medicare+Choice, beneficiaries are guaranteed coverage that is renewable and continuous, and the policy must be issued without considering the beneficiary's health status. Minimum loss-ratio standards apply, and premium refund provisions apply if minimums are not met. Thus, profits are capped, just as Medicare+Choice coordinated-care plans have capped profits through the adjusted community-rate process. Finally, the Medicare+Choice option offers numerous types of provider network configurations. Medicare SELECT is intended only for a PPO and only affects the amount paid by the Medicare SELECT plan for the cost-sharing provisions of Medicare, the deductible and coinsurance. Medicare SELECT plans are exempt from certain antikickback provisions if providers are willing to waive the inpatient deductible or if physicians accept a lower rate of coinsurance.

Although Table 4.4 does not show it, state insurance commissioners enforce significant penalties for restricting the use of medically necessary services, charging excessive premiums, expelling a member except for nonpayment of premium, and withholding required explanation of the workings of Medicare SELECT or marketing inappropriately.

Insurers already in the Medicare supplemental market are ideal candidates for Medicare SELECT. It offers them the opportunity to drive more patients to network providers and reduce or eliminate Medicare cost sharing for their Medicare supplemental enrollees. Medicare SELECT plans can contract with Medicare for utilization review, instead of carrier or fiscal intermediary

	MEDICARE+CHOICE	Medicare SELECT
Qualification	Federal (or state, under limited circumstances)	State with federal oversight responsibility
Guaranteed renewability, continuation, and replacement of Medigap	Required	Required
Limits on profits	Adjusted community rate applies	Minimum loss ratios apply
Exclusions or rating of policy premiums based on pre-existing conditions	Not allowed	Limitations
Network	HMO (with or without point-of-service option), PPO, private fee-for-service network, or medical savings account	PPO only with negotiated payments for Medicare deductible or coinsurance only

TABLE 4.4
Comparison of Medicare+ Choice and Medicare SELECT Features

Managed care lite: Medicare SELECT gives beneficiaries a taste of managed care

review, and share the cost of these reviews with Medicare. For providers, Medicare SELECT offers the potential to enlarge market share, especially for specialists in areas serving Medicare patients predominately.

Bundled Payment for Centers of Excellence

In 1991, Medicare began testing the concept of contracting with high-quality, high-volume medical facilities to provide specific, high-cost procedures. The initial test applied to coronary artery bypass graft surgery. The facilities were paid a fixed, bundled rate for all the facility, diagnostic, and physician services associated with coronary bypass surgery. The tests showed that these centers saved Medicare 12 percent on each procedure while maintaining the quality of care for beneficiaries. After five years of operation, the Medicare Participating Heart Bypass Center demonstration showed that it was feasible for the Medicare program to enter into a negotiated bundled-payment arrangement for complex surgical procedures. Congress authorized expansion of the bundled-payment approach to other procedures in all parts of the country.

This form of Medicare managed care promoted a variety of positive trends. It encouraged cooperation between hospitals and physicians; improvements in quality; more efficient delivery of services; and cost savings for the hospital, the patient, and the Medicare program. The early success of this project led immediately to planning a larger, more complex demonstration to test the concept with more and different procedures at more hospitals. However, because of Year 2000 implementation issues, the expansion was postponed until after July 2000.

The Medicare Participating Centers of Excellence Demonstration for Orthopedic and Cardiovascular Services announced that it will offer individual hospitals and their associated physicians the opportunity to enter a global bundled-payment arrangement for selected cardiovascular and orthopedic procedures. The orthopedic procedures will include total and partial hip and knee replacements.

These procedures were selected, along with the cardiac procedures related to coronary artery disease, for a number of reasons. First, they are established, complex, highly technical, high-volume, and high-priced inpatient procedures; and they tend to have predictable lengths of stay, relatively low mortality, and defined episodes of care. Second, they tend to have immediate benefits in terms of the patient's ability to function. Most important, for the Centers of Excellence concept, they are procedures for which there is a strong correlation at the hospital level between volume and quality and an inverse relationship between volume and cost. The more procedures performed at a particular institution, the better the outcomes and the lower the cost per procedure.

In the bundled-payment approach, participating hospitals are encouraged to market themselves as a Medicare Participating Center of Excellence for either the orthopedic or the cardiovascular procedures. This marketing approach helps persuade beneficiaries and referring physicians to select these hospitals.

Marketing hospitals as centers of excellence is not an attempt to discourage any surgeon from performing surgery in local community hospitals or any other certified facilities. Hospitals and physicians not participating in the demonstration can continue to provide services under the traditional Medicare program. Medicare beneficiaries continue to be free to choose the physicians and hospitals from which they wish to receive services.

When the program is expanded, the criteria for performance will be minimal with respect to volume of services and quality of care efforts. Criteria from the last round of solicitations indicate the level of performance that will be expected. Facilities had been performing at least 250 heart bypass surgeries per year for the cardiac option—of which 80 were performed on Medicare beneficiaries—and at least 50 hip replacements and 50 knee replacements per year for the orthopedic option.

A full-fledged program of bundled-payment facilities nationally could be a relatively select group, with less than 15 percent of all qualified hospitals and physicians currently performing the procedures included in the final cut. For example, in the March 1996 pilot, solicitations were sent to 914 hospitals in selected states. Preliminary applications from 533 hospitals were received. An outside panel reviewed the submitted proposals, and only 152 preapplicant hospitals were invited to submit a final application for the demonstration. Of these, 121 submitted final applications.

The bundled payment for centers of excellence program should soon be reactivated. When it is, it will bear close scrutiny as a possible option for hospitals and doctors wanting to become part of the Medicare managed care field. Although the bundled payment from Medicare is regulated, the transactions between physicians and hospitals or others accepting the bundled payment are not regulated beyond normal fraud and abuse requirements. As a stepping stone along the road to Medicare SELECT and Medicare+Choice, the bundled-payment arrangement can afford opportunities to understand how managed care can work with minimal risk.

Strategic Implications for Your Organization: The Door Is Open

The traditional fee-for-service Medicare program is not the only way hospitals and physicians can participate in Medicare. The door is open to the private side of Medicare in several forms of managed care. Your organization might already be inside with Medicare managed care and exploring other options. Or your organization might be new to the options and deciding which door to enter.

The questions for you are whether to participate more actively in the private side of Medicare and how to participate. The licensure, solvency, and quality requirements that your organization will need to meet will drive your decision. To make this decision, you will have to explore several issues. First, you must examine the relationship between the physicians and hospitals that would be required to serve the Medicare market. Second, you need to identify the source of administrative services that would need to be provided under Medicare+Choice. Finally, you have to determine whether the more modest approaches afforded by Medicare SELECT or bundled payments might be better suited to your organization.

Enrollment is the all-important driving factor for the Medicare+Choice options. A risk-contract Medicare+Choice plan should not expect to break even until it enrolls 5,000 beneficiaries, judging from the successes of other Medicare HMOs. Most plans do not reach steady state, with a chance for financial health, until enrollment of 20,000 beneficiaries.

Ultimately, the level of risk your organization is able to bear answers the question of whether to walk through the door of the private side of Medicare. Normally, meeting the state or federal insolvency requirements answers that question, but coordinated-care plans must be willing to incur losses for some time. A minimum of three years of up to 25 percent losses on the total

Medicare+Choice payment should be budgeted. Marketing, enrollment, and set-up expenses will be significant, more than $2 to $3 million per year depending on how quickly the Medicare+Choice plan scales up and on the size of the market covered. To reach beneficiaries, new entrants must create or develop the provider network through contracts and management services, establish quality assurance staff and procedures, and install plan representatives and marketing and sales staff.

If your organization is not suited to these requirements, examine the Medicare SELECT option as a joint effort with a current Medicare supplement insurer. Although this effort could mean giving up the hospital deductible, it could translate into more patients for your hospitals or physicians, depending on the local market you serve. Finally, the bundled-payment option should be expanded and available for organizations able and willing to accept one payment for physician plus hospital for certain high-cost, high-volume procedures. Bundled payments give your organization the ability to walk through a small door in terms of risk bearing but a large door in terms of realigning incentives between physicians and hospitals.

Strategic Decisions Checklist

Strategic Questions	Strategic Analyses
What Medicare+Choice plan type should you adopt?	You should examine licensure, solvency, and quality requirements. Determine which can be achieved by your organization: • Hospital and physician relationships • Administrative services • Utilization management infrastructure • Performance monitoring and quality improvement infrastructure • Enrollment targets—Medicare+Choice plans need 5,000 to break even and 20,000 to reach financial health
What level of risk can you bear?	First, decide if your organization can absorb losses from accepting the Medicare+Choice payment as a coordinated-care plan. Second, decide what type of coordinated-care plan makes sense from the point of view of network, quality assurance, and beneficiary liability: • HMO • PPO • Private fee-for-service insurer • MSA plan If Medicare+Choice payment is not an option, examine Medicare SELECT as a Medicare supplemental insurer or as a joint effort with one.
What other options are available?	If the risk-bearing Medicare+Choice option is not for you, prepare to participate in the bundled-payment center of excellence option.

Strategic Decisions and Proven Responses

Today's managers of Medicare health plans face a host of strategic decisions and business opportunities. These decisions and opportunities stem from the rivalry that exists among health plans and the ever-present option for beneficiaries to choose another health plan or receive care from the Medicare fee-for-service sector.

The decisions are strategic because of two key economic rules for Medicare managed care plans. The first rule is that government, at a minimum, requires the medical services provided by managed care plans to be the same as those covered by traditional fee-for-service Medicare. The second rule is that the government sets the price Medicare pays. In other words, the government determines nearly all the covered services and much of the price for you.

Because managed care plans are restricted in terms of the services they offer and the prices they charge, their success in the market depends on two interrelated factors. First, managed care plans must purposefully choose to perform activities differently from their rivals, and this is the essence of their strategy (Porter 1998). At the same time, they must meet the needs of Medicare beneficiaries better than other managed care plans in the market or the Medicare fee-for-service sector.

Despite restrictions on services and costs, the size of the Medicare market offers tremendous business opportunities. If you are in the business of providing medical services, you need to be in the Medicare market. Medicare is, after all, the largest single payer of medical services, and it pays providers through the traditional fee-for-service system and the Medicare+Choice prospectively determined, risk-contract system. Participating in one system to the exclusion of the other presents a serious risk. Rivals can take away patients from providers or health plans that do not learn how to use the opportunities available to serve the Medicare market.

Payments In and Payments Out

Figure II.1 is an overview of the economics of a managed care plan in the Medicare market. It illustrates general components of payments into a plan, or revenues and pricing, and the major areas of payments out of a plan, or costs and application of the capitation dollar. The figure also shows ranges for the share of components for an HMO.

Three major sources of pricing establish the payments into a managed care plan: the monthly per-member payment from Medicare for Medicare-covered services, beneficiary-paid premiums, and beneficiary copayments. Co-payments may not be health-plan revenues, depending on the model type of the plan. Pricing and payments into the plan flow through and become the capitation dollar and payments out of the plan.

Four major components of the capitation dollar (or "payments out") exist for any managed care plan. Three are for covered Medicare services and supplementary benefits: institutional, medical, and other. Other services might include prescribed medicines, eyeglasses, and hearing aids—services not covered by Medicare. A certain amount of payments out of the plan are also for administration, including marketing, health services management, and financial controls.

Some of the payments out of the plan can be quite predictable for a group of enrollees in the plan. But some of the institutional and medical portions of payments out of the plan are risky and unpredictable. Managed care plans are required to set aside funds for the more unpredictable portions to protect against large, unexpected financial losses from very high-cost cases.

FIGURE II.1

Pricing and the Capitation Dollar

The money: Payments in and payments out

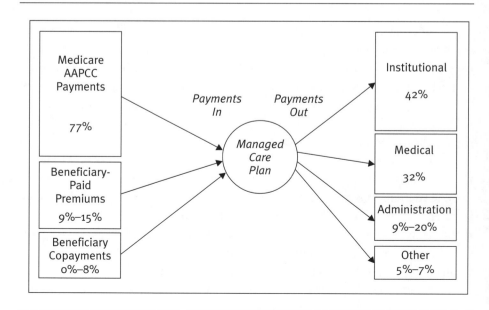

The purpose of Part II is to break down the economic description of pricing and the capitation dollar, specify the unique aspects of Medicare managed care, and identify the strategic decisions that every health plan will face because of those unique aspects. Part II also provides responses to the strategic decisions or suggests a process for making strategic decisions. As in Part I, summary tables of strategic decisions appear at the end of each chapter. These decisions furnish a framework for identifying business opportunities in the Medicare managed care market.

Part II is divided into seven chapters. These chapters discuss the strategic decisions that follow the flow of dollars into and out of a managed care plan. Chapter 5 expands on the payments into and the payments out of a plan, including the predictable and unpredictable portions. The general presentation of pricing and the capitation dollar in Chapter 5 is followed in Chapter 6 by a discussion that expands on the relationship between plan benefit design, marketing, and enrollment.

The remaining five chapters in Part II cover quality, cost, and care management and how the capitation dollar becomes payments out of the plan. An assortment of quality-improvement and cost-control techniques are covered in Chapter 7, followed by a chapter on disease management that addresses the all important high-cost, institutional component of the capitation dollar. Chapter 8 presents three diseases that disproportionately burden older people and that confront any well-managed health plan with strategic management issues.

Chapters 9 and 10 cover the medical services component of the flow of capitation dollars out of the managed care plan. These chapters examine the basic care provided to beneficiaries in the physician's office and offer strategies to help patients manage their own care before incurring costs by inessential use of the medical system.

The last chapter in Part II covers several critical legal topics and the strategic decisions involved. Provider liability, an evolving topic that bears watching, is discussed in Chapter 11 as a strategic management issue without attempting to provide the latest and changing case law in the area.

Taken together, these chapters offer a proposed model for operating a managed care plan. The model plan relies on self-directed physician groups of health professionals to provide optimal care for a defined population. As an ideal approach to health plan management, it offers goals and approaches to adopt conscious decision making at each step to change dramatically the way care is currently provided today in many managed care plans.

PRICING AND THE CAPITATION DOLLAR

Medicare managed care plans are required to accept prices largely set by the government and offered on a take-it-or-leave-it basis. As described in previous chapters, a predetermined, marketwide price is the essence of the competitive model in Medicare managed care. There are some strategic opportunities to managing price, but managed care plans must focus on effectively managing the cost of delivering services while ensuring beneficiary satisfaction if they intend to build cost-effective enrollment levels. Health plans must address many strategic issues on the pricing side, but a multitude of strategic decisions determine success in the market on the capitation dollar side.

To appreciate the strategic decisions, we begin this chapter with a detailed look at **pricing** and how payments flow into a managed care plan. The chapter ends with a profile of the **capitation** dollar and how payments flow out of managed care plans with both predictable and unpredictable components. The presentation of pricing and the capitation dollar sets the stage for how to manage the costs and care of enrollees in managed care plans.

Payments In

When a Medicare beneficiary completes the proper enrollment forms to join a managed care plan, HCFA is notified by the plan through computer linkage to the government computers in Baltimore. The notification triggers a change in the way dollars flow from Medicare. Traditional fee-for-service claims are denied for a newly enrolled beneficiary in a managed care plan after a certain date. At the beginning of the month after enrollment with the managed care plan, Medicare begins to include the beneficiary in the count of plan enrollees for whom Medicare makes a monthly payment—a share of the **Medicare+Choice capitation payment**.

Although the Medicare+Choice capitation payment is controlled by Medicare, administrators of managed care plans must recognize the strategic importance of understanding how the capitation price is set. They must also recognize how best to maximize two other important prices, beneficiary-paid premiums and **copayments**, which are uncontrolled by Medicare. Within limits, both of these elements may be set by the managed care plan. It is the combination of the government-controlled price, the Medicare+Choice payment, and the uncontrolled prices—premiums and copayments—that determines the level of payments into the managed care plan. And these payments

Pricing is the level at which dollars are paid to a managed care plan per member.

Capitation is the dollars per member available to a managed care plan to pay for covered services.

The Medicare+ Choice capitation payment is the basic price for Medicare risk-contracts, composed of three elements that vary for different plans and that directly affect the monthly payment to plans for individual beneficiaries.

Copayments are dollar amounts paid by members in a plan to share the cost of services each time services are provided.

largely determine the success of the plan, especially in marketing to the price-sensitive Medicare beneficiary.

Medicare+Choice Capitation Payments

The Medicare+Choice payment is the most important source of plan revenues. It represents roughly 75 percent of revenues to most managed care plans. Driven by a government formula, three broad ingredients determine the amount of the monthly payment:

1. the geographic residence of a beneficiary;
2. a national actuarial estimate of average payment for Medicare; and
3. the age, gender, and institutional and Medicaid status of a beneficiary.

Medicare payments to managed care plans began in the early 1980s as a basic estimate at the local level of fee-for-service costs to Medicare per beneficiary. The adjusted-average per-capita cost (AAPCC) from 1997 for each county in the country forms the basis for calculating Medicare+Choice payment rates. The Balanced Budget Act of 1997 (P.L. 105-33) changed the law that affected how rates are determined. Rates calculated for 1998 and later can no longer be referred to as being based on fee-for-service costs in the local area. Rather, with the three ingredients above as primary determinants, Medicare+Choice payments are better described as an estimate of what national payments would have been for an enrollee in a managed care plan had the enrollee remained in the Medicare fee-for-service sector with some adjustments for local cost differences and federal budget cost savings.

Managed care plans are paid 95 percent of the Medicare+Choice payment amount. The adjustments made to the monthly premium payment attempt to achieve overall federal budget savings, also known as budget neutrality, or maximum increases as specified by law. A floor payment level ($367 in 1998) also exists for areas with very low AAPCC estimates. But these adjustments are not as important as the three general ingredients that underlie the formula. A description of each ingredient and an explanation for its role in determining strategic decisions follows.

The Geographic Residence of a Beneficiary

From a strategic standpoint, the most important aspect of Medicare managed care pricing is that the payment rates are driven largely by the use and cost of service in a health plan's local market. For this reason, it is vital to understand that the first ingredient in the Medicare+Choice payment represents two factors: a geographic-specific estimate of local average per-capita costs and an adjustment to account for differences between the local geographic area and the nation in demographic characteristics. Together these calculations yield the **standardized county rate** (Fig. 5.1). The standardized county rate is estimated for each county in the country on the basis of an analysis of all fee-for-service claims paid in a county for the

*The **standardized county rate** is the HCFA actuary's best estimate of average*

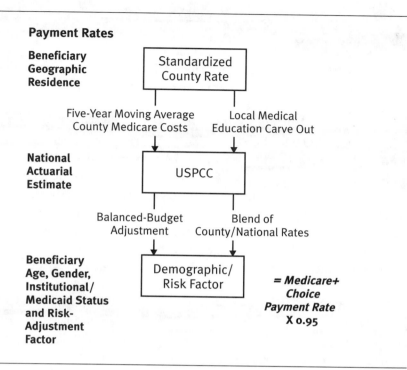

FIGURE 5.1

Medicare+
Choice
Payment Rates

*Complicated but
sound: Payment
rates are derived
from a
well-structured
actuarial process
based on sound
data*

past five years. These claims form the base for calculating the future Medicare+Choice payment. A portion of fee-for-service claims includes payments for graduate medical education. Payments to hospitals for medical education costs are being gradually eliminated from, or "carved out" of, the standardized county rate. Such payments tied to the standardized county rate will end by 2002. At that point, managed care plans will no longer receive payments for medical education through the Medicare+Choice capitation payment.

*county per-capita
costs, assuming the
national
demographic
characteristics of
Medicare
beneficiaries in the
county.*

Another adjustment to rates is also being phased in. Standardized county rates will be blended with a national average-input-price adjustment. The adjustment gradually will reduce the effect of local Medicare fee-for-service costs in determining the managed care payment rate. The provision will be implemented according to a schedule that assigns a 50/50 split to the weight given to local and national cost estimates by 2002. Local fee-for-service costs will account for half of the source of managed care payments even at the end of this blending period.

There is little managed care plans can do about these changes, strategically or operationally. The implication is that fewer dollars will be available for plans through 2002 than would have been available without legislative changes. Nevertheless, these changes determine what each plan ultimately will be paid.

National Actuarial Estimate

The second ingredient that helps set the Medicare+Choice payment is the previous year's average national Medicare payment for all beneficiaries in the fee-for-service sector. This estimated payment is then adjusted to include any actuarial adjustments for next year's increases in provider payments or changes in coverage and benefits. The average national expenditure is called the United States Per-Capita Cost, or **USPCC**.

*The **USPCC** is the Medicare actuary's best estimate of average national Medicare per-capita costs.*

The USPCC is updated each summer on a preliminary basis as part of the federal budget process and published each September 7 in the *Federal Register* on a final basis. Updates can be obtained on the World Wide Web at: http://www.hcfa.gov/stats/. Changes in coverage or benefits during the current year (e.g., the addition of coverage for bone-density screening tests) or changes made by Congress in the Medicare hospital deductible would be factored into the USPCC using actuarial assumptions for the upcoming calendar year. Congressional requirements to reduce the payments to reach balanced budget targets would also be applied in calculating the USPCC.

Beneficiary Age, Gender, and Institutional and Medicaid Status

The third AAPCC ingredient, an enrollee-specific **demographic cost factor**, raises or lowers the payment for an individual beneficiary depending on the personal demographic characteristics of an enrollee. The purpose of the demographic cost factor is to vary the monthly payment to reflect the average expected health risk of a beneficiary. A different demographic cost factor exists for each category of personal characteristics, and these characteristics are defined by age (five categories), Medicaid and institutional (nursing home) status (three categories), and employment status.

*The **demographic cost factors** are 40 numbers used to raise or lower monthly payments to a managed care plan for a beneficiary depending on the beneficiary's personal characteristics.*

There are 40 categories with demographic cost factors for each part of Medicare. Separate Medicare+Choice payments are calculated for Medicare Part A, which covers inpatient hospital services, and Part B, which covers ambulatory physician visits, home health care, laboratory work, and x-rays.

Table 5.1 shows the 1998 demographic cost factors and categories for Medicare Part A and Part B. This set of demographic cost factors is the actuary's answer to the need for payments to health plans that have been adjusted for health risk. Thus, for an 86-year-old male beneficiary who is not institutionalized and not on Medicaid, the managed care plan will be paid 1.35 multiplied by the Medicare+Choice payment for Part A (reduced by 5 percent). A 68-year-old male beneficiary who is not institutionalized and not on Medicaid would garner 0.65 times the Medicare+Choice payment for Part A (reduced by 5 percent). Clearly, a managed care plan is paid less for younger age groups and for females. Long-standing actuarial analysis indicates that such groups cost less for Medicare's fee-for-service sector compared with other groups; they are also less service-intensive.

The managed care plan is paid less for working aged who have private insurance coverage through an employer. The reason for this is that Congress mandates the private employment coverage to be the primary payer. For

Part	Gender	Age	Institutionalized	Noninstitutionalized		TABLE 5.1
			Medicaid	Non-Medicaid	Working Aged	Demographic Cost Factors—Aged, 1997–2001
A	Male	65–69	1.75	1.15	0.65	0.40
		70–74	2.25	1.50	0.85	0.45
		75–79	2.25	1.95	1.05	0.70
		80–84	2.25	2.35	1.20	0.80
		85+	2.25	2.60	1.35	0.90
	Female	65–69	1.45	0.80	0.55	0.35
		70–74	1.80	1.05	0.70	0.45
		75–79	2.10	1.45	0.85	0.55
		80–84	2.10	1.70	1.05	0.70
		85+	2.10	2.10	1.20	0.80
B	Male	65–69	1.60	1.10	0.80	0.45
		70–74	1.80	1.35	0.95	0.65
		75–79	1.95	1.55	1.10	0.80
		80–84	1.95	1.70	1.15	0.90
		85+	1.95	1.70	1.15	1.00
	Female	65–69	1.50	1.05	0.70	0.40
		70–74	1.65	1.15	0.85	0.55
		75–79	1.65	1.25	0.95	0.70
		80–84	1.65	1.25	0.95	0.75
		85+	1.65	1.25	1.00	0.85

Most in one category: Most enrollees are noninstitutionalized and non-Medicaid

example, a 69-year-old female who is not institutionalized and working only brings to the plan 0.35 times the Medicare+Choice payments for Part A (reduced by 5 percent). All the demographic cost factors for the working aged are ≥ 1.0, reflecting the fact that Medicare is a secondary payer for this group.

Only a small proportion of all Medicare beneficiaries who are institutionalized or disabled enroll in managed care plans. But when they do enroll, it means more payments to the managed care plan. For example, an institutionalized female on Medicaid brings 2.1 times the Medicare+Choice payment for Part A (reduced by 5 percent).

Entirely separate factors exist for those eligible because of disability or end-stage renal disease (ESRD). A beneficiary must already be enrolled in the managed care plan and then become eligible for ESRD to qualify for the ESRD categories. Medicare is experimenting with managed care plans that specialize in enrolling ESRD program beneficiaries through a risk contract.

Typical enrollment in an HMO would be about 98 percent aged, 2 percent disabled, and almost no ESRD. Consequently, the factors in the third column under the heading "Noninstitutionalized, Non-Medicaid" are the most relevant and will pertain to the majority of enrollees in a typical enrollment, making the demographic cost factor and the Medicare+Choice payment system much simpler than it first might appear.

Risk-Adjustment Factor

Beginning in 2000, the Medicare+Choice payment was complicated further by minor changes in payments for particular beneficiaries in certain diagnostic categories. So-called risk adjustment, better labeled prior-hospitalization cost adjustment, is based on diagnostic data related to the inpatient hospital stays of enrollees in Medicare+Choice plans. Unlike the demographic rates, risk-adjustment rates use a beneficiary-specific factor that is effective for a calendar year. There are proposals to use other sources of service-use data (e.g., outpatient claims) to make payment adjustments, but all of these are geared toward service use and cost while in the plan, as opposed to the actual health risk of the beneficiaries. All of that is being phased in over a four-year period and will not be implemented fully before 2004.

The way the risk adjustment works is each individual beneficiary with 12 months of continuous enrollment is assigned to one of 15 categories if during the prior year they had been hospitalized for certain diagnoses. For example, a beneficiary who had been in the hospital for congestive heart failure would be placed in one category, and another beneficiary in the hospital for kidney infection would be placed in another category. The payment is unaffected for most beneficiaries—about 88 percent—who were not hospitalized or hospitalized for diagnoses not included in the risk-adjustment system. But those with risk-adjustment hospital stays have their payment rate increased *the following year* on the basis of a risk-adjustment rate book that raises the capitation payment by some factor to account for the hospital stay.

An expert panel advised Medicare on the diagnoses to select. The risk-adjustment system is disconnected and dampens the incentives for plans to remain efficient. Because the risk-adjustment payment is delayed until the following year, it separates the payment from the occurrence of higher costs and does not really make the managed care plan whole until nearly two years later. Efficient plans that are able to avoid hospitalization through disease-management efforts, for example, will not be as eager to put them in place for the 15 designated diagnoses. HCFA has proposed a patch for this problem that would pay extra for outpatient disease management for congestive heart failure. Based on individual risk, as opposed to group risk, the system encourages gaming and might even lead you to encourage unnecessary hospital stays, rather than encourage treatment in less costly settings. As a strategy, you could maximize revenue, but this conflicts with the overarching goal of your plan to efficiently provide the care that your beneficiaries want. Thus, the best plans should probably ignore the risk-adjustment system from a strategic standpoint and focus on good managed care. Ensure that data are being reported accurately to Medicare; but the risk-adjustment system in place, based on hospitalizations and for individual patients, is inconsistent with Medicare managed care.

An understanding of Medicare+Choice payments sets the stage for examining strategic decisions for managed care plans regarding changes in the Medicare+Choice price, the mix of enrollment, and estimates of health plan revenues.

The national actuarial estimates represented by the USPCC play a major role in determining the changes in the monthly payments in future years for any managed care plan that serves Medicare patients. In the 1990s, the average USPCC annual increase has been about 5.9 percent. Most of the increase comes from increases in Part A for hospital services. That reflects increases in admissions for the aged and increases in diagnosis related group payments for hospital admissions (HCFA 1997B; Palsbo 1997).

Managed care plans must watch and understand USPCC updates, especially unexpected fluctuations in the USPCC, and the reason for changes. Health plans must stay abreast of changes in the USPCC that affect the monthly payments to the plan. A reasonable strategy for any managed care plan is to monitor the opinions of experts regarding changes in the USPCC and develop scenarios around the source of possible future increases in the national actuarial estimate. Good information on projected increases is absolutely essential for budgeting and planning.

For example, among the questions one might ask is how much new coverage decisions from Congress will influence the USPCC for the coming year. Will trends in home health care costs, for example, affect the USPCC? How much will overall budget cuts in reimbursement to fee-for-service providers influence the USPCC? The underlying trends and reasons for increases in the USPCC could provide managed care plans with opportunities to gain relative efficiencies for their own enrollees, and they could achieve this through health plan management policy or initiatives that attack the cost increases expected to increase the USPCC. For example, if home health care visits in fee-for-service Medicare are expected to continue to grow at double-digit rates, a managed care plan would be well served to hold their own increases in home health care costs to less than double digit. This might be done with more careful monitoring for unnecessary visits or by negotiating new prices for contract home health care services.

Someone in the health plan needs to be involved with state and national associations and to expect the associations to play a role in monitoring and understanding the trends in the USPCC. Such associations seek to influence national legislation that could affect the USPCC. Thus, the corporate office or a knowledgeable staff person in a managed care plan should track the USPCC and work with national associations to address concerns about the way the rates are set or the assumptions on which rates are based.

The **average demographic cost factor** is critically important for managing revenues and achieving a balanced enrollment. Strategically, health plans will want to take steps to achieve the desired mix of enrollment, especially given the fact that managed care plans themselves are competing for optimal

*The **average demographic cost factor** is the number of members in each demographic cost factor cell multiplied by the cell weight and divided by the total number of members.*

enrollment mix. A vital aspect of achieving optimal enrollment is for the health plan to know the demographic cost factors of the service areas from which the plan draws enrollment. A managed care plan would want to know its own share of enrollment compared to the pool in the market.

Before explaining the strategic decisions about the enrollment mix, Table 5.2 illustrates the calculation of the average demographic cost factor for an assumed 25,000 enrollees in two hypothetical health plans.

The enrollment for Plan A shows a mix of beneficiaries falling dispro-portionately into the lower payment cells. The enrollment for Plan B shows a mix of enrollees falling disproportionately into the higher average (unitary) demographic cost factors. Plan A will receive a fraction of the revenues Plan B will receive.

Experience over many years suggests the average demographic factor is about 0.72, which means most managed care plans only get about 72 percent of 95 percent of the published AAPCC for their area.

TABLE 5.2
Demographic Cost Factors— Aged, Nonin-stitutionalized, Non-Medicaid, 1997–2001

Enrollment characteristics matter: Payments could be 83.9 percent or 105.6 percent of the county Medicare+ Choice payment

Part	Gender	Age	Demographic Cost Factor	Hypothetical Number of Beneficiaries Enrolled	
				Health Plan A	Health Plan B
A	Male	65–69	0.65	2,000	500
		70–74	0.85	2,000	500
		75–79	1.05	500	2,000
		80–84	1.20	250	2,000
		85+	1.35	250	2,000
	Female	65–69	0.55	2,000	500
		70–74	0.70	2,000	500
		75–79	0.85	2,000	500
		80–84	1.05	500	2,000
		85+	1.20	250	2,000
B	Male	65–69	0.80	2,000	500
		70–74	0.95	2,000	500
		75–79	1.10	500	2,000
		80–84	1.15	250	2,000
		85+	1.15	250	2,000
	Female	65–69	0.70	2,000	500
		70–74	0.85	2,000	500
		75–79	0.95	2,000	500
		80–84	0.95	2,000	500
		85+	1.00	250	3,500
	Hypothetical Enrollment			25,000	25,000
	Mean Demographic Cost Factor			0.839	1.056

The fact that enrollment in one set of demographic cost factors is disproportionate to enrollment in the others does not mean the plan experiences biased selection. Each enrollee in each cell could match the relative risk represented by the demographic factor in terms of use and cost of services. Thus, the premium payment from Medicare (plus beneficiary premiums) would match the cost of providing services. The **medical-loss ratio** for each group associated with a demographic cost factor would equal 100 percent—premiums collected match benefits paid. The plan would be **made whole** in terms of dollars into the plan and dollars out of the plan for covered services.

*The **medical-loss ratio** is covered benefits paid as a percent of total premium revenues from Medicare and the beneficiary.*

Ideally, most managed care plans should seek a balanced enrollment unless there are operational approaches to achieving efficiency that target certain groups defined by demographic cost factors; that is, they want the average demographic cost factor to equal 1.0 or to equal the average for the areas served by the managed care plan. A smaller plan, with undeveloped utilization management and little experience in Medicare, might find it advantageous to begin with disproportionately low demographic factors. A larger plan, with well-developed utilization management and extensive experience in Medicare, might find it advantageous to enroll high demographic factor individuals because they have more experience with the higher-risk individual.

*Being **made whole** is insurance terminology for breaking even financially.*

The logic for this approach to enrollment is twofold, and it relates to **biased selection**. First, one school of thought holds that if the lower value demographic cost factors are enrolled disproportionately, the chance of **favorable selection** might be higher. Why? With lower-cost groups, the chance of healthier, active, low service and cost enrollees is higher. At the same time, managed care plan revenues are likewise lower with demographic cost factors <1.0, and the opportunities for efficiencies in care delivery are likewise lower. The second school of thought holds that if the higher value demographic cost factors are enrolled disproportionately, the chance of **adverse selection** might be higher. Revenues would be much higher comparatively, and the opportunities for efficiencies in care delivery are higher. An average demographic cost factor close to 1.0 balances these offsetting factors and means the health plan is enrolling in proportion to the demographic factors in the population. As market share grows for a managed care plan, enrollment in the plan matches the average demographic factor in the local market more closely anyway.

***Biased selection** occurs when enrollees in a health plan have health status or service use and costs different from the expected level for the established premium.*

***Favorable selection** occurs when enrollees have better health status or lower service use and costs than the expected level for the established premium.*

What is the optimal size or market share for a Medicare managed care plan? Costs of caring for Medicare beneficiaries do not become predictable for a managed care plan until 25,000 or more beneficiaries enroll. HMOs with very small enrollment—for example, fewer than 5,000 individuals—historically do not fare well financially in the program, and many Medicare HMOs have ended their contract with very small enrollment. An enrollment between 5,000 and 25,000 beneficiaries yields mixed financial results. It is not until reaching 25,000 beneficiaries that Medicare HMOs seem to reach predictable and sustainable financial results. As it is phased in over the next four years, the risk-adjustment factor should reduce this desirable enrollment

***Adverse selection** occurs when enrollees have worse health status or higher service use and costs than the expected level for the established premium.*

figure by a substantial amount and should remove a large portion of the risk of Medicare managed care when it is fully implemented.

Beneficiary-Paid Premiums

The **beneficiary-paid premium** is the amount paid to the health plan out of pocket by the member to continue monthly coverage and to pay for supplemental benefits.

The **adjusted community rate** (ACR) is a limiting factor on beneficiary premiums that must be calculated by managed care plans according to Medicare rules.

Whereas the Medicare actuaries, and not the marketplace, control monthly premium payments from Medicare, the **beneficiary-paid premium** is highly market driven and has enormous strategic importance. It is also controlled by the managed care plan. Regulated limits on the beneficiary-paid premiums exist, but they are rarely binding on a health plan. An **adjusted community rate** (ACR), calculated by each Medicare managed care plan, is a Medicare-prescribed process to estimate the premium the health plan would have charged its Medicare members on the basis of the premium-setting approach used for its non-Medicare enrollees. Health plans are required to return any difference between 95 percent of the Medicare+Choice payment and the ACR to their Medicare members in the form of additional benefits or reduced cost sharing. They may opt to return the excess to Medicare. Health plans must be able to steer through this final check on excess profits in Medicare and set the beneficiary premiums to grow enrollment.

To persuade beneficiaries to give up their go-anywhere, fee-for-service coverage under Medicare, managed care plans must offer beneficiaries substantial financial incentives to join. The strategic challenge for managed care plans is to set the beneficiary-paid premium low enough so that the plans can compete against traditional Medicare supplemental insurance and other Medicare+Choice plans in the coverage area. The beneficiary-paid premium also has to be set high enough to cover additional benefits that will attract enrollees.

Studies show that Medicare beneficiaries respond to changes in the premium they must pay to join a managed care plan by voting with their feet. Given typical choices in Medicare supplemental insurance and typical network design with no other changes, a 10 percent increase in premiums for managed care plan enrollment will decrease enrollment by 6 percent. A 10 percent increase in the value of the benefits offered will increase enrollment by 5 percent. Thus, beneficiaries are somewhat more responsive to a change in the price than they are to changes in benefits (Marquis and Rogowski 1991).

Figure 5.2 roughly illustrates the trade-offs Medicare HMOs are making today in terms of the combination of beneficiary-paid premiums and number of supplemental benefits.

Using the data available from HCFA on HMO-reported beneficiary-paid premiums and benefits, Figure 5.2 shows the distribution of all Medicare risk-contract HMOs with basic benefit packages. The table summarizes how health plans were marketing in the fall of 1997 in terms of combinations of benefits and premiums. Each type of benefit was counted the same.

The standard in the late 1990s for Medicare managed care plans is to offer a zero-premium product. About two-thirds of all plans offered

Number of Supplemental Benefits	Monthly Premiums					
	Zero $	$20 or less	$20–$39	$40–$59	$60 or more	Total
2	12	1	2	0	0	15
3	7	2	4	3	0	16
4	14	2	7	3	7	33
5	41	3	16	3	3	66
6	51	2	10	6	1	70
7	43	4	4	3	1	55
8	24	2	2	2	0	30
9	15	1	0	0	0	16
10	4	0	0	0	0	4
11	1	0	0	0	0	1
Total	212	17	45	20	12	306

FIGURE 5.2
Beneficiary-Paid Premiums and Number of Supplemental Benefits for Basic HMO Products, October 1997 (Premium median: zero $; benefit median: 6)

Zero-premium rules: Most Medicare+ Choice HMOs offer zero premium

zero-premium products with six different supplemental benefits. All plans offered at least two supplemental benefits of various types. Only one plan offered up to 11 supplemental benefits (the maximum HCFA tracks). The average premium among plans with a premium at the end of 1997 was $35.70.

Business Strategy for the Beneficiary-Paid Premium

The beneficiary premium is probably the most important factor that affects enrollment. The tactics for marketing a plan and its products are covered elsewhere in Chapter 7. But strategic planning involving the beneficiary-paid premium can provide long-term dividends for successfully positioning any products relative to competing managed care plans in the market as well as fee-for-service Medicare.

When it comes to setting premiums, three general strategic decisions present themselves:

1. adopting a **cost-dominant strategy** or **quality-dominant strategy**;
2. planning for premium changes; and
3. managing the influence of beneficiary premiums on biased selection.

First, whether a cost-dominant strategy or quality-dominant strategy makes sense depends on the expectations of the local market. In markets where Medicare managed care is not well known or does not own a very large share of the market, Medicare managed care plans must educate beneficiaries about new options and premium costs. In such markets, quality issues do not matter as much as the answer to "What is this new kind of Medicare plan?" In a more seasoned market, expectations may already be determined by what the competition offers. Good market research on the expectations of the local consumer and their perceptions of competition in the market is mandatory.

Cost-dominant strategy is a conscious positioning of a Medicare managed care product in the market emphasizing lower costs relative to other coverage options.

Quality-dominant strategy emphasizes quality of care and plan or provider amenities.

This research must view the traditional Medicare fee-for-service as one of the competing plans. Focus groups and marketing surveys are a critical, ongoing activity. Moreover, as the managed care market in a specific location matures, the opportunities shift and the marketing strategy must be revised for success.

Experience has proved, even in markets in which the AAPCC is not high compared with the USPCC, that an increasing number of plans have adopted a zero-premium, cost-dominant strategy toward beneficiary-paid premiums. No plan ignores quality in the design of its network and the operation of the plan. But it is difficult to emphasize low cost or zero cost and simultaneously emphasize quality. The first reason for this is that doing so sends too many signals to a group that is easily confused by multiple messages. The second reason is that quality and costs are normally thought to be a trade-off. Although the evidence for this is scant, the perception that you cannot get more for less is common. Thus, it is easier to focus on one dimension, either cost or quality, with cost being the major concern in this group.

The largest, most successful plans in terms of enrollment have used a zero-premium strategy, and these plans have experienced aggressive enrollment results for many years. They tend to be in areas where the AAPCC is very high (Welch 1996). Nevertheless, depending on the premiums offered by others in the local market, the premium established by the plan could be the defining factor in its success or failure in terms of enrollment growth.

It is possible that the cost-dominant strategy will wane in use as publicity about the quality of Medicare managed care plans is disseminated through initiatives that attempt to measure the quality of a health plan and consumer satisfaction. A flood of information about the quality of health plans might affect consumer expectations about the quality of care in their plan, and the plans themselves may react to increased consumer awareness.

The second strategic decision has to do with planning for premium changes. A health plan must understand that it should probably not set premiums one year at a time. A small amount of contingency planning of future changes in the beneficiary-paid premium will avoid rough transition years in which much needed adjustments to benefits or premiums await the next year's roll out of product changes. Premium adjustments might be necessary because changes occur in the following areas:

- the payment to Medicare managed care plans (AAPCC);
- competitor premiums;
- participating provider network;
- the average demographic cost factor for the plan; and
- supplementary benefits.

It will serve the managed care plan well to do some strategic planning when it comes to premiums, looking at several years of potential premium increases. Projected increases in the AAPCC should be considered, as well as competitor premiums for at least the coming three years. When health plans try to achieve the right mix of adjustments to premiums, each market becomes unique.

The third strategic decision requires an understanding of how beneficiary premiums influence biased selection. The package of supplemental benefits and beneficiary premiums influences biased selection within a demographic cost factor category, so enrollment within demographic cost factors requires careful monitoring and planning. The managed care plan's information system should permit an examination of the service use and cost experience of each enrollee. Large health plans should be able to look at each demographic category as a product line and understand whether plan revenues (AAPCC plus beneficiary-paid premiums) exceed costs. Smaller health plans might combine age, gender, and Medicaid/institutional categories to have enough members to analyze revenues for the combined demographic groups relative to costs. Data about service use and costs must be monitored and analyzed constantly so that one can know whether steps should be taken to achieve balanced enrollment. Adjustments to benefits or premiums might be essential to avoid a premium spiral, in which premium increases are used to finance adverse selection. At all costs, a plan should avoid raising premiums to compensate for adverse selection. Higher premiums can discourage average risks and retain the adverse selection group that caused higher costs.

Beneficiary Copayments

Beneficiary copayments tend to reduce the demand for services and can serve as an important tool for managing patient demand. Traditional fee-for-service Medicare relies extensively on beneficiary deductibles and **coinsurance** to control costs by requiring beneficiaries to pay their provider something out-of-pocket each time they receive services. These copayments can be an important source of plan revenues for some types of plans that collect them, or they could be a way to manage costs for other types of plans that expect contracted providers to absorb a copayment and its collection.

Each managed care plan will determine its beneficiary copayments for different services. These copayments will be aligned with the normal copayments for its non-Medicare products and overall management of the provider network. The strategic issue is whether high or low copayments are part of at least a dual offering of so-called **high-option** and **basic-option** products. Such offerings are best understood in the context of traditional Medicare supplemental insurance, which is regulated by the states with federal oversight.

Medicare HMOs and Medicare+Choice policies are free to offer benefits as they wish. Medicare SELECT policies must sell only ten required standard policies. The ten standard policies were developed by the National Association of Insurance Commissioners and incorporated into state and federal law. They have letter designations ranging from A through J, with Policy A being the basic benefit package. Each of the other nine policies includes this basic package plus a different combination of additional benefits. Policy J provides

Beneficiary copayments are dollar amounts paid when services are received. They reduce the demand for services. Most copayments are a nominal amount ($5, $10, $30) per service and are usually paid at the point of receiving the service.

Coinsurance is a percent amount of the fee paid when services are received.

A high-option plan has numerous additional benefits, few or no copayments, and a higher premium than a basic-option plan.

A basic-option plan has some additional benefits, copayments, and low or no premium compared with a high-option plan.

the most coverage. These policies cover specific expenses either not covered or not fully covered by Medicare. Insurance companies are not permitted to change the combination of benefits or the letter designations of any of the policies. With the exception of Medicare SELECT, which in this regard is more like traditional fee-for-service Medicare supplemental insurance, the ten standard policies pay for the various forms of Medicare cost sharing associated with fee-for-service deductibles and coinsurance.

Into the mix of traditional Medicare supplemental standard policies that pay for Medicare cost sharing, managed care plans can add several other types of benefits. About 60 percent of Medicare HMOs offer other benefits, including routine physicals, immunizations, outpatient drugs, foot care, eye exams, and ear exams. A minority of plans offer health education, eye glasses, hearing aids, and dental services. Basic plans have low or zero premiums combined with higher copayments for other benefits. High-option plans have low or zero copayments for other benefits combined with a higher premium.

The high-option plan has fallen from use by most plans in the Medicare managed care market. Fewer than half of all plans offer this option, and evidence suggests that many plans associate the high-option plan with adverse selection (Brown, Clement, and Retchin 1994).

The choice of high option, basic plan, or both depends on what is already in the market. In addition, it should be viewed as a secondary decision after determining the best mix of benefits and premiums. Studies show that the monthly premium and choice of physician or hospital are more important than copayments in determining beneficiary choice of the Medicare managed care option (Langwell and Hadley 1986). Ultimately, the decision may rest more with the type of plan and whether copayments are consistent with the operation of the non-Medicare side of enrollment.

Payments Out

Having covered strategic decisions regarding the components of pricing as revenue sources for managed care plans, we turn now to the flow of the capitation dollar through health plans. Figure II.1 at the beginning of this section showed the components of service—institutional, medical, and other—for which managed care plans take a predetermined flow of dollars per capita and make payments on behalf of members in the plan. Because the dollars are fixed and flow monthly, either as Medicare premium payments or beneficiary-paid premiums, the health plan is at risk for providing the covered services. In other words, if the health plan pays out more than the payments coming into the plan, it must find the money to make up the difference. If it pays out less than payments into the plan, it can keep the difference.

Figure 5.3 shows the capitation dollar as a risk pyramid, in which the entire pyramid may be thought of as the risk transferred to a managed care plan

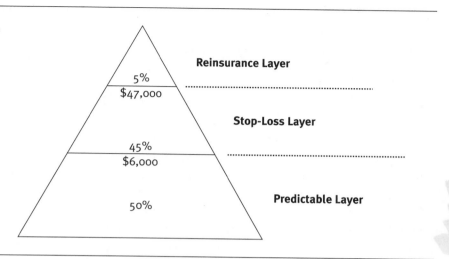

by Medicare and beneficiaries. The total risk transfer breaks down into three basic layers: the predictable layer, the stop-loss layer, and the reinsurance layer.

At the base of the pyramid is a predictable layer of spending for primary and acute care at relatively low levels of spending per capita. For example, half of all fee-for-service beneficiaries have spending of less than $6,000. Even for a relatively small number of beneficiaries—less than 1,000, for example—the costs of the predictable layer can be budgeted and managed. The strategic decisions involved in controlling the cost of this layer and making payments out of the health plan are covered later in Chapter 7.

In the middle of the pyramid is a stop-loss layer of spending for acute care and specialty care at substantially higher levels of spending per capita. For example, about 45 percent of all fee-for-service beneficiaries have spending over $6,000 and less than $47,000. This layer is frequently heavily managed in terms of cost and service use by managed care plans, and it can even have shared risk arrangements in which providers—physicians and hospitals—take on some of the risk themselves. When the risk is shared between the Medicare managed care plan and its providers for this middle layer, it is called provider stop loss. This arrangement is subject to significant regulation, as discussed in the next section.

The top of the risk pyramid is a reinsurance layer of spending. This layer covers the very high-cost acute and chronic care associated with the highest levels of spending per capita. Here, the managed care plan itself may pay a premium and transfer the risk of very high-cost cases to another licensed insurer, meeting requirements of providing reinsurance with a state insurance commissioner. This risk transfer might be for a very small number of beneficiaries who are very high cost.

Figure 5.3 illustrates how this works. The figure shows that 5 percent of beneficiaries in fee-for-service nationally have spending for Medicare-covered services of $47,000 or more. Small to medium size plans—25,000 to 100,000 total enrollment—normally obtain reinsurance for this layer. Reinsurance is discussed in the section following the discussion about provider stop loss.

Provider Stop Loss

Dollar payments flowing monthly from Medicare and beneficiaries enrolled in health plans with premiums assume that Medicare managed care plans will take on financial responsibility for certain insurance risks. In other words, the health plan takes a chance on a patient requiring the high and unpredictable cost of an inpatient hospital stay, the cost of a specialist's fee, or the more pre-dictable costs of primary care. The dollars flowing from licensed and regulated Medicare managed care plans can, in turn, flow downstream to unlicensed and unregulated (for insurance purposes) providers—physicians and hospitals. So-called downstream payments can be associated with downstream risk for providers, depending on the way they are paid, and for which services.

Provider stop-loss insurance is special insurance for physicians that protects them from very large financial losses. A requirement for Medicare managed care plans is that their physicians have such insurance if the physicians are at substantial financial risk.

Providers may be required to have **provider stop-loss insurance** as well as be able to meet certain other requirements in two instances. In the first instance, providers accept downstream risks that directly or indirectly have the effect of reducing or limiting services to enrollees. In the second instance, providers accept downstream risks for services they do not provide directly and must make referrals and pay others. The managed care plan is responsible for reporting to Medicare the extent of downstream risk held by the plan's providers and arranging any necessary stop-loss insurance for them.

The strategic issue, given that the managed care plan meets the regulatory requirements for provider stop loss, is the question of what the expectations are in the market among physicians for assistance from managed care plans to secure provider stop-loss insurance. Some providers may be ready to take on the risk and receive a fixed payment from the plan without provider stop-loss insurance. These providers would handle the administrative tasks of utilization management and quality assurance themselves. Other physicians may expect the health plan to pay the cost or actually provide the stop-loss coverage. How providers respond to this issue varies by local market. However, these responses must be assessed and monitored to keep the managed care plan competitive in terms of its ability to attract valuable physicians and physician groups in its network.

Global capitation payments, partial capitation payments, bonuses, withholds, and other physician incentive plans may place a physician or physician group at substantial financial risk. And as Figure 5.4 summarizes, indirect payments, including the offering of monetary value such as stock options or waivers of debt, may also place a physician or physician group at substantial financial risk. The nature and extent of risk must be determined and disclosed to Medicare and Medicare beneficiaries.

Nearly all current plans comply with these rules and do not place their providers at substantial financial risk. The benefits of placing providers at

Any arrangement or withhold >25 percent of potential payments, defined as maximum anticipated total payments. Payments unrelated to referrals are not counted.

Withholds <25 percent of potential payments if downstream risk exceeds 25 percent of potential payments.

Bonuses >33 percent of potential payments, minus the bonus.

Withholds plus bonuses if the two together equal >25 percent of potential payments.

Capitation payments if the difference between the maximum and minimum possible payment is >25 percent of the maximum possible.

FIGURE 5.4

Physician Incentive Arrangements Considered by Medicare as Substantial Financial Risk, 1998

Too much risk: Medicare has rules about when physician risk is too high

substantial financial risk as defined by Medicare are not worth the costs of meeting the requirements that accompany it.

States often regulate Medicare managed care plans under the McCarran Ferguson Act of 1945, a federal act declaring the right of states to regulate the business of insurance when the federal government does not. Thus, any plan must address the issue of downstream risk according to requirements established by state insurance commissioners for transacting the business of insurance in a state. Every Medicare managed care plan must carefully check these state requirements to ensure compliance.

As a guide for managed care plans, Medicare has laid out some general guidelines for the size of beneficiary panels and the normal limits of dollar amounts of financial risk a physician should assume without stop-loss coverage. The guidelines come from industry experience and they are based on an informal survey conducted for stop-loss insurance. These may serve as a guide for managed care plans that provide or arrange for provider stop-loss insurance regardless of whether they meet the rules regarding physician incentive plans.

In Table 5.3, the limits, deductibles, or attachment points, as they are called synonymously, vary according to the number of beneficiaries at risk for the physician group. Limits vary by beneficiary panel size. A larger beneficiary panel spreads the risk of having a patient with more than the limit in covered expenses over more patients and more revenues from the managed care plan. The limits may apply for all covered services included in the physician incentive plan or they may apply separately for the institutional (hospital or Part A of Medicare) or professional (medical or Part B of Medicare). Given the beneficiary panel size, a managed care plan would want to have deductible limits no larger than those shown in Table 5.3.

Other provider stop-loss provisions can be obtained to cover in-plan network services and especially out-of-network services. There is usually a coinsurance. So once the deductible for the provider is met, the stop-loss insurance pays a percentage of costs exceeding the limits—for example, 80

TABLE 5.3
Provider
Stop-Loss
Limits for
Medicare
Managed Care
Plans, 1998

Beneficiary Panel Size	Single Combined Limit	Separate Institutional Limit	Separate Professional Limit
1–1,000	$6,000*	$10,000*	$3,000*
1,001–5000	$30,000	$40,000	$10,000
5,001–8,000	$40,000	$60,000	$15,000
8,0001–10,000	$75,000	$100,000	$20,000
10,001–25,000	$150,000	$200,000	$25,000
>25,000	None	None	None

*Beneficiary panel size too small. Provider stop loss not recommended.

Suggested limits: Medicare has suggested limits for physician risk

or 90 percent. Emergency out-of-area stop-loss insurance is available with variable limits and coinsurance. Provider stop-loss insurance can also be had with a maximum payable once enough is paid through the coinsurance.

The advantage to a health plan for offering its providers stop-loss insurance is the linkage and relationship that emerges between the plan and its physician network. Not providing stop-loss insurance can be an ongoing point of dispute if the physicians think the premium for coverage is excessive or if there are problems paying claims. But only physicians and physician groups with the ability to assume the downstream risk should accept it. Every plan needs to take a sound approach to provider stop-loss insurance, and this approach must be appropriate to the market.

Reinsurance

Having taken care of the stop-loss needs of its own providers, a managed care plan must itself meet the requirements of contracting with Medicare and its state insurance commissioner in terms of risk. Many current Medicare managed care plans, especially those with enrollments greater than 100,000, have sufficient reserves and financial strength to **self-insure**, or be at full risk for covered services with catastrophic costs. But to protect against the high financial risks of Medicare contracting, small to midsize Medicare managed care plans often purchase **reinsurance**. Reinsurance represents an agreement between a reinsurer and a licensed Medicare managed care plan. In the agreement, the managed care plan pays a premium to a licensed insurance company. The insurance company, in turn, agrees to cover the managed care plan for certain losses it experiences as a result of providing care to a beneficiary.

Technically, reinsurance only exists between two insurers, although the word is frequently used to describe individual or aggregate stop-loss insurance when a managed care plan provides stop-loss insurance to its providers. Individual, or single, stop-loss coverage refers to coverage for an individual patient. Aggregate stop loss refers to coverage for all high-cost patients for a particular time period, usually a year.

Self-insure means a managed care plan alone retains the catastrophic risk of Medicare coverage for plan members following insurance requirements.

Reinsurance is insurance purchased from an insurance company by another insurance company.

A managed care plan buying reinsurance will benefit in a couple of distinct ways. First, reinsurance spreads the risk of loss. And second, having spread the risk, the contractor increases its capacity to accept new business because some risk has been passed on to another insurer, which modifies minimum capital, surplus, and reserves under most state insurance laws.

The most common form of reinsurance is **nonproportional stop-loss insurance,** or excess loss insurance. With nonproportional stop-loss insurance, the reinsurer typically pays a percentage of the difference between (1) the high-end costs incurred by a managed care plan in rendering covered services to a particular patient over a defined time period and (2) some predetermined deductible amount.

Nonproportional stop-loss insurance is purchased by insurance company from another to pay a percent of high costs for a case above some minimum dollar amount.

For example, assume that a particular nonproportional stop-loss insurance policy has an annual deductible of $50,000 and 60 percent cost sharing. If a managed care plan incurred $140,000 in costs attributable to a patient during the plan year, the reinsurer could pay $54,000 [($140,000 − $50,000) × 0.60]. Costs may be defined as Medicare fee-for-service costs or actual costs that might be calculated from a cost-to-charge ratio. Such issues are operational concerns that should be defined in the reinsurance policy. In practice, however, they are subject to interpretation on both sides. Selecting the reinsurance company carefully and checking its claims processing and premium experience will serve a managed care plan well. But the issue of reinsurance is more than just operational issues.

From a strategic viewpoint, a plan wants to minimize the cost of reinsurance and manage the health services risk of high-cost cases because of the effect they have on health plan costs and premiums. The cost of reinsurance can run between 3 and 8 percent of total costs. Lowering this cost means the premium or benefits offered can be marketed more attractively, and this in turn can increase enrollment. Reinsurance should not be viewed as a fixed cost of participating. Rather, it should be viewed as another component of the capitation dollar to be managed in a way that distinguishes one's health plan from the competition.

Medicare managed care plans have access to two major sources of reinsurance. First, many health plans are supplied reinsurance by an affiliated company. For example, statewide or regional Blue Cross and Blue Shield plans often supply their HMO subsidiaries with reinsurance. Second, national reinsurance companies offer another source. The cost of reinsurance from these national companies is often combined with the purchase of reinsurance for the commercial (non-Medicare, non-Medicaid) lines of business.

Whether the reinsurance is supplied by a parent company or a national reinsurance company, the managed care plan will be well served to shop for alternatives on an ongoing basis. At least every year, the health plan should issue a request for proposals or work with a broker to review the current market and the alternatives. A health plan that is buying reinsurance from a parent company might find this type of shopping useful for setting internal transaction prices between affiliated companies prudently and fairly.

Another approach to managing reinsurance is to establish a stop-loss insurance reciprocal or cooperative. Reinsurance supplied by national companies, although sometimes appropriate for very large risk contractors, may not be the lowest cost alternative for small to medium size Medicare risk contractors. Four points support this position.

1. *Noncompetitive pricing.* As limited and specialized suppliers of Medicare reinsurance, national companies charge higher prices (premiums) than would be expected from more competitive markets.
2. *Claims from states with high healthcare costs.* National suppliers of Medicare reinsurance base premiums on national claims costs. As a result, premium payers from states with generally lower healthcare costs subsidize premium payers from states with generally higher healthcare costs.
3. *Underwriting.* Premiums from national suppliers of reinsurance reflect poor-risk health plans, with inadequate or nonexistent risk management, as well as good-risk health plans.
4. *Profits.* Part of the premium to national reinsurance companies includes profit. Moreover, the national reinsurers retain any interest earned from funds they maintain because of the way cash flows from premium revenue held before claims are paid.

All four points suggest that Medicare managed care plans that use national reinsurance companies pay higher premiums than they should. If rivals are using the same national reinsurance companies or paying similar reinsurance premiums, these health plans do not distinguish themselves in the market in terms of costs when they design and price their product.

Competitive pricing is crucial because the cost of reinsurance can be a key segment of the total capitation dollar. If reinsurance is not low cost, it could be the source of higher beneficiary premiums for plans. Higher premiums affect a contractor's ability to successfully market the plans to beneficiaries, making that portion of the premium cost no lower than what is available nationally.

Ultimately, excessive reinsurance costs can affect the overall financial success of the plan. A well-operated plan, with low costs or a cost-conscious provider network, does not want to be thrust into a reinsurance pool with high-risk, high-cost plans. It will pay too much for the risk coverage and could take several percentage points off of its bottom line. Although it seems relatively small, it could be the difference between success or failure.

A stop-loss insurer represents an effective, low-cost alternative to national reinsurance companies. This approach to reinsurance, patterned after the familiar medical liability captive, reciprocal, or stock insurer, represents a viable alternative for a select few health plans in any state that have entered or plan to enter the Medicare managed care market.

A stop-loss insurer arrangement allows owners or subscribers of the stop loss to pool risk. The ability to pool risk has definite appeal for plans with fewer than 25,000 beneficiaries. For new plans entering the Medicare risk market and small plans alike, the stop-loss insurer enables them to create a more predictable risk pool. Figure 5.5 illustrates how four plans, each with fewer than 25,000 Medicare beneficiaries, can benefit from the arrangement.

Figure 5.5 illustrates four Medicare managed care plans, each with 6,250 Medicare beneficiaries in enrollment. Less than 25,000 beneficiaries indicates low, unpredictable enrollment, and reinsurance is recommended. The four plans can pool their risk through another entity. The stop-loss insurer would be created by the four member plans as a separate company, depending on state insurance laws and assuming each of the four members meets the insurance requirements for the enrollment each has individually. Not only can these plans share risk, but the pooled stop-loss arrangement allows them to share management responsibility. They can also share information about best practices to control risk and data on high-risk patients, which are likely to be only a few for each plan. Pooled data across all four plans, in the example, are likely to yield more useful analysis of how to improve quality and reduce costs. Establishment of such a stop-loss insurer must meet the requirements of individual state insurance commissioners.

Whether you decide to obtain self-insurance or reinsurance, the reinsurance risk must be managed. Even if reinsurance is purchased, the premium next year will be tied to the current catastrophic experience. Thus, good risk management of health services (not liability) is crucial. The general topic of care management in Chapters 7 through 9 address the use of case management, disease management, and high-cost case management. But the most important responses a plan can take are to continually collect data on high-cost cases, develop approaches to lowering costs while maintaining quality, and build an information database on best practices.

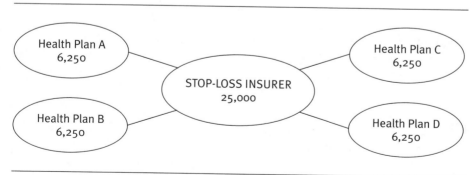

FIGURE 5.5

Illustration of Stop-Loss Insurer Reciprocal Model with Four Health Plans

Health plans can stop-loss: Pool risk until you can bear risk alone

Strategic Decisions Checklist

Strategic Questions	Strategic Analyses
How do you prepare for annual changes in the USPCC?	First, you monitor the national actuarial estimate carefully and constantly.
	You develop targeted responses to the reasons for changes in the USPCC.
	You maintain close links with national associations who are supposed to have their proverbial fingers on the pulse of nationwide changes.
Are you achieving optimal enrollment in terms of demographic groups?	You need to know the average demographic cost factor of the service area.
Are you achieving optimal enrollment in terms of risk adjustment?	You should decide whether you want to treat differently those beneficiaries likely to fall into the 15 risk-adjustment categories.
	Develop managed care quality and efficiency programs for non-risk-adjustment beneficiaries.
How are you generating conservative and accurate estimates of the projected revenues from a Medicare risk contract?	Most managed care plans only get about 72 percent of the published Medicare+Choice payments for their area, which is further reduced by 5 percent.
	You need to track the average demographic factor each month.
How do you support your choice between a cost-dominant or quality-dominant strategy?	You need to analyze market expectations.
	Conduct ongoing competitor analysis of Medicare supplemental products in the market as well as fee-for-service Medicare.
How much can you plan for current and future changes in beneficiary-paid premiums?	To properly plan premiums, you might be required to project premiums for three years.

continued

Strategic Questions	Strategic Analyses
Are you enrolling an unbiased selection of beneficiaries?	You need to constantly monitor and analyze service use and cost data compared with revenues.
	You need to make adjustments to benefits and premiums to avoid a premium spiral, in which premium increases are used to finance adverse risk selection.
Are you making an ongoing assessment of self-insurance or reinsurance?	You need to conduct ongoing comparison shopping regarding coverage and price.
	You could establish a reinsurance reciprocal or cooperative with others.
How are you conducting and improving health services risk management, especially for high-cost cases?	High-cost cases are of less concern now with risk adjustment being phased in, but information system decision support to identify high-cost cases early and to intervene is essential.
	You should have a process to identify and adopt best practices.

BENEFIT DESIGN, MARKETING, AND ENROLLMENT

Benefit package design is a precarious concern for Medicare managed care plans and requires watchful market research. Marketing your benefits to relatively complacent beneficiaries reporting high satisfaction with traditional Medicare can be costly and require patience. The enrollment process is vital because beneficiaries can switch plans today with less than a month's notice, although they will be locked-in for six months beginning in 2002. What happens immediately after a beneficiary signs up for your plan is important also for retaining new enrollees. Those issues are all in this chapter. Whether you are new to the Medicare managed care market or have served it for a long time, you will want to develop a business plan around benefit design, marketing, and enrollment procedures. The three are interrelated, each with implications for the other.

One theme in this chapter is that marketing Medicare managed care is not the same as marketing commercial managed care. Managed care companies predominantly concentrate commercial marketing today on employment-based groups. Commercial marketing is geared toward obtaining group contracts with employers either through brokers or with a company sales force. Often the group administrator or employer defines the requirements in terms of benefit package and provider network. Enrollment is handled through central employer offices. The employment-based market and the whims of employers influence decisions. As working employees, the enrollees are generally healthy compared with the entire population.

Marketing in Medicare managed care is quite different. The marketing is concentrated on individuals. The marketing is geared toward signing up an individual through brokers or a company sales force. Individuals make decisions differently from group plan administrators and give different weight to entirely different factors. Nevertheless, Medicare is more than just an individual insurance market; it is older Americans with a rather large, clear alternative—traditional Medicare with or without a traditional supplemental policy. The rules are subject to Congressional whim. The beneficiaries generally have lower health status than the general population, and it is more changeable than the commercial employer market. This important distinction between the traditional activities of managed care companies and the requirements of participation in the Medicare market implies altered marketing strategies, materials, and, possibly, different marketing staff and organizational relationships (Langwell and Hadley 1986). One link between the employment-based and Medicare markets is the growing ranks of retirees who are already enrolled in and comfortable with the managed care plan from their former place of work.

This chapter begins with a discussion of benefit design. Because the market environment drives the benefit package, making it impossible to describe the ideal package for every market, this section describes a process for developing the benefit package year after year. The next section covers marketing and describes what most health plans use today for marketing with a content analysis of current marketing materials. The final section covers enrollment issues, all the way from implementing the enrollment rules from HCFA to managing first contact with a new enrollee.

Benefit Design

Benefit design is the process of establishing the beneficiary-paid premium; copayments; the amount, duration, and scope of benefits; and the managed care physician–hospital network that will grow enrollment.

Managed care plans must offer substantial financial incentives in their **benefit design** for beneficiaries to join a Medicare+Choice managed care plan. Traditional fee-for-service Medicare offers a tremendous choice of hospitals and physicians for beneficiaries with almost no financial implications from selecting one provider over another. For a beneficiary to accept a limited network of hospitals and physicians, a managed care plan must offer attractive benefits at a reasonable or low-cost beneficiary-paid premium. Medicare managed care managers should not delude themselves that price does not matter if they only market heavily and offer a good network of well-known hospitals and physicians. The large number of zero-premium plans (presented below) documents the need for managed care to be the low-cost option.

Being forced to be the plan in the market that offers the low-cost option means having the lowest cost premium with respect to the type and level of Medicare supplemental benefits generally available. Thus, benefit design refers to both the choice of benefits to be offered and the level and mix of premiums and copayments in the package. Benefit coverage must be defined in terms of amount, duration, and scope for the supplemental benefits offered by the plan (see Table 6.1). There can be limits on the number of supplemental services, the days of supplemental coverage, or the package of supplemental services covered by the plan. The flexibility in benefit design extends only to the supplemental portion of coverage. All Medicare+Choice plans must cover the basic Medicare package of services shown in Chapter 1.

A good business plan for Medicare managed care might provide for annual critical examination and modification of the benefit package. The choice of package is conditional on the express desires of the population served and the offerings of competing plans. Thus, benefit design starts with an environmental analysis, including a competitor analysis. The design cannot be considered static as time goes on. Therefore, some scenario planning around

Amount	The number of visits, procedures, prescriptions, treatments covered
Duration	The period of time (number of days) covered
Scope	The package of supplemental services covered

TABLE 6.1
Factors in
Benefit Design

*Benefits
controlled by
three factors:
Amount,
duration,
and scope
characterize the
benefit coverage
package*

possible reactions in the market to the benefit design is necessary. Finally, the strategy for using the benefit design should be understood.

This approach to benefit design, marketing, and enrollment is called strategic cycling (Begun and Heatwole 1999). A singular strategic plan for benefit design and marketing can stifle creative responses to the marketplace and be conducive to adherence to outmoded strategies. Health plans with multiple markets should adopt strategic cycling to allow the managers in each market to develop dynamic plans tailored to their situation. A strategic cycling model facilitates continuous assessment of the goals and primary strategies from benchmarking analysis and understanding of the effects on beneficiaries (Fig. 6.1).

It works in four steps, starting with development of the overall mission and values of the Medicare+Choice plan. Most managed care companies enter the Medicare market counting on doing well financially. But beyond the fiscal considerations, what is the mission of the organization overall and how does

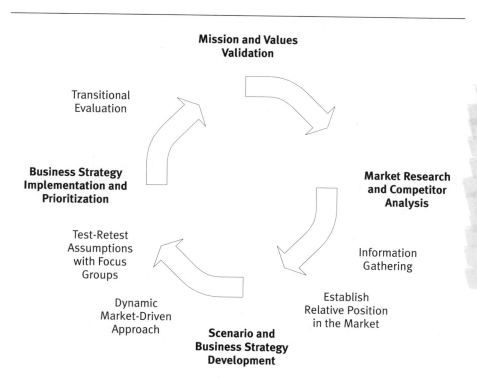

FIGURE 6.1
Strategic
Cycling Model

*Four steps to
strategic benefit
design: Strategic
cycling model
offers a
continuous
assessment
approach to
changing
market
dynamics*

the Medicare market validate that mission? Medicare managed care could be important to you because your health plan wants to serve all population segments of the geographic market. It might be a logical market to enable you to negotiate contracts with your hospitals and physicians for other lines of business. Your ability to deliver Medicare+Choice enrollees to them might encourage the loyalty of these hospitals and physicians to your health plan. An overall mission to serve large employer groups who would like to enroll their retirees in the same managed care plan serving their regular employees may be a reason for further loyalty. The mission and values statement for serving the Medicare market with a Medicare+Choice contract should be spelled out clearly and reassessed every year or so.

The second step involves market research and competitor analysis. In the past, strategic planning involved gathering data and analyzing all strengths, weaknesses, opportunities, and threats (SWOT). While still a useful tool for strategic planning and product development, a continuous analysis of customer needs and wants might facilitate the third step, as discussed below. Customers can be beneficiaries, affiliated physicians and hospitals, or the Medicare program itself.

The third step is scenario and business strategy development. Alternative market scenarios are warranted in terms of potential new competitors, changes in the managed care plan's hospital and physician network, or government policy.

Business strategy is a rational pattern in a stream of decisions.

The final step is **business strategy** implementation and prioritization. This is perhaps the most important step. Often too much effort is put into the development of the plan, but too little effort is spent on implementation. People need to be assigned responsibilities, and resources must be devoted to the effort. Setting priorities among competing needs in implementing the plan is also important. To ensure a dynamic, responsive model, there needs to be an evaluative step that gives feedback and informs the mission and values of the organization.

The model suggests these four major portions of strategic cycling for benefit design, marketing, and enrollment. Each is discussed in more depth in the following sections.

Market Research and Competitor Analysis

This first step should start with coordination among other divisions of the managed care plan. For example, market research might include detailed data analysis of the number and characteristics of Medicare beneficiaries in the targeted geographic markets. This information might already be available to your plan through another planning process. You will want to seek input and participation from the key members of the managed care plan's management team. People left out of the loop may have insights and information that can help to avoid duplications. In addition, if they have input early on in the process, they are more likely to support the ultimate plan and its implementation.

Ask others in the plan about opportunities to influence enrollees and how they think beneficiaries obtain information about Medicare+Choice and your health plan. You will have a better understanding of your colleagues' assumptions in the health plan and perhaps of what you must do to change them.

Much of the information needed for market research is available on the World Wide Web at the home pages of HCFA. Go to www.medicare.gov and find the geographic areas for which you are interested in identifying competitors. Medicare Compare is an interactive database that includes detailed information on Medicare's health plan options. It is designed to allow Medicare beneficiaries to "comparison shop" by the costs of premiums and benefits offered. These pages will include all of the current Medicare+Choice health plans approved for marketing, their enrollments, their benefits, and a summary of beneficiary perceptions about and satisfaction with each plan. Your plans for benefit design can be benchmarked against the other plans available in the market as a reality check. You can expect other plans to change their benefits next year, and you must anticipate the kinds of changes they might make. Thus, we will discuss scenario development and contingency planning to consider that possibility.

Information Gathering

What are not shown on the Medicare Compare web pages are the details of the hospital and physician network. The SWOT analysis may be useful for analyzing enrollment, benefits, beneficiary perceptions, quality measures (from the Medicare Compare web page), and the provider network (features of your network compared with others). Make a list of these in a table and summarize the strengths, weaknesses, opportunities, and threats for each one for your health plan as compared with your competition.

A summary of benefits found on the Medicare Compare web pages for all plans is shown in Table 6.2. One of the distinctive features of the Medicare+Choice market over the years has been the large number of plans with zero-premium benefits. The percent with zero-premium benefits has actually grown over the years, reflecting the primary characteristic that prompts beneficiaries to switch to Medicare managed care. About two-thirds offer prescription drugs with a limited amount of coverage. Almost all offer preventive services that traditional Medicare does not. A majority cover eye exams and ear exams. A minority cover foot care, glasses lenses, hearing aids, and dental services. The traditional Medicare copayment is covered by nearly all plans for a physician office visit, as is customary in HMOs. About half of all plans offer at least one other richer benefit package, at a higher premium, with more generous amount, duration, and scope of benefits.

Having evaluated your comparative position in the market and determined the elements of SWOT, examine your performance in the market critically. You should have a clear game plan to improve, relative to other plans, in premiums, benefits, or your network of hospitals and physicians. You can mimic the best practices in your market or elsewhere that lead to success for others. But you

Establishing Your Relative Position in the Market

TABLE 6.2
Trends in
Premiums and
Supplemental
Benefits,
Medicare+
Choice Health
Plans,
1987–1998
(Basic Option)

*Zero-premium is
the norm: The
percent of
Medicare
HMOs with
zero-premium
and high benefits
has grown in the
1990s*

Percent Offering	1987	1990	1994	1995	1996	1997	1998
Zero Premium	10	18	33	51	65	69	70
Outpatient Drugs	43	35	38	50	61	68	67
Routine Physicals	80	87	97	97	97	97	97
Immunizations	—	77	90	86	88	89	89
Health Education	—	31	30	24	24	37	38
Foot care	—	28	31	33	37	30	30
Eye Exams	60	83	83	90	90	92	83
Lenses	—	12	20	5	7	15	1
Ear Exams	35	54	68	71	76	78	72
Hearing Aids	—	1	6	3	4	10	1
Dental	11	22	28	36	37	39	37
Visit Copayment in Basic Package?	—	80	95	95	97	96	93
Offer High-Option Package?	—	4	33	40	42	47	51

Source: Mathematica Policy Research. 1999. MPR Analysis of December 1 Medicare Managed Care Reports for indicated years. Washington, DC: Mathematica.

need a clear plan of the steps to take now that will improve your performance and relative position in the market.

You will want to be able to implement change in the plan for improvement so that the next round of premiums and benefits betters your position. In too many plans, premium setting and benefit design are an annual grind of the actuarial experience in a formulaic process. The strategic cycling approach offers a way to overcome the normal process and build in plans and activities that overcome your weaknesses and threats while building on strengths and opportunities.

For example, if the reports of plan satisfaction from Medicare show your plan to be an underachiever, conduct your own patient satisfaction survey. Uncover the reasons for low plan satisfaction. Take the steps to correct the problems and target a change in satisfaction that will improve your reported satisfaction levels the next year or the year after. You have to take steps today to solve the problem or be prepared to find a repeat of the same results the following year.

Market positioning for the next year of Medicare+Choice marketing begins the previous year. If you foresee a zero-premium package difficult to maintain because of cost considerations, start immediately to plan changes in the amount, duration, and scope of benefits to bring costs in line. Review the network of physicians and hospitals to channel patients toward the more cost-effective providers. But do not let another year go by when the upcoming benefit design and premiums are due to HCFA for posting and you have not consciously developed a position in the market.

Scenario and Business Strategy Development

Strategic planning has been associated with singular approaches that need to be accomplished according to a well-articulated schedule. As an example, the plan using a singular approach would have the same benefits plans have always had. The plan would have no way of knowing what beneficiaries thought about the plan and the benefits. The singular approach would have no budget for finding out what beneficiaries thought. A budget for gathering information is not necessary because a singular approach would wait for enrollment to drop to find out that there is a problem. Strategic planning has been criticized for overreliance on this singular approach and possibly faulty assumptions.

There is no crystal ball for the state of the market in the future. You must always test your assumptions about the number and type of competitors, and what they are offering. Scenario planning helps you do this. **Scenarios** are a means of learning. It means development of ideas, analysis, and financial projections that contemplate events different from those that may have been considered most likely. They help you and the other managers in your health plan "color outside the lines" and think about the unexpected. So much of Medicare managed care is defined by the Medicare program itself. Scenario planning can help get you out of the comfort zone you may find yourself in when preparing for annual benefits and premium changes.

Scenarios are the development of ideas, analysis, and financial projections that contemplate different events than those that may have been considered most likely.

For example, is it safe to presume that the current number of plans offering enrollment to compete with you will always be the same? Imagine each of your competitors merging. Whom would they merge with, and how large would that make the new plan? What is the list of the most likely new market entrants from outside your market? Are there markets similar to yours, and what changes are influencing the health plans in those markets? If total enrollment grows by 5 percent next year, for example, who is likely to get most of that growth in enrollment? Who has gotten the growth in total enrollment in the last three years? These changes are likely to have implications for your network of physicians and hospitals, and the same market scenario development can be applied to them as well.

Continuously evaluate and consider all possible environmental changes, adverse outcomes, and how you might respond. Monitor the market through beneficiary surveys, focus groups, and frequent talks with people involved with your plan offering. Include a broad spectrum of people familiar with your health plan. Talk to current members, but also check with your hospitals and physicians and determine what they are hearing. Your contacts with the Medicare program also can share insights. Ask them how you are doing in terms of

Dynamic Market-Driven Approach

compliance and timeliness. An honest critique could be very instructive. Create charts and tables that track year-to-year changes in premiums, benefits, patient satisfaction, and major policy changes in the Medicare+Choice program. Use this information to think of changes in the market that could influence your strategic choices. This type of thinking can extend to subgroups of your populations as well. Analyze the effects of premiums, benefits, and patient satisfaction by income, geographic location, and regular source of care.

Computer simulations using "what if" options are always useful for modeling dynamic market characteristics. Define the local geographic market as the metropolitan area or a logical collection of counties. Compute the market share of all plans in the local Medicare managed care market. Calculate how fast the Medicare managed care market has been growing the last year or so. Compute your enrollment next year, if you grew as fast as the market had grown recently. What would your enrollment be if you grew as fast as the fastest growing health plan? Could you double the average or fastest rate of growth? Imagine what would have to happen to attain that rate of growth.

Factor in changes in the market in terms of demographics, the economy, development of new housing options for people, and so on. Ask yourself if any of these will have an effect on your assumptions.

Make a list of potential new market entrants. Research them and know their tactics for entering the market. Understand how they position their product and how they develop their physician and hospital network. Have a written plan, even if it is one-half page long, of how you would respond to a particular new market entrant.

Test and Retest Assumptions and Focus Groups

The essence of the strategic cycling approach is never to allow plans become stagnant and linear. A healthy dose of skepticism about your assumptions regarding the market will lead to continual reassessment and information gathering. You should have a process for obtaining formative research about the market and your place in it. That includes some affirmation that the approaches to benefit design, marketing, and enrollment have worked in the past and you have developed some confidence about the tactics you are using and the message you are delivering. Once you have a working business strategy, you will want to test it.

One of the best methods of reassessment is the focus group. Focus groups are excellent for testing the positioning you have assumed or are planning. They are most effective when the details of the approach to the market are identified and you want to discern how your plan will be received.

Focus groups can be insourced and done on your own, but most people do not have the time to pull together what it takes to run a focus group. Although they can be costly, it is better to outsource to focus groups experts. They bring a level of objectivity to the process because they are generalists in all fields and help you maintain a fresh examination of assumptions. The marketing firm running the focus group will need to work with you to develop a discussion guide to ask the right questions. They will know how to recruit people, but you will want to help identify the right types of participants. Focus groups can almost never be statistically representative because the number of people is just too small. As such, the findings cannot be generalized and should be handled with care. Nevertheless, focus groups can provide very intensive, qualitative insights and ideas that you would not normally obtain from a survey, for example. That is exactly what you would require to test and retest your assumptions.

Barrett (1996A) offers the outline of a script for a focus group. The focus group outline in Figure 6.2 begins with welcome and introductions of the leaders and a brief explanation for why people have been invited to participate. A brief icebreaker exercise at the beginning gets each person to talk and understand that their voice needs to be heard. Most focus groups begin with global questions and become progressively more specific as the session goes on. About two hours are an adequate amount of time to have a good discussion, and perhaps a group of eight to ten participants is workable.

The discussion can start with comments on where managed care fits within the Medicare program. You can obtain general perceptions of managed care and managed care companies. The discussion in the Barrett outline then turns to each person, their current coverage, and why they selected that coverage. The likes and dislikes of their current health insurance are important, as is the likelihood of changing coverage. You can get a sense of the depth of feeling about different factors that make people change insurance, although there is great persistence in the choice of insurance once the choice is made.

A discussion of competitors and relative name recognition should give you a good idea of whether your health plan is advertising enough and in the right way.

Finally, the focus group can sharpen the perceptions on specific benefits that are of most importance to the participants. These would include low-cost premium, benefit coverage, and the network of hospitals and physicians.

Several other methods exist for challenging your assumptions about the market. Beneficiary surveys are an excellent way to take some of the ideas you may have uncovered in the focus groups and test them statistically. In other words, an opinion expressed in a focus group is only a sample of one or a few people. You may want to see whether the views or ideas expressed hold up in the broader market, which can be accomplished with a member survey by mail or phone. To see which health plan has the best name recognition, for example, or whether the impressions offered in the focus group of your plan are consistent with the general population, conduct a survey. The other benefit of a survey is that it can be conducted periodically, and changes in attitudes and perceptions can be tracked over time. In contrast, focus groups and other qualitative research techniques, such as interviewing leaders, can help you understand the forces that might be emerging to create change in the market. Qualitative methods can be more open ended and lead in surprising directions.

FIGURE 6.2

Outline for Typical Medicare Managed Care Focus Group

Test assumptions by asking: Focus groups can be an invaluable method of tracking a dynamic market

Welcome	Introduce yourself and tell a little about yourself. Thank the group for coming.
Purpose	Need to make sure we are meeting your needs. Want your input into what you think health insurance should be about and what you want most from your health insurance. Stress confidentiality. What you say will not affect your individual benefits or the type of care you are receiving.
Agenda	Talk generally about what is important to you as far as healthcare, health insurance, and benefits. There are no right or wrong answers.
Group Introductions	People introduce themselves. Icebreaker exercise is done so that everyone has a chance to speak at the outset.
Perceptions of Medicare Managed Care	How do you feel about the coverage you receive from Medicare? Have you heard about Medicare HMOs? What have you heard? The first thing comes to mind when I hear "managed care" or "HMO" is....
Current Coverage	Do you have insurance in addition to Medicare? Why did you choose that particular health plan? What went into your decision to choose that health plan?
Likes and Dislikes	What do you like best about your health plan? What do you like least about your health plan? If you could change one thing about your current health coverage, what would it be? If you were in the market for a new health plan, what would be the three most important factors in your decision?
Competitor Recall	Besides your current health plan, what other companies or products come to mind when you think about a health plan? What are your perceptions of each of these other health plan companies? Have you ever heard of our company?
Benefits	What health benefits are most important to you? Why? How important to you is freedom of choice regarding primary care physicians and specialists? Why? Is access to your physician more important to you than the cost of the plan?

continued

FIGURE 6.2
Continued

Benefits *(continued)*	A card sort exercise with well-known benefit features could be done to reach consensus among the group on the priority order of benefits.
Marketing	What is the most common way you hear about other health insurance plans? How involved are your children in helping you decide on health insurance issues?
Conclusion	Do you have any other comments? Thank you for your participation.

Source: Adapted from D. E. Barrett, in *Implementing A Successful Medicare Managed Care Product*, edited by D. Mlawsky. 1996. Washington, DC: Atlantic Information Services, Inc.

Finally, some health plans have standing advisory committees made up of members. These committees can be a very low-cost method of staying in touch with your membership. If the committees meet monthly or quarterly, that can be a useful vehicle for testing your assumptions about how well you are doing and for trying out new ideas before they are fully developed.

Business Strategy Implementation

Once all the data are collected and analyzed, a more intuitive approach must be applied to devise the business strategy. Although a plan faces a stream of decisions made about marketing, operations, financing, and network development and the pattern they create to define how the business is operated, you will want to gravitate toward one dominant business strategy. Your business strategy defines how your managed care plan participates in the market to be competitive.

For Medicare managed care plans, the business strategy is executed in the benefit design. Although it probably oversimplifies the complexity of enrollee decision making, some research exists on the importance of basic types of benefits for Medicare beneficiaries. You must choose which one will embody your business strategy.

One study suggests the type of benefit is important (Marquis and Rogowski 1991). Medicare beneficiaries seem to place particular emphasis on benefits that protect them against high out-of-pocket expenses or catastrophic expenses, especially for long-term care (which is not covered under Medicare except under particular circumstances related to a hospital stay.) They appear to have less attachment to preventive benefits, whereas many HMOs place emphasis on preventive services in their advertising.

Every study of beneficiary satisfaction with Medicare managed care satisfaction finds costs are a major concern. Beneficiaries join managed care plans because they are concerned with the competitive premiums they pay in traditional Medicare supplemental policies. Thus, from the research done, there are two broad strategies—a benefits-dominant positioning and a costs-dominant positioning. You must decide the way in which you will describe the health plan to the market, the features to stress, and how you will be defined differently from competitors. Although there are two basic approaches in this market, as discussed below, there are other approaches and factors to consider in designing the benefit package and marketing strategy.

Benefits-Dominant

Benefits-dominant means the health plan emphasizes coverage, network features, and quality in the design of the plan and its marketing.

To some extent the **benefits-dominant** approach is dependent on the model type of the health plan. Newer health plans with broad, unmanaged physician and hospital networks might be best suited to emphasize benefits. There is a trade-off between a lavish benefit package and the premium that can be charged. As more benefits are included in the package, the premium is going to be higher. But a health plan could choose purposefully to be the rich benefit plan in the market and use that as a strategy. Markets where Medicare managed care is new or total enrollment is relatively low are good candidates for the benefits-dominant approach because beneficiaries will be attracted to the nontraditional benefit package that goes beyond normal Medicare coverage. It may be more effective to offer a generous package given the competition.

Costs-Dominant

Costs-dominant means the health plan emphasizes lower costs in the design of the plan and its marketing.

The other way to go is a strategy that describes the plan and its features placing primary dominance on costs. Low plan premiums, small copayments, and little paperwork are all features of plans that can portray **costs-dominant** business strategy. Older plans with narrow, well-established hospital and physician networks under tight control are good candidates for this strategy. They must deliver what they promise, however, and be the lowest or one of the lowest plan premiums in the market. Large, for-profit health plans are better able to take this strategy, compared with regional, not-for-profit health plans unless they have narrow, well-established networks of physicians and hospitals. Staff- and group-model HMOs are also good candidates for the costs-dominant approach. This approach, over the years of Medicare managed care, has become the principal strategy in large part because major national players have adopted it, and they dominate the Medicare+Choice enrollment.

Figure 6.3 offers two illustrations of the polar choices for positioning around costs or quality. Ad A from Keystone shows an active, middle- to upper-class couple presumably enjoying their retirement. The phrase, "Medicare Made Simple. And Simply Better", sends a clear message that you can get high-quality, coordinated care from this plan. Ad B shows a pleasant scene with one individual with the suggestion that she is worried about the "high cost of medical care." Ad B incorporates another sentiment about having earned the right to not have to worry about costs. Note the contented, rather youthful appearance of the persons depicted in both ads. The same themes and positioning appear in all the promotional materials on the market.

FIGURE 6.3
Two
Illustrations of
Positioning
Around Cost or
Quality

Ad A

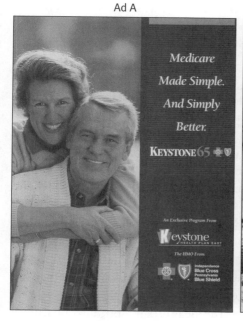

Ad B

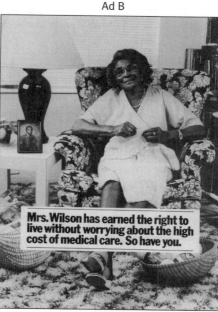

Source: Independence Blue Cross. Keystone Health Plan East marketing brochure.

Another quite reasonable approach is simply to follow the leader in the market. This is sometimes called **shadow pricing** or mimetic behavior—if a large competitor already exists, it might be reasonable, perhaps even cost less in terms of marketing research, to match what the leader is doing in the market. It can work for a while, especially if your health plan can better *implement* the same business strategy. For example, if a costs-dominant strategy is the rule, match the strategy in the market, and then work to distinguish your plan on other features. Match the lowest price and then deliver better than prevailing quality by offering a better size or better characteristics of the provider network, or better member relations. You must study each market and decide what the market is demanding. Although it might seem logical to offer a benefits-dominant position, if a major player already offers a costs-dominant plan, the "can't beat 'em, join 'em" rule may apply if the market is demanding lower-cost options.

A discussion of benefit design must focus on the premium paid for the scope of covered services, but the location of services is a vital dimension of benefit design. If the plan covers one pair of eyeglasses, but only when ordered by mail from across town, the perception of the coverage changes. If the Part A deductible is covered only when the patient is admitted to the health plan's

Follow the Leader

Shadow pricing is when a smaller, less dominant health plan follows the lead of a larger, more dominant health plan, particularly in premium pricing and benefit design.

Location, Location, Location

owned hospitals, that will influence beneficiary views of the benefit design. Borrowing the old real estate phrase, there are three threshold issues for benefit design: "location, location, and location." Because of the personal nature of receiving healthcare services, the location of services is a vital aspect of its benefits to the beneficiary.

Location in this context means the geographic location of health centers, physicians, and hospital facilities germane to the Medicare population. Most health plans serving predominantly the healthy, employed population will need to reassess their network constantly. They will need to contrast the location of current enrollees and potential enrollees. Some may want to add new service sites, for example, if the former sites were for healthy, employed members and now the health plan requires more locations geared toward the elderly.

One option in this regard is a phenomenon that started with the Medicare HMO program in 1983. It goes by various names, one of which is Senior Health Centers. Senior Health Centers offer a way to market aggressively through visible locations for facilities specifically designed for enrollees. They offer not only convenient office locations for primary care physicians (perhaps with practices owned or not owned by the health plan) but also pharmacy, exercise, day care, and community activity and education rooms. Pioneered specifically for the Medicare managed care enrollees in Long Beach, California, in the mid-1980s by FHP, a large Medicare HMO at the time, the notion was to offer to the community a location to receive the benefits of the health plan that specialized in caring for the Medicare managed care members of the plan. The services could be controlled closely and better managed by the health plan, and they could be combined with other offerings such as exercise, community or support groups, and social activities that not only helped in the marketing of the plan but also attracted a broad spectrum of beneficiaries from the neighborhood served.

There must be a concentration of beneficiaries in the local area to make a Senior Health Center viable. But it can provide an intensive marketing and promotion option, especially if new Senior Health Centers can expand the locations for the health plan and make the benefit package more attractive.

Marketing and Promotional Materials

Marketing and promotional materials are the primary sources of information to new and current enrollees that describe your health plan and how you differentiate yourself from others. They represent the results of the strategic cycling process and reflect how your health plan positions itself in the market. In addition, they are regulated closely by HCFA. In fact, HCFA requires its own review of the final proof, or blueline copy, that will be used by the printer to make the plates before the printing. In cases where the health plan makes its own reproductions of a document rather than use a printer, a final copy of the document that will be used as the master for the reproductions must be reviewed by the HCFA Regional Office. Table 6.3 lists the major items considered to be **Beneficiary Notification Materials** requiring final marketing approval by HCFA. The marketing review includes required wording, size of typeset, the types of pictures used, and other matters. Once you understand what is expected, the marketing requirements are not difficult to meet. You must allow time for the review. And there is ample latitude to position your plan for success within the marketing materials review.

To see how current Medicare+Choice health plans position themselves, in 1998 we repeated an earlier content analysis study of marketing and promotional materials used by Medicare+Choice plans (Langwell and Hadley 1986) (Table 6.4). We obtained and reviewed new member inquiry mailings sent by nearly 183 HMOs in the Medicare market at the time. We wrote plans in existence for more than two years with more than 5,000 enrollees, from all parts of the country with enrollment, requesting a packet of information, just

***Beneficiary Notification Materials** are regulated marketing materials used to explain benefits and services, or any communication documents used to relate or obtain needed information from potential or existing members.*

---

1. Enrollment Applications

2. Enrollment by Mail Forms

3. Enrollment Letters, e.g.,
   - Proposed Enrollment Effective Date
   - Receipt of Medical Services under Medicare Fee-for-Service Prior to Enrollment
   - Confirm Enrollment-Effective Date

4. Denial of Enrollment/Disenrollment Letters, e.g.,
   - Sending out Disenrollment Form
   - Disenrollment Confirmation
   - Confirmation of Disenrollment Date
   - Failure to Pay Plan Premium
   - Involuntary Disenrollment
   - Confirmation of Involuntary Disenrollment

5. Summary of Benefits

6. Evidence of Coverage

7. Annual Notice of Change Letters

8. Member Handbooks

9. Provider Termination Notices

10. Claims Denial Notices

11. Service Area Reduction Notices

12. Nonrenewal Notices

TABLE 6.3

Examples of Items for Beneficiary Notification Marketing Materials Reviewed by HCFA, 2000

HCFA wants to see it all: Final verification of Medicare and managed care beneficiary notification marketing materials is required for at least 12 items

Source: Health Care Financing Administration. 2000. Medicare Introduction. [Online information; retrieval 9/25/00]. http://www.hcfa.gov/medicare/intro.htm.

TABLE 6.4
Percent of
Medicare+
Choice Plans
That Mention
Selected
Features in
Advertisements,
1997

Low costs rule:
Promotional
materials
overwhelmingly
mention the low
costs of Medicare
managed care

Feature Mentioned	Percent
Low Costs	74
No Paperwork	50
Many Physicians	47
High Quality	46
Age of Plan	30
Convenient Location	19
Hospital Affiliation	15
High Enrollment	4
Short Waiting Time	2

as a potential new enrollee might do. The responses were reviewed by a team of reviewers, trained in content analysis of such materials, using a checklist format to look for certain items. The data collection instruments are available from the author upon request.

Overwhelmingly these marketing and promotional materials emphasized low costs as a benefit to joining. Fully 74 percent of the time, low costs relative to Medicare and other traditional Medicare supplements were named. The second most frequent feature mentioned was "no paperwork" involved with plan membership. However, mentioned nearly as much was having many physicians and the high quality of care offered by the plan. Low cost, no paperwork, many physicians, and high quality were the four most frequently mentioned features. These were not mutually exclusive in our content analysis and any feature was counted if it received at least one mention. In other words, a feature was counted each time it was mentioned.

Features mentioned less often include the age of the plan (30 percent), convenient location of facilities (19 percent), hospital affiliations with well-known hospitals (15 percent), and high enrollment (e.g., "we are the largest plan in the area"), and short waiting times to see healthcare providers.

In terms of the benefits covered by the plan, several services or benefits mentioned were almost always mentioned and others were not (Table 6.5). Obviously, Medicare+Choice plans cover the same services as Part A of Medicare, primarily inpatient hospital care, and Part B physician care. Naturally, these are the two most frequently mentioned services in promotional materials. The third most frequent benefit was prescription drugs followed by vision care (82 percent) and home health care (76 percent).

In the 1990s, mental health care, eyeglasses, lab services, preventive care, dental care, and physicals or checkups, were all mentioned in a majority of promotional materials. In sharp contrast, the earlier study from the 1980s (Langwell and Hadley 1986) found no mention of mental health services. A collection of services, including routine foot care, diagnostic services (already covered by Medicare), nursing home care, homemaker services, and private duty nursing were mentioned by some health plans, but all in the minority

Service or Benefit Mentioned	Percent
Inpatient Hospital Care	89
Outpatient Physician Care	86
Prescription Drugs	86
Vision Care	82
Home Health Care	76
Other	76
Mental Health Care	72
Eyeglasses	63
Lab Services	63
Preventive Care	59
Dental Care	56
Physicals or Checkups	54
Diagnostic Services	40
Nursing Home Care	39
Routine Foot Care	33
Homemaker Services	2
Private Duty Nursing	2

TABLE 6.5
Percent of Medicare+ Choice Plans That Mention Specific Services and Benefits, 1997

Service offerings vary: Some services are predictable and others are not

of plans. Most of these are not associated with coverage for medical care, but coverage for long-term care, which is very limited coverage under Medicare, and Medicare+Choice plans are not obligated to provide them, except as a supplemental service.

More than 90 percent of Medicare+Choice plans operate in markets with competitors, and nearly two-thirds of all beneficiaries have the choice of two or more health plans in their area. To examine the competitive nature of the market, we studied the promotional materials for comparative claims. As shown in Table 6.6, only 5 percent of marketing materials we reviewed made any comparison specifically to another Medicare+Choice plan. This type of advertising might be viewed as too aggressive for this market, but it may also reflect the fact that most plans are competing with traditional fee-for-service Medicare. They make comparisons to traditional Medicare as the major competition for comparison, rather than another private plan.

HCFA has a Standardized Summary of Benefits requirement with a format that attempts to standardize the information beneficiaries receive comparing Medicare+Choice plans to traditional Medicare. A common language and standard format for all plan benefit summaries is required. There are three sections to the standard format:

1. *Beneficiary Information Section* includes the highlights of participating in the Medicare+Choice program;
2. *Plan Benefits Comparison Section* contains a ten-page matrix that describes each benefit and compares each specific health plan offering to traditional Medicare benefits; and

TABLE 6.6
Percent of
Medicare+
Choice Plans
That Engage in
Comparative
Advertisements,
1997

No comparison:
Promotional
materials
overwhelmingly
make no
comparative
claims

Mentioned	Percent
No Comparison Made	95
Compares to Other Unspecified Plan	5
Compares Specifically with Another Plan	0

3. *Plan Information Section* accommodates up to four pages in which health plans can describe themselves or further explain their benefits.

The information provided by each managed care plan is used by HCFA to create the Medicare Compare web pages operated by the agency for beneficiaries to shop for plans. The standardization is such that the costs-dominant or benefits-dominant approach is not revealed readily by these standardized reports. Thus, health plans must have further dissemination of their own marketing materials, approved by HCFA, to position themselves in the market.

In a 1999 government report, the Government Accounting Office challenged the accuracy and usefulness of health plan literature in Medicare managed care (GAO 1999). As of January 2000, participating plans must adhere to new standard reporting. Health plans do not need to advertise or promote their benefit differences, the Medicare program itself will do this according to standards for making comparisons. Nevertheless, from our survey, discussed previously, of the promotional materials mailed by most plans in 1997, we found plans made specific comparisons (e.g., eyeglasses) if they did not make general comparisons (e.g., lower cost), and only about 9 percent made no comparisons in the promotional materials sent to prospective enrollees (Table 6.7).

Table 6.8 tallies the percent of health plans that mentioned selected features, benefits, and services. More than half the promotional materials sent through the mail to prospective new enrollees mentioned low cost as the core benefit of enrollment. Following low cost were two other cost concerns for beneficiaries in terms of transaction costs for obtaining services. The second feature mentioned most often was no paperwork, followed by convenience of location of services. A little more than 10 percent of health plans mentioned quality and choice in terms of the number of physicians. Two other factors mentioned were the age of the health plan, or how long it has been serving the Medicare market, and high enrollment to induce a bandwagon effect to potential enrollees.

Branding
any name, term,
color, or symbol
that distinguishes
one health plan
from another.

To distinguish the health plan from government-run Medicare and to distinguish themselves in the market, many plans use branding. **Branding** is any name, term, color, or symbol that distinguishes one health plan from another. Many Medicare+Choice plans have a national presence and have well-known names (Blue Cross Blue Shield, Aetna, Cigna, PacifiCare). Others

Mentioned	Percent
Specific Comparison to Traditional Fee-for-Service Medicare	49
General Comparisons to Medicare	42
No Comparisons to Medicare	9

have more local names that might be considered brand names (University of Pennsylvania Health System, Mayo Clinic, Cleveland Clinic). Branding has become an important part of the Medicare managed care market, with 87 percent prominently displaying a brand name in their promotional materials. These brand names have become an important signaling device to beneficiaries that the health plan is a well-known name in the insurance business. It would appear that branding has become the standard in Medicare managed care, as shown in Table 6.9.

Finally, we analyzed the contents of the entire package of promotional materials and determined whether the primary focus was on cost, quality, or something else. Nearly two-thirds of plans focused on cost as the major feature emphasized in the plan. Less than a third focused on quality for positioning their product. Approximately 9 percent had a collection of positioning focus on comparative benefits, location, and brand name (see Table 6.10).

Feature Mentioned	Percent
Low Costs	55
No Paperwork	20
Convenience	16
High Quality	13
Number of Participating Physicians	13
Other	12
Age of Plan	2
High Enrollment	2

Eligibility Communications and Enrollment

In fact, marketing, benefit design, and enrollment are inextricably linked because of the ease in switching plans for beneficiaries. That will be modified in 2002 with a minimum six-month lock-in period, but it still connects the three. There can be friction at the point of enrollment (for the beneficiaries) surrounding eligibility, completing the proper documents, and especially understanding the new rules of accessing care in the managed care plan. Your success in the managed care market is in part dependent on quick mail and telephone response times, timely and accurate answers to beneficiary

TABLE 6.9
Percent of
Medicare+
Choice Plans
That Use Brand
Name in
Promotional
Materials, 1997

Branding:
Promotional
materials
mentioning a
brand name
dominate

Feature Mentioned	Percent
Brand Name Mentioned	87
No Brand Name Mentioned	13

questions, and the use of people trained especially to communicate with older beneficiaries. It is so important that many marketing and sales directors in Medicare managed care plans do not count enrollment, for example, for a sales force bonus, until the beneficiary has been enrolled six months. Focus on minimizing any discrepancy between the promise of enrollment in the health plan and the experience with the care delivered, right at the start.

Approximately 20 percent of new enrollees change their mind in this six-month window after enrollment and disenroll. Thus, the intersection between marketing and sales on the one hand and plan operations and delivery on the other hand is the source of many complaints. If done poorly, the gains from many dollars spent on marketing and sales quickly can be eroded with errors and problems at eligibility and enrollment.

Beginning January 2000, enrollments and disenrollments made on or before the 10th day of the month is effective the first day of the next month. All enrollments and disenrollments made after the 10th day of each month are effective the first day of the second calendar month after the election is made. Detailed and clear rules from HCFA describe the eligibility determination and enrollment process. Both are managed care plan responsibilities. The details in the form of operational policy letters are available at www.hcfa.gov/medicare. But the eligibility determination can be summarized as shown in Table 6.11. From a strategic standpoint in the marketplace, you will want the eligibility and enrollment determination to be as fast and easy as possible because it is the first exposure to the health plan for the new enrollee.

TABLE 6.10
Percent of
Medicare+
Choice Plans by
Overall
Strategic Focus
in Promotional
Materials, 1997

Strategic focus
comes down to
cost or quality

Feature Mentioned	Percent
Cost Focus	62
Quality Focus	29
Other	9

First, there are a small number of beneficiaries who for a variety of reasons are not enrolled in Part B of Medicare covering physician services. Medicare managed care has always required both Part A and Part B coverage because, after all, it is designed to be comprehensive, integrated care for hospital and physician services. Thus, the first eligibility rule is that beneficiaries must be eligible for both.

1. The beneficiary is entitled to Part A and enrolled in Part B (certain exceptions apply).

2. The beneficiary has not been medically determined to have end-stage renal disease prior to completing the enrollment form (certain exceptions apply).

3. The beneficiary resides in the service area of the Medicare+Choice plan.

4. The individual or his/her representative signs an enrollment form that is complete and includes all the information required to process the enrollment.

5. The individual is fully informed of and agrees to abide by the rules of the Medicare+Choice plan that were provided during the election process.

TABLE 6.11
Medicare+
Choice
Requirements
for Enrollment,
2000

Eligibility is exacting: Eligibility for Medicare+ Choice plans requires meeting five tests

The second pertains to persons with end-stage renal disease (ESRD) who have a separate coverage available if they already have ESRD. The Medicare+Choice program includes payment categories for people who do not have ESRD when they enroll but have it after enrollment.

Third, with some exceptions, beneficiaries must reside in the approved service areas served by the health plan.

Fourth, the beneficiary or his or her designated proxy must complete and sign the enrollment form with information required to change the master files at Medicare and make the assignment to the proper Medicare+Choice payment category. When the health plan submits this enrollment information, the computers at HCFA are programmed to deny future service claims for payment in the fee-for-service side of Medicare.

Fifth, and perhaps most important, the beneficiary or their designated proxy must sign specific statements warranting that the beneficiary understands that with managed care the beneficiary can no longer go to just any provider. HCFA has required wording for these statements. This must be explained at every step of the marketing, sales, eligibility determination, and enrollment process, as well as at intake. Since the start of the Medicare program in the mid-1960s, beneficiaries have been accustomed to go-anywhere Medicare. Frequent, clear communication about how managed care limits choice cannot be overdone. Table 6.12 summarizes the key points that beneficiaries must understand. They need to read the materials provided by the plan and approved by Medicare that explain the lock-in provisions with regard to both enrollment and choice of hospital or physician. They need to authorize disclosure of information. They need to attest that they understand they can only be enrolled in one plan at a time.

These required enrollment forms must be processed during an appropriate election period, which is summarized in Table 6.13. Each new beneficiary to the Medicare program may elect Medicare managed care three months before initial eligibility or the first month of eligibility, whatever month of the year that may be (*Initial*). In addition, Medicare+Choice plans

TABLE 6.12
Key Points New
Enrollees
Should
Understand at
Enrollment,
2000

*Understanding
is the key: New
enrollees have
responsibilities
and rights they
need to
understand*

1. Agrees to abide by the membership rules of the managed care plan as outlined in material provided to the member, including the lock-in provisions

2. Authorizes the disclosure and exchange of necessary information with HCFA

3. Understands that enrollment in the managed care plan automatically disenrolls the beneficiary from any other managed care

4. Understands that enrollment in more than one plan with the same effective date will cancel all the attempted enrollments

5. Knows the date to begin receiving care through the managed care plan (i.e., the effective date) and knows of the right to appeal service and payment denials made by the plan

TABLE 6.13
Election
Periods and
Effective Date
of Coverage for
Beneficiaries
Switching to
Medicare+
Choice or
Managed Care
Plans

*Four chances to
switch:
Medicare+
Choice offers
four times to
switch plans or
sectors*

Election Period	Effective Date of Coverage
Initial Coverage Election Period	First day of the month of entitlement to Medicare Part A and Part B
Open Enrollment Period	First day of the month through the 10th day of the month the health plan receives a completed enrollment form
Annual Election Period	January 1 of the following year
Special Election Period	Varies

may decide to have continuous or selective open enrollment throughout the year (*Open*). But all Medicare+Choice plans must have an annual election period (November) in which Medicare itself informs the beneficiaries about the choices, and any plan that is not already at capacity enrollment must accept all enrolling beneficiaries (*Annual*). Finally, there are times throughout the year (*Special*) that beneficiaries may elect a different plan.

There are also times when a beneficiary may return to traditional fee-for-service: when the beneficiary permanently moves, the contract with the health plan is terminated, not renewed, and other special circumstances. These elections are called voluntary and involuntary disenrollment.

*Voluntary
disenrollment is
when a beneficiary
leaves a
Medicare+Choice
plan outside an
election period and
returns to
traditional
fee-for-service
Medicare or another
health plan for a*

Voluntary disenrollment by a member of a Medicare+Choice plan is required when the beneficiary leaves the service area, loses Medicare coverage, or dies or when the contract between Medicare and the managed care plan ends. **Involuntary disenrollment** may occur and be initiated by the health plan if the beneficiary fails to pay premiums to the health plan, exhibits disruptive behavior, or is associated with fraud and abuse on the part of the beneficiary.

In summary, a common challenge facing Medicare+Choice plans is ensuring a smooth transition from the marketing and sales function to the membership function in the form of eligibility determination and enrollment. One writer (Wood 1996) estimates as many as 35 percent of new enrollees in some plans confront problems with their enrollment because of inattention to the process. To manage the process, you will want a comprehensive database to track all potential enrollees in the market, the type of mailing or contact they may have had with the plan, whether they are in the process of being enrolled, and whether they are already a member. You do not want to waste time or money communicating solicitation materials to existing members. A well-trained, attentive staff of plan representatives is also essential. Some plans have established separate toll-free help lines for Medicare beneficiaries to facilitate the intake process. Enrollment should be a part of the overall benefit design and marketing strategy.

reason. Voluntary reasons include leaving the service area, loss of Medicare coverage, death, or the plan no longer contracts with Medicare.

***Involuntary disenrollment** reasons include failure to pay health plan premiums, among others.*

Appointments and Scheduling Member Communications

Any **prior screening** of potential enrollees is not permitted and severely sanctioned by HCFA. It is not possible to use any sources of patient information regarding prior claims or self-assessment of health status to evaluate the heath or expected costs of beneficiaries before they elect a plan. However, the moment the enrollment starts, health status assessment tools can be used and can be very helpful to quickly achieve a new level of medical management that did not exist while the patient was in traditional fee-for-service Medicare. A rapid intake process that includes health risk assessment, after enrollment, gives the health plan a management opportunity as well as the chance to reinforce the communications about the new rules of managed care and answer any questions. Thus, many plans quickly contact the beneficiary and engage in a number of appointment and scheduling activities, which are summarized in Figure 6.4.

*****Prior screening** is using sources of patient information regarding prior claims including knowledge or medical records of any physician or self-assessment of health status to evaluate the health or expected costs of beneficiaries before they elect a plan. Such prior screening is strictly prohibited under Medicare+ Choice rules and severely sanctioned with civil and monetary penalties.*

Print materials prepared for new members should be prepared especially for the elderly with large print and clear instructions. Many plans prepare instructions that include tips on how best to use the managed care plan and list the physicians and hospitals to get needed care. Most designers recommend 12-point type at a minimum, large amounts of white space in the copy, nonglossy paper, and high-contrast graphics and colors.

FIGURE 6.4
Strategies for
Effective Com-
munication
with Members

*Can't do
enough:
Transition from
marketing and
sales to
appointments
and scheduling
member
communication
needs to be
seamless*

Print Materials Attuned to Older Members: Large, clear print pictures and graphics, and simple step-by-step instructions are all standard. As a marketing rule of thumb, most beneficiaries consider themselves ten years younger than they really are. Use of terms like senior citizen, elderly, and disabled must be done carefully. Older persons or older members are preferred.

Medical and Social Workup: Initial phone call at enrollment to ensure plan card has arrived and member knows where to receive care. Schedule two immediate appointments — (1) to meet with a geriatric nurse practitioner to prepare a full medical and social workup and (2) to meet with primary care physician to review treatment plan based on workup.

Brown Bag: Enrollees are asked to bring all the medications they are taking in a brown bag. Medication reviews by community pharmacists in collaboration with a nurse practitioner or primary care physician are done to derive maximum benefit of medicines, identify medication-related problems, and reduce waste and expensive medicines. In one study, 12 percent of cases had problems that could have resulted in a hospital admission. Beta-blockers, NSAIDs, and Verapamil were identified with the greatest clinical problems (Nathan et al. 1999).

Prevention Passport: Put the "Guide to Clinical Preventive Services" (DHHS 2000) recommendations for older persons into a booklet that your enrollees can keep with them. As they receive scheduled preventative services, their booklet is stamped or checked, much as a passport is stamped or checked.

Internet: The informed patient should become an integral part of any managed care plan strategy for changing fee-for-service patterns of care for new enrollees. Review all forms in your health plan and put them on the Internet. The elderly are the fastest-growing segment of the population using the Internet, and new Internet devices will enable you to manage patients at home, communicate with them, and allow them to educate themselves about their care.

Self-Care: Devise lifestyle plans for Medicare enrollees that identify barriers to change and initiate a lifestyle change. Social support, tailoring strategies, self-monitoring medication, and cue restriction have been shown to be effective (Timmerman 1999).

Sensitivity to Ethnic and Racial Differences: Experts identify several domains of concern: communication (general clarity, responsiveness to patient concerns, explanations, empowerment); decision making (responsiveness to patient preferences, consideration of ability and desire to comply); and interpersonal style (friendliness, respectfulness, avoidance of discrimination, and showing cultural sensitivity and support) (Stewart, Napoles-Springer, and Perez-Stable 1999).

Personal Service Program: Based on the idea that people would rather have a relationship with one person instead of a phone bank. Personal service representative makes call to new enrollee and serves as enrollee representative throughout membership.

Toll-Free Nurse Advice Line: Get new enrollees immediately using a 24-hour nurseline for health tips and brochures about better lifestyle.

continued

Benchmarking: Compare yourself in terms of print materials, call-center performance measures, etc. Do satisfaction surveys to compare yourself to other health plans in the same company or to other industries.

Beneficiary Advisory Committee and Workshops: Listen to your new enrollees, ongoing enrollees, and old-faithful enrollees. Understand what concerns them by having standing committees to provide advice and ideas for improvement. Conduct workshops on specific topics or health concerns and use them as focus groups to find out what your enrollees are thinking.

FIGURE 6.4
Continued

Strategic Decisions Checklist

Strategic Questions	Strategic Analyses
What dynamic process can you use to have effective benefit design?	You must have market competitive financial incentives to join Medicare managed care. You should have an ongoing strategic cycling process of: 1. mission and values validation; 2. market research and competitor analysis; 3. scenario and business strategy development; and 4. business strategy implementation and prioritization. You can still employ traditional strengths, weaknesses, opportunities, and threats as a useful adjunct.
Are you conducting market research and competitor analysis?	Begin by coordinating with other divisions in your health plan. Use *Medicare Compare* for up-to-date competitor analysis. Be able to describe your relative position in the market.

continued

Strategic Questions	Strategic Analyses
Do you conduct scenario planning as a part of business plan development?	"Color outside the lines" by creating scenarios to develop a dynamic view of the market.
	Track year-to-year relative changes in premiums, benefits, and patient satisfaction for your health plan and your competitors.
	Create contingency plans around new market entrants.
	Conduct focus groups or have an ongoing formal advisory board. Some other research is needed to gauge changes and test the message.
Do you have a conscious business strategy?	Make the stream of decisions in Medicare managed care follow a rational pattern.
	Your choices are not large and probably fall along some basic options. You need to decide among: • benefits-dominant; • costs-dominant; • follow the leader; and • location, location, location.
What is the content of your marketing materials?	Decide whether to feature low costs or high quality.
	You will need to make comparisons to traditional Medicare, but you must refine and sharpen those distinctions in your own communications.
	Brand your health plan.
Are you operating a superb enrollment and beneficiary communication effort?	You absolutely must have a comprehensive marketing database to tailor your message to the information needs of the beneficiaries.
	It is essential to have a well-trained, attentive staff of plan representatives.
	Do as much as possible on the transition from marketing and sales to appointments and scheduling member communication.

QUALITY REALLY CAN COST LESS

If you're trying to provide affordable, high-quality healthcare, you'll find plenty of advice on how to do it. Entire books address the subject. They offer an abundance of techniques for moderating the service use and costs of a health plan, and they list a range of factors that determine success (Heinen, Fox, and Anderson 1990; Gabel 1997; Gabel et al. 1997; Remler et al. 1997; Robinson 1997). Although these techniques and determinants of success are often presented as being effective on a universal scale, local situations dictate their effectiveness.

This chapter doesn't pretend to be a cookbook of successful techniques for balancing quality and cost in a managed care plan. Instead, this chapter details the quality and cost issues that are particular to Medicare, and it describes strategies that contribute to the success of a managed care plan.

With this limited goal, Chapter 7 offers an overarching organizational and management framework with an economist's view of quality and costs. At the heart of this view is the need to understand a fundamental management concept: **transaction costs**. Chapter 7 explores the cost of transactions within organizations and markets.

Transaction costs are the costs to someone in the economic system of performing an economic exchange, or the benefits given up when an efficiency-enhancing exchange is not performed.

Throughout recorded history, human interactions have assumed the form of transactions, and these transactions occur so that those involved can meet economic objectives. Transactions have their own set of costs, which the well-run managed care plan will want to minimize. They also involve prices, which can be used by the managed care plan internally and externally for coordination and motivation. For example, it costs a health plan a great deal of money to conduct utilization review. However, this review, costly though it may be, can save other transaction costs by reducing unneeded services. Here is another example. There is a cost reduction associated with having a physician serve as a primary care case manager to regulate referrals, yet the managed care company must compensate someone for this activity. In short, higher transaction costs in one area of a health plan mean lower costs in another.

The concept of transaction cost explains why managed care exists today. The transaction costs of unbridled fee-for-service became excessive and dissociated from the perceived satisfaction those services provided. Managed care represented a way to dramatically reform transactions costs in healthcare. The excess supply of physicians and the declining cost of obtaining and using information to make coverage decisions fueled the growth of managed care.

Viewed in this way, managed care companies that can simultaneously address the issues of quality and cost have enormous potential as they enter a Medicare market still dominated by a fee-for-service orientation. If these companies can leverage information technology and bring out best practices among the clinicians in their networks, they will wrest much lower transaction costs from the system, offer better quality at lower premiums than their rivals, attract enrollment, and succeed in the market. In short, quality really can cost less.

In an effort to lower overall costs and improve quality, well-run managed care plans must take a series of actions. First, they have to build a managed care process and culture. This includes promoting physician leadership, constructing teams of self-directed clinicians, and advancing learning and education programs to foster professionalism in the clinical team. Second, these plans should operate according to evidence-based quality assurance, which rests on good management information systems and squarely addresses compliance with fraud and abuse regulations. Perhaps the most important thing a managed care plan should do is put in place effective physician incentive systems with good strategic partners.

The bulk of the chapter is devoted to these three actions: building culture, establishing evidence-based quality assurance, and implementing a physician incentive system. But before reviewing these issues with you, the next section sets the stage by discussing some basic organizational management issues regarding the economics of transaction costs. Because none of the three actions will transpire without the resources that come from a fiscally sound budget, this topic is covered at the end of the chapter along with three other timely and controversial issues: utilization review, drug benefits, and the contribution of prevention and wellness programs.

Economic Organization and Management Issues

Managed care plans, physician groups, hospitals, and indeed Medicare—all the actors in the Medicare market—are economic organizations. Economic organizations are created by human beings for interacting as they work toward individual and collective goals (Milgrom and Roberts 1992). During these interactions, people exchange goods and services. If there are no interactions, there are no economic organizations.

With Medicare, interactions work in the following manner. The public pays taxes and the beneficiaries pay premiums to the Medicare program. The Medicare program then exchanges Medicare+Choice payments for health benefits coverage. The beneficiary exchanges premiums for supplemental health benefits coverage. The managed care plan exchanges revenues either internally with clinical employees in the case of integrated health plans or externally with clinical suppliers of physician, hospital, or other services. One person's expenditure is another person's revenue. All these expenditures and revenues require coordination. The coordination is geared toward meeting the common goal that quality and cost are acceptable to beneficiaries.

Necessary coordination in these economic organizations is normally accomplished with a nexus of contracts, which are legally enforceable agreements involving a quid pro quo—this for that. When this type of trade is involved, "this" and "that" must be carefully defined or at least well understood. Alternatively, the parties to the transactions trust each other to conduct the transaction honestly and to meet the terms of the agreement.

Thus, Medicare needs to know what it is purchasing in the form of health services and what quality it can expect from its contracting managed care plans. Beneficiaries must be reassured that their premium payments will provide the kinds of services they want or need. Managed care plans need to know they will be paid a fair price and what amount and quality of care they can expect from their suppliers of clinical services. Physicians, hospitals, and other clinicians affiliated with the managed care plan have to know what prices they will be paid and how, in turn, they will pay their suppliers. The smooth flow of information and communication promotes effective transactions that run according to plan so that all parties are satisfied.

Two organizational methods can help you coordinate transactions better among parties. The first is command and control, and the second is markets and prices. There are many variations between these two extremes. Your health plan must decide what type of organizational culture to adopt and how to organize your plan so that you conduct transactions sensibly.

The **command and control** approach works well when transactions are highly predictable and uniform. When standard rules and procedures apply to achieve standard results, command and control produces results. There is a central authority with a well-defined communication hierarchy throughout the health plan. Divisions within the health plan make logical sense for what must be accomplished and the same approaches work in most or all situations. When this occurs, command and control can accomplish goals. This approach might work well, for example, in the claims-processing function in which hundreds of thousands of individual payments to physicians and hospitals must be processed quickly and accurately across the country for a multistate company. Or it might work best for marketing your plan in order to meet strict expectations from HCFA for legal and appropriate contact with beneficiaries.

Command and control refers to a way of organizing economic transactions that relies on hierarchy and rules to give directions to participants.

The **markets and prices** approach to organizing transactions, on the other hand, is more useful in uncertain situations, especially those when coordination and internal processes of the organization are complex and unpredictable. The ways of doing things in one market served by the health plan may not work in any other market. A central authority, if it exists, doesn't have the specific knowledge or information required to devise solutions that meet a particular need in the health plan. In this case, more of a pay-for-performance approach is needed for coordination. For example, instead of rigorous and burdensome utilization management, a health plan might set out quality and cost-performance goals for affiliated specialists and annually

Markets and prices refers to a way of organizing economic transactions that relies on autonomy and freedom to give directions to participants.

review continued participation with the plan. These are strong and powerful motivators that rely on the market and prices for achieving goals.

Normally, performance measurements are laid out to external suppliers, physicians, and hospitals, and prices are established to pay when the performance is achieved. Markets and prices can exist for internal suppliers as well. In this case, health plans establish performance expectations for internal divisions of the health plan and identify expected outcomes. If expectations are met, the plan offers bonuses or budgets. On the other hand, if expectations go unmet, the division could be eliminated and work could be sent to an outside supplier.

Stock ownership for external or internal suppliers can be a particularly strong market incentive to urge all parties to work together for the maximum benefit of the health plan. Failure to reach health plan goals in terms of enrollment, quality, or cost carry a heavy price through falling share value when stock ownership is involved.

One reason investor-owned managed care plans dominate the Medicare+Choice market to date is that the requirements of caring for the elderly are more complex than any other type of care, and the approaches must be tailored to the situation in each local market. The science of managed care for the elderly is not standardized by any means. Thus, a market and prices approach—in the extreme represented by the stock-ownership organization—may be best suited to Medicare managed care at this time. Medicare is risky business. Although the rewards for successfully competing against traditional fee-for-service can be great, there also a tremendous financial price to pay for those unable to succeed.

Whether organized in a command and control framework or a markets and prices framework, the organizational form must grapple with transaction costs. Transaction costs take two forms: coordination costs and motivation costs.

A managed care plan cannot account for all contingencies. For example, suppose two hospitals suddenly merge, a new managed care plan enters the market, or Medicare revises its regulations. These actions have an aftereffect on your plans, and solutions can be costly. Communicating the needed changes or protections against contingencies usually cost something. These are the **coordination costs** of running a managed care plan.

At the same time, a managed care plan cannot have all the relevant information needed to carry out a potential or actual transaction. For example, the quality of care provided by a hospital or physician is normally not well known. The track record of shirking duties or of dishonesty may not be known for employees. These transaction costs include the fairness of the transaction on both sides and whether the terms are being met as a contract moves forward. These are the **motivation costs** of running a managed care plan. Commitment to complete the terms of a transaction can wane as time goes on, and it's sometimes necessary to police against deception. These policing functions cost something.

Coordination costs result from the need to overcome the bounds to rational action. Not all contingencies can be known in setting prices for transactions, identifying the buyers and sellers, and communicating and negotiating the arrangements.

Motivation costs result from the need to install safeguards against opportunistic behavior. People do not always behave with esteem or confidence and may even renege on a contract.

Prices coordinate and motivate the participants in a managed care plan. When applied to *external* suppliers, they can take the form of withholds, bonuses, risk-sharing arrangements, payments for performance—all economic in nature. But even *internal* to an organization, price is an issue. These so-called **transfer prices** coordinate activity and motivate performance by offering a common currency for rewarding favorable results inside the organization. Internal bookkeeping systems allow one division of an organization to negotiate and pay for the performance of another division. For example, if the enrollment department successfully retains 98 percent of the new enrollees recruited by the marketing department, both departments get a bonus. Such approaches for organizing can surmount transaction costs—bungled communication, noncooperative behavior, shirking—within a managed care plan. Lowering transaction costs allows a health plan to improve quality and lower costs at the same time because doing so frees up the resources needed to provide the desired healthcare efficiently. Given that 80 percent of transactions for services covered by Medicare involve a physician, one logical place to start in lowering transaction costs is the practice of medicine.

Transfer prices are internal organizational mechanisms for budgets or bookkeeping to negotiate and reward divisions for desired results.

The Medical Group and Self-Directed Groups

The dominant form of medical practice in the United States is the medical group. A medical group is four or more physicians sharing practice expenses, income, or both. There are around 20,000 medical groups in the United States today with an average size of 10.4 physicians (Havlicek 1999). Approximately 206,557, or almost half of physicians in 1996 were in groups, and this figure has been growing for many years (Havlicek 1999).

As a collection of professionals with common interest, the medical group offers great potential to improve care. Early studies found little evidence for economies of scale—that is, the group is more efficient or lower cost as it gets larger (Reinhardt 1979). Economies of scope may be more likely—that is, the group is more efficient or lowers costs as it adds more specialties (Pauly et al. 1992). He posits that interaction among the professionals in the provision of services should lead to efficiencies. There is a learning-by-doing effect and fewer transaction costs to practicing together. Patients can be handed off to another specialist physician more easily in a group when patients need to be referred for different types of care.

However, Pauly finds the economies of scale seem to be exhausted in the range of six to ten physicians. The cost benefits of a larger group is offset by difficulties of coordinating complex activities of physicians in moderately sized multispecialty groups. The threshold is around ten physicians. Conrad and colleagues (1996) suggest the multispecialty group and the physician group owned by a hospital are natural responses to market demands for risk-bearing contracts. This type of vertical or horizontal combination is done to reduce the coordination costs of operating under all-inclusive contracts that pay one flat rate for all covered services provided by the group.

In addition to the growth of medical groups, another trend is for physicians to be employed rather than to operate as independent solo practitioners (Kletke, Emmons, and Gillis 1996). The number of employed physicians has risen from 24 percent in 1983 to 42 percent in 1994, as the percent of self-employed solo practitioners has fallen from 41 percent to 29 percent (Kletke, Emmons, and Gillis 1996). Employed physicians work fewer hours and earn lower incomes than do self-employed physicians. The primary employers of physicians are medical groups (34 percent), medical schools or universities (20 percent), hospitals (16 percent), and staff-model HMOs (10 percent) (Kletke, Emmons, and Gillis 1996). Markets and prices are probably needed to maintain or boost productivity with significant portions of the profession in group practice.

Short of being employed by them, physicians may have certain integrated arrangements with hospitals. Sometimes they share revenues, expenses, or both. Physician-hospital organizations, in which another entity represents the hospital and some or all of its physicians in negotiations with managed care companies, represent one integrative arrangement. Management services organizations do the same and carry out physician practice management functions such as billing. Burns and colleagues (1998) found little evidence that these integrating arrangements had an effect, but it may be too early to measure whether the process of integration affects quality or costs. Arrangements between hospitals and physicians have focused primarily on managed care contracting. Once the contract is won, little is really done to alter the basic relationships between hospitals and physicians.

Burns and colleagues suggest that to improve performance, managed care plans should integrate eight *processes* rather than eight *structures*. These processes include:

1. economic integration (salary and ownership);
2. economic integration (networks and joint ventures);
3. administrative integration (physicians in governance and management);
4. management services provided to physicians;
5. sharing of cost information;
6. information system integration;
7. product line integration; and
8. clinical guideline utilization.

Transaction costs can be lowered as your health plan moves up the list of eight integrative processes. Each one may not have the same effect on transaction costs, and each may have different effects in different circumstances. They are listed in order of most integrative and highest impact to least integrative and lowest impact.

Medicare managed care plans with their own internal integrated physician-hospital relationships, or external contracts with more integrated organizations, should be able to gain better control over quality and cost with some or all these features. Few local hospital systems with multiple hospitals and various arrangements with physicians have achieved the full list of eight processes identified by Burns and colleagues. This may account for the lack of involvement from integrated delivery systems in the Medicare+Choice PSOs discussed in Chapter 1.

In economics, the notion of group production implies contributions to a complex, joint product from several members of a group. Such production means it is difficult to attribute contributions to one individual. Hard to define and measure, this sort of group contribution leads to one of the main sources of opportunistic transaction costs—shirking. **Shirking** can be overcome if each member of the group receives a residual payment proportional to that individual's contribution. There might even be a set of property rights associated with the group that would reward members for joint success of the relationship. However, measurement of the residual and establishment of the property rights is rarely found in practice.

Shirking is wasting time, loafing, evading.

Figure 7.1 shows a highly idealistic, but potentially logical, extension of the integration of physicians, hospitals, and other health professionals representing the self-directed group. The first representation is the multidisciplinary. Each member (represented by the arrows) interacts with the group (represented by the circle) yet maintains its own interest. With a multidisciplinary group, transactions occur but with no common direction or result. The second representation is the interdisciplinary. Each member of the group joins with different interests and emerges from the group transaction with a new interest, generally in the same direction, but still separate and distinct. The third representation is the transdisciplinary. Each member comes to the

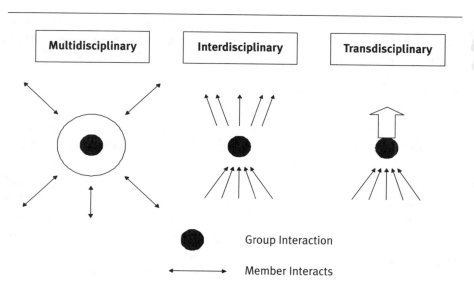

FIGURE 7.1

Three Ideal Types of Group Involvement

Wish upon a star: Achieving the self-directed group may hold the promise of lower transaction costs

group with different interests and emerges undifferentiated with a common direction or result. Quality and costs should improve as your health plan moves from multidisciplinary to interdisciplinary and transdisciplinary interactions.

Most transactions within medical groups and among medical groups and hospitals or health plans are multidisciplinary. The advanced transactions, the most integrative type identified by Burns and colleagues, are interdisciplinary. The third type is probably nonexistent. Identifying the types of relationships in your health plan or medical group may help you reduce transaction costs. There are a variety of ways to achieve disciplinary relations: adopting clinical guidelines, integrating product lines, improving information systems, sharing cost information, creating a management services organization, putting physicians in governance and management, pursuing joint ventures, and managing salary and ownership.

Building a Managed Care Process and Culture

Group culture is an imprecise term, but it's a helpful concept for assessing the mission, vision, and values of an organization. Organizations often have mission statements hanging on the wall or printed in annual reports. More often than not, however, they do not represent the real mission. Organizational culture represents the customary way things are done, the values the members of the organization exhibit, and what must be learned by new members of the organization (Duncan et al. 1992). Some pundits say organizational culture is difficult to manage. They believe it is not real because the bottom line can be influenced in more concrete ways by deploying resources and making strategic decisions. This attitude is rejected here based on years of visiting Medicare managed care plans and immediately knowing the culture after only two days on a quick visit.

For a self-directed medical group, an integrated hospital system, or a Medicare+Choice plan, a managed care culture is real and unmistakable. There are three ways you can accomplish a managed care process and culture: learning, sharing, and externalizing (Duncan et al. 1992).

Managed Care Culture Is Learned

You create the managed care culture for your organization by what employees or clinicians new to the organization learn. New employees or affiliated clinicians should learn about the principles of managed care. They should be able to define it with ease and experience it firsthand. In a good managed care plan, the notion that patients must select from among a network of affiliated providers should be value proposition because the plan selects the best possible physicians and hospitals to be available to patients. Financial incentives for enrollees in the plan should be designed, enforced, and supported as a way to encourage personal responsibility for one's healthcare. Quality assurance and utilization review systems should be continuously improved and appreciated by the people who use them. The leadership should set the tone for supporting the essential aspects of managed care and point out the history of useful processes and how they have been updated. In this connection, the employees or clinicians affiliated with the organization should also learn about care for the elderly and their special needs.

Managed Care Culture Is Shared

To share organizational culture is to have the opportunity to voice your understanding and meaning of the way things work in the organization. More than a suggestion box, sharing can be accomplished by separate meetings in which strategic vision and mission are discussed and where people have a chance to say what they think. This sharing of vision should drive your organization. Even with locations in different parts of a market or the country, an organization can create opportunities to share. Medicare managed care organizations need ample opportunity to discuss what it means to serve an older population of enrollees and how to focus its vision on meeting their needs. Granted, this input may not always affect decisions but it certainly won't result in any changes if it never reaches the discussion stage.

Managed Care Culture Is Externalized

The learning and sharing of the process of managed care and culture should naturally lead to a witnessing outside the organization. Successes should be identified, recognized, and publicized. Clinical heroes or administrative heroes should be acknowledged through ceremonies and rituals. Even Medicare enrollees with success stories to tell need to be identified and publicized to others. Externalizing the culture will provide useful internal reinforcement.

Physician Control of the Process

Under the law, physicians are the sole professional group entrusted with diagnosing disease and prescribing medicine. Unless the law changes, physicians must now play a major role in controlling the process of managed care. At present, they can play three broad leadership roles. In the first, physicians can serve on the board of directors in a controlling manner or on powerful advisory groups to the health plan. In the second, they can serve as medical director. In the third, they can serve as team leader in the clinical site of care.

The physician leadership role in the structure of the health plan can be important in establishing the culture of the organization. If the quality of patient care is important, clinicians, not administrators, will be involved in all the major decisions. A physician as the chairman of the board or a physician majority ownership sends a message internally and externally.

A stereotype of the medical director is that of a "Dr. No" who denies care to patients he has never even seen (Bodenheimer and Casalino 1999). But good medical directors also take control of the quality improvement apparatus of the health plan and induce changes that improve care to patients. Day-to-day duties include reviewing individual medical charts and determining medical necessity, which can take between 50 percent and 60 percent of a medical director's time. This is complemented by time spent reviewing patient appeals and grievances, reviewing literature, consulting with outside experts, tracking trends in hospital days per thousand, and measuring other kinds of service use. Medical directors also make policy decisions about treatment protocols, such as which medical treatment guidelines to use and whether certain specialty types can perform particular procedures for the patients in the health plan. Other important functions of medical directors include participating in the budgeting process, creating and maintaining the physician network, profiling physicians, determining how physicians are to be paid, and serving on advisory groups for patient and payer groups.

To achieve the interdisciplinary or transdisciplinary group, you need a leader from within the clinical team. Physicians can play an important role in disease management, demand management, policy setting and implementation for wellness and prevention programs, and as a member of an interdisciplinary team. They may need to be reimbursed for their time away from patients. But their role as facilitator and source of authoritative information plays a vital role.

Commitment to Education

Lowering transaction costs, taking the medical group to the next level as an interdisciplinary or even transdisciplinary entity, infusing the organization with a managed care culture, and empowering the professions, especially physicians—achieving all this means creating change. Change only occurs when people learn to do things differently. If you want everyone in your organization to make yours a well-managed health plan, you need to make a commitment to educating the medical groups affiliated with your plan.

The goals of a well-run Medicare managed care plan are to minimize transaction costs to deliver high-quality patient care that produces favorable outcomes and avoids the use of expensive settings such as inpatient hospital services, emergency room, and unnecessary treatments.

The goals of a well-run Medicare managed plan should be to minimize transaction costs in the course of delivering high-quality care. Such care produces favorable outcomes and avoids unnecessary treatments and the use of expensive settings, such as inpatient hospital services and the emergency room. To achieve these goals, managed care plans should use internal and external markets and prices. Rather than contract with vendors of computerized utilization review and prior authorization systems or build them internal to the health plan, managed care plans should adopt the right incentives and delegate authority. Vest existing affiliated professionals with the responsibility to improve health outcomes, and lower costs should follow.

To offer this type of incentive and delegate professional authority requires education. Education is key to your success. Employees and affiliated physicians and hospitals need to learn new rules and meet new expectations. They need to be educated about the tools and guidelines that allow them to provide better care. As a Medicare managed care plan, you need to invest in an education division or purchase top-flight educational interventions for your clinical network.

To be successful, however, the education program for a managed care plan must do the following.

- Encourage professionals to accept the effort by making sure leaders in the health plan and the community being served are involved in the effort.
- Invest in professional skills development so that health plans are seen as partners with an interest in providing high-quality care to Medicare patients.
- Use Medicare databases to study and identify the problem areas for high-priority efforts.
- Adopt targeted clinical intervention strategies that can be tracked through time for their effect on health outcomes.

An integral part of the educational program is the use of real patient-level data with full protection of confidentiality. Physicians and others who see patients all day long every day are more likely to understand and appreciate problem-based learning that uses their own patients as illustrations. Talking heads or Internet-based packaged programs will not work. The training also needs to emphasize the unique needs of older enrollees in terms of the complex set of diseases they may have and their special communication needs. These special needs are discussed more fully in Chapter 8—Disease Management—and Chapter 10—Demand Management.

Structure of Quality Assurance

Enrollees in Medicare managed care plans expect high-quality healthcare. If this isn't a good enough reason for you to have a sound structure for quality assurance, then here is another. Federal regulations require an ongoing quality assurance program for all Medicare+Choice plans as authorized by Section 1301 (C) (7) of the Public Health Service Act, at 42 CFR 422.152. The strategy for any Medicare managed care plan is straightforward. Have a good **total quality management** (TQM) program following Medicare guidelines for quality assessment and performance **continuous improvement**.

TQM has been critiqued by some (Senge 1990; Tompkins 1995; Deevy 1995) because of notable failures in other industries. The failures probably stem from implementation, not the concept of TQM. W. Edwards Deming, Armand V. Feigenbaum, Kaoru Ishikawa, and J. M. Juran are among the leaders in the field.

With TQM, the aim is to create an attitude at all levels of the organization that encourages people to reach new performance levels by improving relationships with employees and suppliers alike. Deevy (1995) stated that three core conditions for TQM need to be in place. First, each person in the

Total quality management (TQM) is a management approach to achieving long-term results through continuous customer satisfaction.

Continuous improvement is the ongoing betterment of services or processes through incrementalism and new breakthroughs.

organization is allowed to know what is going on. An open-book management style gives everyone who can affect performance access to the business data of the organization. This openness fosters communication and trust. Second, the organization must be completely customer-oriented. In Medicare managed care terminology that means **patient-focused**. Everyone in the organization must be patient-focused, not just some people with that function or certain specialists. Emphasizing simplification and encouraging better processes are essential to being patient-focused. Ideally, every contact with a patient should be the best it can be with no mistakes. Making that happen is being patient-focused. Third, people should be motivated by being given a stake in the outcome. Incentives and compensation should be tied to the business strategy for the people who have control over the business strategy. A strategy of quality and costs that relies on markets and prices will be more successful than other approaches.

Patient-focused means delivering services with complete attention to exceeding patient expectations.

Table 7.1 offers a quick reference for applying the TQM model to the structure of quality assurance in your health plan. It begins on the right with the objective of TQM. Reflecting the customer or patient focus of the program and Medicare's objectives as one of the customers, the overriding objective should be to have a beneficial effect on health outcomes and enrollee satisfaction. Naturally, this should foster enrollment and help you retain new members, both of which offer the promise of financial success. Enrollment growth and financial strength are secondary objectives; however, that should flow from meeting the primary objective: listening to and caring for patients.

To support this primary objective, the guiding philosophy is continuous quality improvement. Either by leapfrogging current methods or by doing things in an incremental fashion, the goal is to do things better. If you can adopt this philosophy, you should have no trouble meeting the Quality Improvement Standards for Managed Care (**QISMC**) promulgated by HCFA (http://www.hcfa.gov/quality/3a.htm). The elements of a structured system are shown in Table 7.1:

QISMC project is an intervention or initiative to assess performance in one or more focused areas.

- management commitment;
- total participation;
- internal and external customers;
- internal and external suppliers; and
- systematic analysis.

Here's a description of what each element means:

Management commitment is perhaps the most essential to continuous improvement. If there is management commitment and involvement, not just lip service, the rest of the elements follow. HCFA also enforces this element of TQM by requiring that each plan have a clearly identified individual or organization component responsible for quality. There also should be clear participation by a policymaking body to oversee quality. Most boards of directors of a health plan would receive a report on the financial status of

Objective	Philosophy	System Elements	Element Description
Beneficial Effect on Health Outcomes and Enrollee Satisfaction	Continuous Quality Improvement Meet Standards and Goals	Management Commitment	• Clearly identified individuals or organizational components responsible • Policymaking body oversees • Designated senior official • Annual formal evaluation
		Total participation	• Health-plan-wide involvement • Internal surveillance • Complaints • Clinical and nonclinical services
		Internal/External Customer	• Meet QISMIC standards • Show demonstrable improvement • Involve enrollees in selection of topics and goals
		Internal/External Suppliers	• Conducts performance improvement projects • Acute conditions • Chronic conditions • High-volume services • High-risk services • Continuity and coordination of care • Monitor physician incentive plans
		Systematic Analysis	• Standard methods (e.g., HEDIS, FACCT, CAHPS) • Continuous data collection • Include change in health status or functional status or proxy • External benchmarks • Approved sampling methods

TABLE 7.1

Framework and Elements of TQM

First things first: The TQM framework can help meet the elements of the quality improvement system for managed care

the health plan. They should also receive a similarly valued report on the quality status of the health plan. The buck has to stop somewhere, so you should designate a senior official in your health plan to assume responsibility for taking corrective action when errors occur. The quality assessment and improvement program itself should be evaluated annually. That can be done by an external evaluator or through a formal committee or team internally with a checklist of items to review. The QISMC provides just such a checklist.

Total participation in the context of continuous improvement is important, and your efforts should involve every employee and every physician and hospital in the health plan. Quality should not be something that another group does within the health plan. Everyone needs to be involved, as demonstrated by HCFA's requirement for health-plan-wide involvement. Internal surveillance systems to identify and track errors or complaints should be in place. Both clinical and nonclinical areas should be addressed. For instance, the time it takes to answer questions from a beneficiary could be a measure of quality, though one unrelated to the clinical quality of care. HCFA expects you to meet standard measures established by the agency each year and go beyond these as much as possible into all aspects of your health plan.

Internal/external customers, in the parlance of TQM, refer to the employees of the health plan and the network of affiliated physicians and hospitals in Medicare managed care. The primary external customer is HCFA, which expects Medicare managed care plans to meet the QISMC. For these standards a Medicare+Choice plan is expected to do the following.

- Carry out individual QISMC projects to undertake system interventions to improve care.
- Monitor the effectiveness of those interventions.
- Continuously monitor its own performance on a variety of dimensions of care and services for enrollees.
- Identify its own areas for potential improvement.
- Take timely action to correct significant systematic problems that come to its attention through internal surveillance, complaints, or other mechanisms.

Your health plan is expected to demonstrate improvements and involve your enrollees in selection of topics and goals. A member advisory committee is an ideal mechanism for getting input from enrollees and reflects the patient focus that should be the mark of TQM.

Internal and external suppliers are the physicians and hospitals in your managed care network. These must be involved in a way that shows **demonstrable improvement**, which is a minimum level set by HCFA in a focused area. These areas, which are shown in Table 7.1, include acute conditions, chronic conditions, high-volume services, high-risk services, continuity and coordination of care, and anything that monitors physician incentive plans you may have in place.

Demonstrable improvement is a quality assessment measure that meets or exceeds the minimums expected from HCFA each year.

Systematic analysis is the final element of TQM. With this, you should use established methods for the continuous collection of data. For example, HCFA currently recommends certain standard methods available at these Internet sites: www.ncqa.org, www.facct.org, and for the CAHPS, www.ahcrq.gov. You can use these standards to collect information for analyzing the bad, the good, and the best. Your analysis should involve minimizing variation in processes. HCFA also expects you to track functional outcomes among your beneficiaries and benchmark your analysis against external sources of the same data or other health plans. HCFA will want to approve your sampling methods as well. Keep in mind that samples are perfectly acceptable, if not recommended, techniques for TQM and should be used to maximum advantage to lower the resource costs of collecting and analyzing data.

Types of Managed Care Information

In perhaps his best-known aphorism, W. E. Deming said: "If you can't measure it, you can't manage it." All the structure and standards for total quality improvement in the world will not work without reliable, relevant data and analysis to bring forward information that can be used for managing care. Regrettably, most managed care plans, even in this information age, remain tethered to legacy systems designed to pay claims. Figure 7.2 illustrates the types of files often available for total quality improvement. Legacy systems are existing, older systems for information processing. Claims-based data have records on eligible enrollees in the health plan so that everyone with access to the data knows at any point whether an individual is enrolled. The largest files are for claims of all types. Another coordinating file contains information on the physicians and hospitals associated with the health plan. Figure 7.2 is an oversimplification, but it illustrates the basic file structure for a traditional claims file.

Claims-based data can be converted to a more useful format, as illustrated in Figure 7.3. Sorting through the claims types allows the creation of a claims-based definition of a patient with a disease (see Chapter 8). International Classification of Diseases codes and diagnosis related group codes can

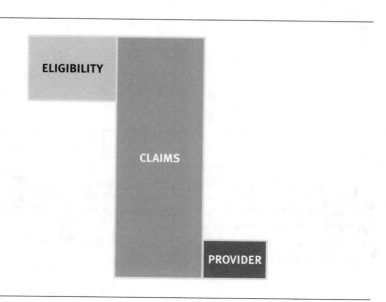

FIGURE 7.2

Basic Structure of Traditional Claims Files

The legacy of the past: Transaction-based systems are only good for one thing—paying claims

FIGURE 7.3

Claims by Type Converted to Profile of Service Use and Costs by Disease to Create Managed Care Information

The power of information technology: Disease-structured database from claims files

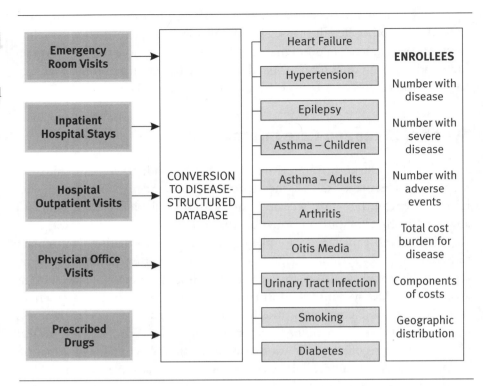

be used to create the disease-structured relational database. You must select a period of time the definition of a disease will apply and the period of time claims will be tracked (normally one year) to create the definition. The beauty of the disease-structured database is that you can track the number of enrollees with a disease, with severe disease (based on the pattern of claims), and with adverse events. Then, you can measure the total costs burden for the disease by major component of costs. The geographic distribution of the enrollees with a disease can be obtained. The best disease-structured databases allow you to associate patients with diseases to the physicians and hospitals treating those patients. As a result, you have a benchmark for comparing one clinician with another. You can use this sort of profiling to generate gentle suggestions for improving feedback on the patterns of care a provider generates. You can also use it to eliminate a provider from your network who is performing poorly and then reassign that patient to a better provider.

Both of these information systems for managed care spring from the head of the fee-for-service sector. The ideal system for the future of fully integrated health plans receiving capitation payments is one that is Internet based and that collects patient outcomes over time and space (Fig. 7.4). Systems are evolving toward this approach. Nevertheless, the transition from the legacy fee-for-service systems is complex. It is difficult to maintain the old claims system and implement new outcomes monitoring systems, especially

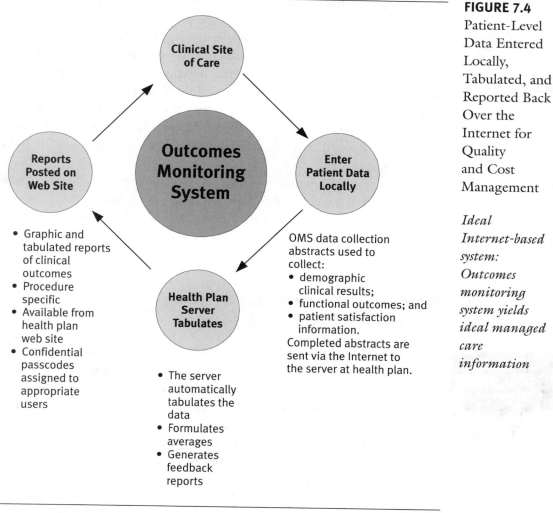

FIGURE 7.4

Patient-Level Data Entered Locally, Tabulated, and Reported Back Over the Internet for Quality and Cost Management

Ideal Internet-based system: Outcomes monitoring system yields ideal managed care information

if the network of physicians and hospitals continues to operate in a mixed capitation and fee-for-service environment.

The ideal system assumes that no physician or hospital is paid on a fee-for-service basis. Rather, clinicians and suppliers are paid on a performance basis that rewards physicians and hospitals that improve treatment for patients, health outcomes, and patient satisfaction.

The ideal system connects diverse and geographically dispersed clinical sites of care. Either data abstraction from paper medical records, scanning devices, or electronic medical records provide information at the local site of care on demographics, the clinical results of care, the patient's functional outcomes, and patient satisfaction. This information is sent over the Internet to the health plan server, which automatically tabulates the data and generates feedback reports. These reports can take many forms, including profiles of patients or providers, benchmarks of one provider versus all providers, and summaries of health outcomes. These are all posted on the health plan web site for the appropriate people to access. These people can then use the findings to support their decisions regarding improvement. The type of feedback reports, by disease or procedure, are illustrated in Chapter 8 on Disease Management.

When this type of information on outcomes monitoring is disseminated along with recognized medical treatment guidelines, clinicians that see patients everyday will respond as a team to improve the care. If the feedback reports are developed with the buy-in of clinicians and used as gentle reminders to look out for opportunities for improvement, they can be a powerful tool for quality improvement.

This type of Internet system is not without cost, but the cost is falling rapidly as Internet technology expands it reach. The great functionality of the system exceeds any costs. But the question is clear. Can plans afford not to move toward this type of system if they are serious about managing quality and cost?

Management Information Systems and Medical Informatics

Medical informatics is the science that studies the use and processing of data, information, and knowledge in medicine.

Management information systems and **medical informatics** are moving to the Internet (Table 7.2). Medicare managed care plans must prepare and invest for the new age of connectivity between enrolled beneficiaries and their network of physicians and hospitals. The Physician Internet Campaign lists seven ways that the Internet can benefit physicians.

First, physicians can increase their productivity by saving time on paperwork, communications, and journal reading using the Internet. The Internet provides easy access to clinical guidelines and disease management protocols, and it also allows convenient e-mail with colleagues. Managed care companies can ease their communication with physicians by providing online access to referrals, formularies, coverage policies, and claim status in a secure environment

TABLE 7.2

List of Topics in Informatics

Overload: There is an explosion of topics in management information systems and informatics

Information and Communication
Data Processing
Database Management
Telecommunication, Networking, and Integration
Coding and Classification
The Patient Record
Strategies for Medical Knowledge Acquisition
Predictive Tools for Clinical Decision Support
Structuring the Computer-Based Patient Record
Human–Computer Interaction in Healthcare
Costs and Benefits of Information Systems
Security in Medical Information Systems

on the Internet. Busy staff time can be reduced by shifting patient education to resources on the Internet. Giving patients information sheets that point them to relevant Web pages for their medical condition can improve patient education and reduce phone calls to staff with questions. But experience also has shown that this information can lead to increased frequency of questions by enrollees for their physician, and many physicians are frustrated by the time these more informed beneficiaries are taking. To the extent office staff use the Internet, which may be the main source of hits from the physician office, it might increase office staff productivity if they can reduce holds on the phone. Many vendors are giving discounts or free shipping for ordering supplies on-line. Finally, a number of organizations and universities now offer continuing medical education over the Internet, which can reduce travel time and costs.

There are a large number of emerging topics for managed care plans to become involved in now and in the future. You must assess your readiness to change and decide if it makes sense for your health plan to become involved in leading or following in these areas. You will want to invest heavily in data processing and database management, which are the core functions of a managed care plan. But telecommunications, networking, and integration in most markets do not makes sense if your network of physicians and providers has multiple loyalties.

Physicians have not yet embraced coding, classification, and electronic medical recordkeeping. One recent study found that computer experience, computer anxiety, and perceptions of organizational support predict the degree to which physicians and other clinicians embrace electronic medical recordkeeping. The systems are also enormously expensive at this time (Dansky et al. 1999). These authors suggest a checklist of usefulness for determining whether computerization might improve quality of medical care (Table 7.3). Any new computerization should contribute to work productivity and have a payback on the investment. It should save time somewhere in the organization. If it helps in the delivery of patient care and improves the quality of care in clinical settings, then it's worthwhile. It should be rewarding, if not fun. Sometimes technical or administrative systems can be deadly serious. There should be a concerted effort to make them attractive to visit. Humorous art or graphics, contests, and exciting information help. As an integral part of the TQM effort, information systems are a vital strategic tool for your health plan.

Compliance with Fraud and Abuse Regulations

A total quality improvement effort should encompass the total acquiescence of your health plan to the federal regulations that govern managed care plans. Table 7.4 summarizes these regulations. Too often, a cavalier attitude toward reimbursement creeps into day-to-day activities in Medicare traditional fee-for-service and managed care plans. It's crucial that you avoid an organizational culture that, under the banner of reimbursement maximization, thinks

TABLE 7.3

Items in Perceived Usefulness Scale

Does it click? Checklist for the usefulness of computerization

Will Computerization . . .
- √ contribute to work productivity?
- √ be worth the investment?
- √ save time?
- √ assist in the delivery of patient care?
- √ be a valuable aid in clinical work?
- √ improve the quality of patient care?
- √ be rewarding?
- √ enable people to set higher performance standards?

Source: Dansky, K. H. et al. 1999. "Electronic Medical Records." *Journal of Healthcare Management* 44 (6): 440–55.

TABLE 7.4

Elements That a Medicare Managed Care Plan Should Address in a Compliance Program, 2000

Comply or die: For well-managed Medicare+ Choice plans, compliance programs are easy to run and send a message to all customers

- √ Implement written policies, procedures, and standards of conduct
- √ Designate a compliance officer and committee
- √ Conduct effective training and education
- √ Develop effective lines of communication
- √ Conduct internal monitoring and auditing
- √ Enforce standards through well-publicized guidelines
- √ Respond promptly to detected offenses and develop corrective action

it is shrewd, even tricky, to push the rules or circumvent regulations without being caught. Nationwide conferences and newsletters tout consultants and experts with the latest methods—including computer programs—for getting the most money out of Medicare. Certainly, Medicare should pay health plans, physicians, and hospitals appropriately. However, some healthcare managers who have followed overly aggressive advice have confronted multimillion dollar settlements with the Office of the Inspector General of the Department of Health and Human Services (DHHS) when tricky reimbursement maximization goes awry.

Millions of elderly and disabled Medicare beneficiaries and their families rely on resources of the Medicare program for some of the most basic personal needs of their lifetime, especially at the end of life. The taxpayers—all of us—insist that these funds be used carefully. Although managed care plans seek to maximize revenues, such efforts must be conducted within the bounds of prudent behavior. The well-managed health plan must establish a compliance program that touches almost every part of the plan operations.

DHHS's Office of the Inspector General has suggestions for establishing internal controls and monitoring to correct and prevent fraudulent activities. A compliance program is not mandatory. Nor is it the only thing you need to do in addition to meeting the conditions of participation in the contract between a Medicare+Choice organization and HCFA. But just as promotion of a wellness program can improve the care of patients and lower costs, a good compliance program can be a mechanism for improving the quality, productivity, and efficiency of your managed care plan. As with a total quality improvement program, the program begins at the top. The officers and managers of your health plan should provide ethical leadership. They must ensure that adequate systems and resources are in place to promote ethical and legal conduct. All the actions and words, including the resources devoted to compliance, indicate the seriousness you give to compliance. Superficial programs that do not involve senior management are obvious to employees, the government, and perhaps even beneficiaries. The elements in Table 7.4 should be a useful guide to establishing an effective program on compliance.

Write down the policies and procedures of your compliance program. These do not need to be created from whole cloth. Take them from consulting groups, professional associations, or other health plans and modify them to fit your needs. Appoint a compliance officer. Establish a compliance committee with broad representation, including Medicare enrollees. This committee should follow a checklist of internal monitoring and auditing functions as part of its work. This group should meet regularly and have written minutes of each meeting. The minutes do not need to be lengthy, but they should indicate the major topics discussed and any decisions made.

A compliance training program is essential for virtually all employees. Many consulting groups offer preestablished programs that can be effective and useful. If top executives fully support the compliance program, there should already be effective lines of communication. But spell out these issues in the policies and procedures. Generate credible, frequent, and broad publicity for the compliance guidelines and what you expect each employee or provider to do. Have an understanding in the lines of communication involving top management who is supposed to respond to problems and promptly deal with them.

Marketing Materials and Personnel

Marketing materials and personnel continue to be one of the most violated aspects of the Medicare managed care program. Marketing personnel and contractors are normally not accustomed to having their copy and claims regulated by the government. The rough and tumble of the marketplace in most products and services leads to a fine line between grandiose marketing claims and false and misleading claims.

As a Medicare+Choice organization, your health plan serves as the agent of the Medicare program, and inconsistent communication to beneficiaries can quickly become confusing to elderly and disabled beneficiaries. Many years ago, Medicare required approval of almost every aspect of marketing materials and election forms. This extended to almost every form of communication, including general circulation brochures, leaflets, newspapers, magazines, television, radio, billboards, Yellow Pages, Internet pages, slides and charts, and anything distributed by providers.

You do not want to be accused of distributing anything that could violate the fraud and abuse provisions. Submitting everything to the government for review will protect against this. The notion of a clear, consistent approved message should carry over to the sales force. Brokers are discouraged for Medicare+Choice organizations because experience shows that brokers are hard to control and instances of inaccurate information are common. Table 7.5 summarizes the major federal fraud and abuse provisions as of early 2000. You will want to consult your attorney or the cited sections of the Code of Federal Regulations (CFR) or the United States Code (USC) for complete provisions.

Selective Marketing and Enrollment

It is forbidden to ask medical questions before enrollment because it is assumed the questions are designed to selectively market and enroll, which is forbidden. Any Medicare beneficiary can join a Medicare+Choice plan without prior underwriting. Significant penalties exist for selective marketing. The marketing should be broad based and not targeted at places where persons healthier than average for their demographic category are likely to be found. Continuing enrollment must be broad based and never dependent on an analysis of prior service use and costs in the health plan.

Disenrollment

The same fraud and abuse considerations pertain to disenrollment as to enrollment. Neither the health plan nor the network of physicians and hospital representatives in the health plan should at any time encourage someone to disenroll because they face costly procedures or chronic illness. Disenrollment rates are carefully monitored by HCFA and investigated if they increase without explanation or are too high. Your compliance program should be able to show that you have taken preventive steps to check any selective disenrollment.

Underutilization and Quality of Care

A total quality improvement program should have no trouble meeting the next fraud and abuse rule in Table 7.8 regarding underutilization. Of course covered services, including specialist services, should be available on a reasonable basis. "Gag rules" are prohibited. Physicians certainly can be involved in incentive plans, but these should not make payments to reduce or limit medically necessary care, especially if the payment is linked to a particular beneficiary rather than a group of beneficiaries. Normally, physician incentive payments that reward cost-conscious behavior should be combined with payments that reward good-quality care. Physician incentive payments involving excessive risk are discussed in more detail in Chapter 5. Health plans should check out all providers to ensure they are who they say they are (www.npdb.com).

Data Collection and Submission Processes

The Office of Inspector General has found apparent instances of knowingly or carelessly submitting information to Medicare that is used to then make

MARKETING MATERIALS AND PERSONNEL, 42 CFR 42280

❏ Marketing materials and election forms must be approved by HCFA.
❏ Marketing personnel must present clear, complete, and accurate information.
❏ Contract brokers and physicians are discouraged as marketing personnel.

SELECTIVE MARKETING AND ENROLLMENT, 42 CFR 422100

❏ Asking medical questions before enrollment is prohibited.
❏ Marketing only in places where healthier enrollees are more likely to be present is prohibited.
❏ Target marketing reenrollment based on prior cost experience while in the plan is prohibited.

DISENROLLMENT, 42 CFR 42274

❏ Disenrolling or requesting or encouraging disenrollment is prohibited.
❏ Policies for appropriate medical personnel discussions with beneficiaries about disenrollment should be in place.

UNDERUTILIZATION AND QUALITY OF CARE, 42 USC 1395w22

❏ Covered services must be available in standing contracts, geographically reachable, provided without delay, and made on reasonable referral.
❏ Policies that prohibit interference with professional advice to enrollees are illegal.
❏ Physician incentive plans must:
  • make no payments to physicians to reduce or limit medically necessary services;
  • not put physicians at substantial financial risk (see Chapter 5); and
  • disclose certain information to the public about the physician incentive plans.
❏ Procedures for selection of providers must verify valid license to practice, clinical privileges in good standing, and appropriate educational qualifications.

DATA COLLECTION AND SUBMISSION PROCESSES, 42 CFR 422 60(c)

❏ CEO or CFO must certify the accuracy, completeness, and truthfulness of relevant data, including enrollment data, encounter data, and information provided as part of the adjusted community rate process.
❏ An information collection and reporting system must be in place reasonably designed to yield accurate information for claiming capitation payments and calculating ACR.
❏ Adequate controls for reporting institutional status should be in place.

ANTIKICKBACK STATUTE, 42 USC 1320a 7b(b)

❏ Knowingly and willfully offering, paying, soliciting, or receiving remuneration to induce the referral of Medicare or Medicaid services is prohibited.
❏ A safe harbor protects Medicare+Choice health plans except if the managed care financial arrangement is linked to a broader agreement to steer fee-for-service beneficiaries for referrals.

ANTIDUMPING, 42 USC 1395dd

❏ Notwithstanding the terms of any managed care contract to seek prior authorization from the health plan, the provisions of the antidumping statute govern the obligations of hospitals to screen and provide stabilizing treatment to any presenting patient at an emergency facility.

TABLE 7.5
Summary of Major Fraud and Abuse Prohibitions, 2000

Rules are rules: Most Medicare+ Choice plans and affiliated hospitals and physicians should have no problem meeting Medicare fraud and abuse rules payments. This information includes beneficiary institutional status and residence. When data are submitted to determine the amount of payment received from HCFA, the management of the health plan must certify that such data are accurate, complete, and truthful. You should not view this as certifying an absolute guarantee of accuracy. Rather, it means that you have done the best you can to submit accurate information. The Office of the Inspector General conducted a limited study on some Medicare+Choice plans and found sloppy data-submission efforts.

That is unacceptable. Health plans must insist on protections as a part of their overall compliance program. Draw monthly samples of beneficiary data and verify manually what you are submitting. Correct mistakes, track the results of your validation, and report them to the leadership of your plan. This is just one approach to help ensure accurate data.

Antikickback Statute

From the very start of the Medicare program, remuneration to induce the referral of services that raise Medicare costs has been illegal. It is only in the last few years, however, that new Medicare laws and regulations have clearly articulated the types of arrangements that are safe for providers and health plans and those that are strictly forbidden. Still, there is a huge gray area between safe activity and strictly prohibited activity, and cases falling within this area are addressed by the Office of Inspector General or the Justice Department on a case-by-case basis. For managed care plans, there is a broad safe harbor protecting remuneration between risk-contract health plans and physicians and hospitals that could influence referrals. The antikickback provisions pertain to fee-for-service arrangements that *raise Medicare costs*. Because referrals under a risk contract cannot raise Medicare costs, they are protected. But managed care plans must ensure they do not link remuneration under a risk contract with a separate fee-for-service arrangement. The law prohibits a connection between the two in which one arrangement depends on incentives in the other.

Antidumping

Finally, as covered in Chapter 10 on demand management, the reasonable layperson rule applies to access to emergency services. Prior authorization is not permitted for emergency care. To make doubly sure Medicare beneficiaries receive emergency services, the antidumping provisions governing all hospitals also pertain to the managed care plan and its hospitals.

Controlling Costs Through Physician Incentive Systems

To lower transaction costs, enforce market incentives, and establish competitive prices, managed care plans always have a select network of physicians and hospitals that attempt to coordinate care closely. Most health plans rely on self-imposed markets and prices to manage their networks. The most compelling incentive for any health plan is to not allow every physician or hospital in its network unless they accept prices the health plan is willing to pay. A national study done by an agency of the U.S. Congress (Gold et al. 1997) examined mechanisms used for selecting physicians in Medicare HMOs. Table 7.6 reproduces the results for 108 plans that participated in the study's survey.

Economic Incentives and Selection

All health plans said they verify licenses and credentials. That is the right answer given because it is required that health plans conduct this verification. Nearly all respondents said they consult the National Practitioner Data Bank.

CONTRACTING WITH INDIVIDUAL PHYSICIANS	Percent
Verifies License and Credentials	100
Consults National Practitioner Data Bank	92
Visits Physician Office, Review Facility, and Screen Care Through Medical Records	
Percent All Three	43
Percent None	27
Reviews Quantitative Data from Claims	37

SELECTION DECISION	
Requires Board Certification or Recent Board Eligibility	29
Requires Existing Privileges at Network Hospital or Ability to Obtain Them	82
Commitment by Agreement to Take Predetermined Size Panel or Not to Practice Outside Plan	37
Stated Effect of Cost or Utilization Experience on Decision Large	13

EXTENSIVE EMPHASIS ON ORIENTING NEW PHYSICIANS*	
Percent with All Four Elements:	
None	30
One	4
Two	17
Three	23
All Four	26

TABLE 7.6
Mechanisms Used by Managed Care Plans to Select Physicians, 1994

Broad versus selective contracting: Medicare+ Choice plans report a minority use economic credentialing

Source: Gold, M. et al. 1997. "Disabled Medicare Beneficiaries in HMOs." *Health Affairs* 16 (5): 149–62.
* Plan has orientation meetings specifically for medical staff, 75 percent or more of physicians participate, top management is involved, and less than 75 percent of time is devoted to administrative issues.

Approximately 43 percent visit physician offices, review the facility, and audit the care given through a review of medical records. Twenty-seven percent of plans reported they do none of these things. Thirty-seven percent review the claims history of their physicians and decide whether to include them on the basis of the plan's criteria for cost-conscious patterns of claims.

Only 29 percent of survey respondents said they require board certification or eligibility. A total of 82 percent require existing privileges at the hospitals affiliated with the health plan. Only 37 percent agree to limit the practice either by agreeing to accept a certain number of patients or agreeing to make their relationship exclusive. Thirteen percent said they heavily weighed the cost and service use experience heavily in their decision to include the physician in their network.

Thirty percent have orientation meetings specifically with their new affiliated physicians, and these plans have 75 percent or more of physicians participate, involve top management in the meetings, and devote less than 75 percent of the time to administrative matters.

In the mid-1990s, the most recent that data have been available for Medicare managed care plans specifically, most were not vested heavily in one of the strictest financial incentives: the decision to include or not to include a physician or hospital in the health plan network. Their networks would seem to be fairly wide open with few onerous provisions to join the plan as an affiliated physician. Economic credentialing involving the profiling of service use and cost claims experience was not the norm.

Economic Incentives and Payment Methods

Table 7.7 examines the next level of economic incentives, the payment method. Many Medicare+Choice plans are independent practice associations and pay physicians fee-for-service out of the capitation payment the plan receives from Medicare. In the mid-1990s, about one-third of plans paid fee-for-service with no withhold or bonus. Around 12 percent paid with a withhold payment. In the past six years there are anecdotal reports that the percentage of primary care physicians being paid capitation has increased dramatically and may have doubled from the 37 percent shown in Table 7.7. The largest Medicare+Choice HMOs pay their physicians on a capitation basis, so the number of Medicare beneficiaries receiving care from capitated primary care physicians is probably much higher than Table 7.7 indicates. Nearly 20 percent of physicians are paid on a salary, and about one-half of those receive a bonus.

Capitations for specialist physicians seem to have peaked in the late 1990s and may not be much different from the figures shown in Table 7.7 and the 1994 survey. Fee-for-service medicine still dominates the specialist market with around 70 percent paid in this way. Capitation is less than 20 percent. In percentage terms, specialists are half as likely to be salaried compared to primary care.

PRIMARY CARE PHYSICIANS	Percent 1995
Fee-for-service (Total)	43
With withholding or bonuses	12
Without withholding or bonuses	31
Capitation (Total)	37
With withholding or bonuses	29
Without withholding or bonuses	8
Salary (Total)	19
With withholding or bonuses	11
Without withholding or bonuses	8
SPECIALIST PHYSICIANS	
Fee-for-service (Total)	70
With withholding or bonuses	19
Without withholding or bonuses	52
Capitation (Total)	18
With withholding or bonuses	7
Without withholding or bonuses	10
Salary (Total)	11
With withholding or bonuses	6
Without withholding or bonuses	6

TABLE 7.7
Basic Physician
Payment
Methods by
Plan Type,
1994

Capitation is tops: Many Medicare+ Choice plans use capitation payments for physician payments

Source: Gold, M. et al. 1995. *Arrangements Between Managed Care Plans and Physicians*. Washington, DC: PPRC.

Economic Incentives and Performance

Performance-based capitation payments with a **withhold** or **bonus** offer Medicare managed care plans great potential when it comes to improving quality and doing better than fee-for-service at managing patient care. Two prominent programs have been used in the Medicare program for more than ten years: PacifiCare Health System and Aetna U.S. Healthcare. These plans allow physicians to earn as much as 30 percent above the capitation payment. PacifiCare Health System, with the largest Medicare managed care enrollment, uses a multidimensional rating system to identify the best physician groups that it capitates. The system has two major components—clinical measures and service measures. Each capitated group receives an overall score based on HEDIS measures of required screenings and prescription drugs for heart failure. There is also a customized measure of optimal outpatient care to avoid the need for hospitalization. The service measures include member satisfaction with the group and the individual physician, member satisfaction with referral process, several measures of complaints, and overturned appeals (see www.pacificare.com). Those practices performing best

Withhold is a percentage of payments or set dollar amounts that are deducted from the service fee, capitation, or salary payment. This money may or may not be returned, depending on specific predetermined factors like productivity and utilization.

after all the scores are summed receive a bonus payment in addition to the capitation.

Aetna U.S. Healthcare has long used a performance-based system with five dimensions of performance (see www.aetnaushc.com). The first is a risk adjuster. It estimates the prevalence of patients with certain conditions expected in the practice based on claims history and size of the practice. The next has access measure, including number of visits per period. The third is a series of process measures very similar to the HEDIS measures of types of screenings. Several outcome measures follow in the form of emergency room rates for conditions that should not require an emergency room, and these are considered adverse outcomes. Finally, there are satisfaction measures, including overall satisfaction, appointment time satisfaction, and emergency care satisfaction.

Ideal Economic Incentives?

From the standpoint of transaction costs and balanced economic incentives, an ideal model of physician incentives is shown in Figure 7.5 for a hypothetical BestCare HMO. Average Medicare+Choice capitation payments of $440 are assumed per enrollee per month to cover all operating costs. The enrollee is considered to be of standard age, gender, and Medicaid status (see Chapter 5—Risk Payments—for details on calculating the Medicare+Choice payment). Out of this premium, $56.31 per member per month (13 percent) is retained by the HMO for administration (9.8 percent), reinsurance (2 percent), and contribution to reserves (1.2 percent).

The remainder is allocated between a medical services pool and a risk-sharing pool. The medical services pool is the amount of money paid monthly to the capitated primary care medical group for each enrollee. The $186.82 medical services pool capitation rate is paid at the beginning of the month and is the only payment for covered services rendered to an enrollee. If the enrollee does not utilize any medical services during the month, the medical group simply retains the capitation payment. If, on the other hand, the enrollee uses medical services that cost more than the capitation, the medical group must absorb the additional cost. Because the catastrophic illness of a single enrollee could seriously affect the financial condition of BestCare HMO, an individual stop-loss provision is activated once hospital inpatient services costs for an individual enrollee reach $30,000 during a contract year. BestCare HMO will pay for any further inpatient services out of reinsurance proceeds. The medical group assumes all risk for professional medical services, including outside referrals, rather than purchasing medical stop-loss insurance.

Incentives and Medical Services Pool

Through this capitation mechanism, the medical group accepts a significant amount of the risk for providing care to enrollees for a predetermined, prepaid amount. Such an arrangement fosters a financial incentive for the physicians

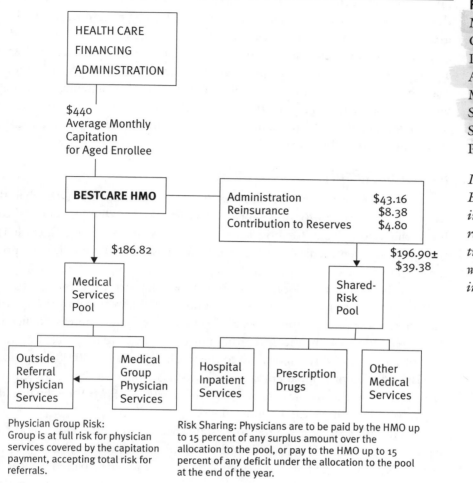

FIGURE 7.5

Medicare+ Choice Payment Allocation to Medical Services and Shared-Risk Pool

Ideal incentives: Everyone involved faces reasonable transaction costs with economic incentives

HEALTH CARE FINANCING ADMINISTRATION

$440 Average Monthly Capitation for Aged Enrollee

BESTCARE HMO

Administration	$43.16
Reinsurance	$8.38
Contribution to Reserves	$4.80

$186.82

$196.90± $39.38

Medical Services Pool

Shared-Risk Pool

Outside Referral Physician Services

Medical Group Physician Services

Hospital Inpatient Services

Prescription Drugs

Other Medical Services

Physician Group Risk: Group is at full risk for physician services covered by the capitation payment, accepting total risk for referrals.

Risk Sharing: Physicians are to be paid by the HMO up to 15 percent of any surplus amount over the allocation to the pool, or pay to the HMO up to 15 percent of any deficit under the allocation to the pool at the end of the year.

Source: Adapted, with permission, from a case that appeared originally in H. L. Sutton and A. J. Sorbo. 1982. *Actuarial Issues in the Fee-for-Service/Prepaid Medical Group*. Denver, CO: Center for Research in Ambulatory Health Care Administration.

who take seriously the management of the healthcare of HMO enrollees. The managed care plan rewards the medical group for providing effective preventive medicine and health education, detecting disease in its earliest stages, and providing necessary healthcare in its most appropriate setting when it is cost effective to do so.

Capitation payments for medical services provide incentives for physicians to offer their own services to enrollees in a cost-effective manner. Nationally, however, physician fees represent a relatively small portion of the healthcare dollar. A more significant portion, estimated at 80 to 90 percent, is spent through physicians acting as agents for their patients by prescribing hospital services, prescription drugs, and other medical services. Because the physician is in such a powerful position as gatekeeper to the health system, the HMO's risk-sharing arrangements were established to reward the medical group for appropriate and cost-effective selection of healthcare services for its patients. Conversely, the risk-sharing arrangements impose financial loss if a plan selects wasteful and inappropriate treatment. If physicians consistently make cost-effective treatment decisions for their HMO patients, then they will receive a financial reward. If, however, the physicians consistently select unnecessary, ineffective, and high-cost treatment modalities for their patients, then they stand to lose financially.

Shared-Risk Pool

The mechanism by which BestCare provides physician incentives is the shared-risk pool. Monthly, $196.90 is allocated to this pool for each HMO enrollee. From this pool, claims for hospital services, prescription drugs (included), and other covered medical services not encompassed in the medical group's capitation will be paid by the HMO. If, at the end of a given year, a surplus exists in the shared-risk pool, BestCare will pay the medical group up to 50 percent of the surplus. This payment is limited to 15 percent of the budgeted allocation to the pool during the year. If, on the other hand, there is a deficit in the shared-risk pool, the medical group must pay BestCare 50 percent up to a limit of 15 percent of the allocation to the pool. Again, the $30,000 stop-loss provision for hospital inpatient services costs is included in this arrangement so that neither the medical group nor the BestCare HMO are financially jeopardized by a single catastrophic illness.

The risk-sharing arrangements established between the HMO and the medical group do, in fact, provide real economic incentives for the physicians to provide, or arrange for, cost-effective healthcare for their patients without jeopardizing the group's financial position. The risk-sharing arrangements also significantly enhance the potential for BestCare to become a financially secure organization.

Although such financial incentives could impact quality of care negatively, there are countervailing influences at work. Quality of care is protected because the physicians have their own professional standards and educational requirements to retain a license. The state and federal governments also regulate the quality of care. Most important, perhaps, is that physicians recognize that if enrollees perceive that they are receiving poor quality healthcare, they will drop out of the HMO and choose another health plan offered in the area. Not only would physician reputation and their ability to attract HMO enrollees be threatened, but there also could be a negative impact on the fee-for-service business.

Incentives and Performance

As a final twist, BestCare has instituted a new outcomes management department. The staff in this department analyzes the hospital claims associated with the medical group, conducts patient satisfaction and health status surveys, and does medical record–check surveys, using explicit criteria for quality reviews on select diseases.

The amount of risk assumed by physicians under the current arrangement has left the physicians wondering whether or not they're doing enough to manage their own risk. They have instituted a disease management effort by selecting certain diseases, disseminating guidelines, and collaborating with BestCare to monitor outcomes. Quarterly bonuses are tied to various performance measures like the ones in Table 7.8.

Patient satisfaction ranks at the top measure of performance, and the indicators are from nearly all perspectives: patients, support staff, peer physicians, and managers. Complaints are included as well. Various measures are used to assign a point score with highest scores shown, and these measures

TABLE 7.8
Summary of Components for Physician Incentive Plan

High-performance incentives: Five components with multiple measures determine performance payments

Component	Highest Score
PATIENT SATISFACTION	
Patient Satisfaction Survey	4
Support Staff Assessment of Physician	3
Peer Assessment of Physician	3
Complaint Rate of Physician	2
Physician/Manager Comments	2
	14 points
GROUP INVOLVEMENT	
Participation in Committees	4
Peer Assessment	5
Current CPR Certification	1
	10 points
PRODUCTIVITY	
Encounters	4
Capitated Charges	4
FFS Charges	4
	12 points
UTILIZATION	
Lab Utilization	1
Radiology Utilization	1
Peer Assessment	3
Special Efforts	2
	7 points
PATIENT OUTCOMES	
Improvement Basic Care	4
Improvement Diabetes Patients	4
Improvement Hypertension Patients	4
	12 points
TOTAL	55 points

are based on surveys and interviews. Some credit is given for participation in the group as a member of a self-directed team of health professionals. Committee participation, peer assessment, and current CPR certification are also counted.

Productivity counts toward performance, and this includes both encounters seen during the time the performance is measured as well as contributions to sources of revenue. Service use and costs are factored in along with lab use, radiology use, and peer assessments. There is also a special efforts score that the managing physician assigns based on perceptions about each physician's ideas and actions.

Finally, patient outcomes for three basic measures (Chapter 8, Disease Management, and Chapter 9, Basic Care) are included. Points are awarded based upon improvements on these measures of patient outcomes.

The total points add up to 55, and a bonus is paid for all those meeting a threshold level of points, with the highest bonus paid to those with a perfect score. Management, depending on how much money is available for bonuses, arbitrarily sets the threshold of points for a bonus. Each component has an explicit weight in the overall scheme of performance-based payments. Patient satisfaction is the highest, adding up to 14 points. Utilization adds up to 7 points and is weighted exactly half as much as patient satisfaction. It is also the least-weighted component. In a capitation scheme, one needs to strike a balance between disincentives to provide services that inherently stem from the capitation with incentives to reward components of care that improve patient satisfaction, reward good group behavior, encourage productivity and cost consciousness, and enhance patient outcomes.

Strategic Alliances

Vertical integration occurs when two or more successive stages in producing and distributing a good or service are brought under common control.

Business alliances arise when two entities need some strategic advantage the other has, and they develop special arrangements to access those advantages from each other.

The BestCare HMO illustration of an ideal managed care incentive system not only highlights certain incentives and their relationship to cost and quality, but it also shows a very special arrangement between the HMO and the medical group. These are almost vertically integrated entities because they work in a close partnership to manage the medical services pool and the shared-risk pool. The HMO purchases the reinsurance used to protect the medical group in the shared-risk pool. The HMO also collects and analyzes the data and helps the medical group administer the performance-based system. The medical group helps the HMO manage the shared-risk pool, and significant positive and negative rewards can be made to the medical group for its trouble.

Vertical integration either in the form of outright ownership or, in the case of BestCare HMO, as a **business alliance** can significantly lower transaction costs and improve cost and quality. This integration relies on trust for smooth functioning—the BestCare HMO must trust the medical group and vice versa. If your health plan or your medical group can find partners to form an alliance based on mutual trust and strong incentive reward systems, you can greatly lower the transaction costs in the system. This relationship can result in better quality at lower cost.

Most alliances are successful because each partner has a distinctive competency the other needs, and together the payoff is better than apart. One risk to an alliance is that one of the entities would learn the distinctive competencies of the other and become proficient in them, thus making the alliance less beneficial to at least one party. Frank and honest communication is the best cement for maintaining any strategic partnerships.

Building a Fiscally Sound Budget

The budget for your organization can be based on a constant set of factors, yielding a strict blueprint for the coming year. Alternatively, you can base it on a variable set of conditions modified throughout the budget period. Variances of actual budgeted amounts help you identify problems early and act to correct them either by cutting the budget in the affected area or elsewhere or addressing the reason for the budget shortfall.

Table 7.9 illustrates this principle based on the case involving the medical group in the BestCare HMO. As you recall, the medical group was at risk for $186.82 per member per month. In this form of cost budgeting, benchmark figures on the number of full-time equivalent (FTE) physicians required to care for elderly and disabled Medicare beneficiaries are available from the medical group's previous experience. These factor out to a dollar amount per member per month. And on the basis of past experience, the medical group knows what it spends on supplies, x-rays, and other line items in the budget. The cost of office space is allocated per member per month. An expected profit is factored in depending on financial goals. All this adds up before outside physician referrals to $154.83 in costs per member per month. This is well below the capitation. Once the outside physician referrals are factored in, the cost-based budget is $168.72, which yields a $18.10 margin, or 9.6 percent of the capitation amount. This is a comfortable amount for flexible budgeting and would allow any of the line items to change during the course of the budget year without going over the capitation amount. This surplus, if it exists at the end of the year, also could be put to future growth and development capital expenditures or special projects.

Utilization Management

Published studies in the 1970s, 1980s, and 1990s have long revealed that managed care substantially reduces the use of hospital services, but it either increases or does not affect physician visits (Luft 1981; Manning et al. 1984; Feldman et al. 1990). Nelson and Brown (1990) looked at the effects of hospital use among the early Medicare HMOs and found hospital admission

TABLE 7.9
Determining
Cost per
Member per
Month for
Medical Group
Prepaid Services

*A budget
to manage
against:
Bestcare HMO
illustration of
cost method*

Medical Services Pool	Cost per Member per Month (PMPM)
Primary Care: 1.7 FTE per 1,000 members	$32.08
Average Total Compensation = $275,000[a]	
Cost/Member/Month = .7 × 275,000/(1,000 × 12)	
Specialty Care: .4 FTE per 1,000 members	$10.00
Average Total Compensation = $300,000[a]	
Cost/Member/Month = .2 × $300,000/(1,000 × 12)	
Support Staff: 6.0 per FTE physician	$31.25
Average Total Compensation = $70,000[a]	
Cost/Member/Month = 0.9 × 3.0 × $70,000/(1,000 × 12)	
Medical Supplies[b]	$5.84
Assume 7.0 visits per member per year	
Average cost/visit = $10.00	
Cost/Member/Month = 3.5 × $10.00/12	
X-Ray Supplies	$5.24
Lab Supplies	$6.60
Depreciation of Equipment[c]	$16.84
Occupancy[d]	$17.34
Assume 1 square foot/member	
$104 per square foot per year	
Cost/Member/Month = $104/12	
Miscellaneous Overhead[e]	$15.56
Total Direct Cost	$140.75
Profit, Capital Allowance (10% of Total Direct Cost)	$14.08
Subtotal	$154.83
Outside Referral Physician Services	$13.44
Total Cost per Member per Month for Medical Group Services	$168.72

Note: The cost of referrals assumes outside providers are willing to negotiate a discount from their normal charges.
[a] Includes base compensation, fringes, retirement and profit-sharing plan, individual malpractice, continuing education allowance, memberships, and dues.
[b] Includes cost of disposable medical supplies and medical records.
[c] Assumes $1,000,000 of medical equipment and furniture depreciated over seven years. Assume equipment can handle demands of 30,000 patients.
[d] Includes depreciation on building or lease, amortization or improvements, utilities, taxes, insurance, and janitorial/maintenance.
[e] Includes malpractice insurance for group, telephone, memberships for group, administrative staff expenses related to prepaid operations, postage, office supplies.

rates among enrollees fell by 8 percent. They detected a start-up effect in which hospital service use was actually higher in the first year enrollment, followed by a sharp drop in the range of 14 to 28 percent in the second year.

Managed care plans should heed these findings. Too often, utilization management is couched in terms of simply driving down inpatient hospital days per 1,000 enrollees. New enrollees differ from continuing enrollees. The intensity of the impact of managed care on Medicare beneficiaries probably depends on the average demographic factors of your enrollees. Do they come from the lower-weighted demographic factors or the higher-weighted ones? Hospitalization rates have been falling since the early 1980s, providing efficiency gains for the Medicare fee-for-service sector as evidenced by 1999's first-ever drop in Medicare spending. Medicare managed care may no longer be able to achieve the same percentage reduction in hospital utilization relative to the fee-for-service sector that it had in the past.

A single-minded approach to utilization management that only looks at one piece of healthcare is component management. If all your health plan manages in terms of utilization is hospital days per 1,000, you are doing **component management**. You are not coordinating across disease states, care settings, or types of services. Among a healthy, employed population of enrollees, a utilization management program that only focuses on hospital days may be sufficient. Elderly and disabled Medicare beneficiaries have chronic conditions, characterized by persistent and recurring health problems lasting for extended periods. Their needs are more multidimensional and interpersonal, requiring a more integrated approach across components of care than do commercial enrollees.

Component management is a focus on utilization management of just one piece of healthcare at a time.

Table 7.10 illustrates what studies have found to happen to service use and costs when beneficiaries join an HMO (Brown et al. 1993). These studies are based on the experience of the Medicare managed care program in the 1990s, and they were done with a very large number of enrollees and health plans from all parts of the country. All the dollar figures have been adjusted to the estimated 2001 USPCC. The percent distribution is taken from the original studies for illustrating the after effects of Medicare managed care from a system perspective.

We estimate that the average beneficiary costs fee-for-service Medicare $5,280 per year (which takes into account demographic factors and geographic location across the country). As discussed in Chapter 6, the average enrollee in a Medicare+Choice organization costs less because these beneficiaries tend to be younger. The Medicare+Choice payment rate makes adjustments on the basis of the younger age groups and, therefore, lowers costs comparatively. For illustration, and based on the available studies, $4,398 is a reasonable estimate of the fee-for-service equivalent cost of an enrollee in managed care. Table 7.10 shows the dollar distribution and the percent distribution across the components of care.

Sophisticated regression analysis examining tens of thousands of claims calculated the HMO effect shown in Table 7.10. The best information available for the average plan suggests that, when a beneficiary enrolls, inpatient hospital days on average fall by 16.8 percent or $29 per year from the enrollee fee-for-service equivalent cost. Outpatient hospital days fall less than one percent. Visits to physicians rise nearly 5 percent and cost the plan $57 more per beneficiary per year. Skilled nursing home days and home health visits fall. Skilled nursing home days fall 24 percent. Home health visits fall 53.6 percent.

TABLE 7.10
HMO Effects
on Medical
Care, Valued at
Medicare Prices

*Systems, not
components:
Care
management
for the elderly
should replace
single-
component
utilization
management*

Component	Average Fee-for-Service Reimbursements[2]		HMO Effect on Service Use	Implied Effect on Costs at MEDICARE Prices
	Non-enrollee	Enrollee[3]	Percent	Dollars
INPATIENT HOSPITAL DAYS			−16.8	−$429
Dollars	$3,110	$2,555		
Percent of Total	58.9	58.1		
OUTPATIENT HOSPITAL DAYS			−0.7	−$41
Dollars	$428	$387		
Percent of Total	8.1	8.8		
VISITS TO PHYSICIANS			+4.6	+$57
Dollars	$1,352	$1,236		
Percent of Total	25.6	28.1		
SKILLED NURSING HOME DAYS			−24.4	−$27
Dollars	$158	$110		
Percent of Total	3.0	2.5		
HOME HEALTH VISITS			−53.6	−$59
Dollars	$232	$110		
Percent of Total	4.4	2.5		
TOTAL			−10.5	−459
Dollars	$5,280	$4,398		
Percent of Total	100	100		
DRUGS[1]				
Dollars	—	$475		
Percent of Total	—	9.7		
TOTAL WITH DRUGS[1]				
Dollars		$4,873		
Percent of Total		100		

Source: Brown, R. S. et al. 1994. "Care of Patients Hospitalized. . . ." In *HMOs and the Elderly*, edited by H. S. Luft et al. Chicago: Health Administration Press.
[1] Drug costs were not available in original study and have been estimated for this illustration for a benefit with substantial cost sharing.
[2] All dollar figures have been adjusted to estimated 2001 USPCC. Percent distributions and percent effect are the same as the original study.
[3] For each cost aggregate, enrollee Medicare fee-for-service reimbursements were predicted from regression models estimated for nonenrollees, with Medicare reimbursements as the dependent variable.

The net change in costs is about 10.5 percent savings over what fee-for-service would have cost at Medicare prices, or around $459. If the managed care plan is able to pay lower fees than what Medicare pays, that would lower costs to the plan further.

To illustrate all of the components, Table 7.10 also shows an estimate for drug coverage. Some health plans provide this at no additional charge, but many now charge a premium. Fee-for-service Medicare does not cover drugs, so these figures are estimated separately from the studies that supply the other figures in the table. Drugs cost nearly 10 percent for a plan, or $475 in our illustration. This just about offsets the savings the plan derived from hospital and the other services.

This illustration raises several systems questions. What accounts for the reduction in inpatient hospital costs? Is it restrictive prior authorization and utilization management, or is it the fact that drug coverage is included and coordinated with the other components? Does increased use of physician services mean there is a substitution between inpatient hospital days and visits to physicians? Why would the studies estimate such a large effect on reducing skilled nursing home days and home health visits? Could a Medicare managed care plan spend more in these categories, instead of less, and further reduce the inpatient hospitalization rate? Alternatively, does the drop reflect the excesses of an unbridled fee-for-service sector, as the estimates are computed as a change from expected fee-for-service costs? Like a hydraulic system in which pressure at one point can cause changes to occur at another point in the system, care management for the elderly is complex and can benefit greatly from better coordination.

Primary care gatekeeping, preadmission screening for hospital stays, and financial incentives to control service have been hallmarks of utilization management for managed care plans (Nelson et al. 1990). In a thorough case study of 13 Medicare managed care plans (Hurley and Bannick 1993), the process by which successful plans attempt to manage service use goes beyond relying on financial incentives. In their interviews, Hurley and Bannick found that Medicare managed care plans believe that the key to effective utilization management lies in building cooperative relationships between the plan and the physicians. Effective utilization also means emphasizing educational rather than control strategies. Plans focus on managing inpatient hospital use because of its high cost and the fact that hospitals will not negotiate financial risk-sharing arrangements.

Many plans still struggle with different approaches in the amount of risk sharing that is considered necessary to motivate physicians to be effective resource managers. Most managed care plans promulgate medical treatment guidelines, but they do not necessarily use them aggressively to manage care. Either they have not figured out how to do that, or their patient base is spread too thinly among too many physicians to make any worthwhile investment in medical treatment guidelines as a method of changing behavior.

Some managed care plans broadly delegate utilization management. Others centralize the function. You should assume that if you transfer to Medicare what you are doing with the commercial enrollment in your health plan in terms of utilization review, it will cost two to four times more per member per month. The corresponding costs for Medicare versus commercial enrollees will be that much more because of the complexity and comorbid conditions.

Physician Practice Patterns

Because there are frequent, irreversible personal consequences to the application of modern medicine, it is among the most scientific of all professions. Evidence of the safety of what is done to patients and clinical effectiveness are integral to being a physician. Consequently, physicians are naturally drawn to data and information about their patients.

Managed care companies are using this mark of modern medicine to build a cooperative relationship with their network physicians. Data that examine physician practice patterns, when presented to physicians about their own care patterns, can help reduce variation, identify possible areas of improvement, and lower transaction costs by dealing with unnecessary costs. An approach to physician profiling done in a collaborative mode sets up an exchange relationship. If the managed care plan can give the practitioner useful, understandable profile data with incentives to change, it is likely to be much lower in transaction costs than investing in a monitoring and authorization system.

There are a number of common rules about effective physician profiling. First, start simple and pilot methods of profiling. Keep the effort small so the costs of doing the profiling do not outweigh the benefits in costs, quality, or productivity. Figure 7.6 illustrates how profiling can be made easy. This is outcomes assessment for ambulatory surgery in which an executive dashboard has been created to show where the ambulatory surgery center has been, and where it is going in terms of indicators of outcomes. At a glance, one can gauge patient outcomes and know where to focus attention. The dark circles indicate where the practice is more than two standard deviations below the average performance. The circles with a dot indicate average, within two standard deviations. The open circles indicate above-average performance. The arrows indicate how the practice performed against itself in the previous quarter.

This example focuses on clinical indicators of quality and cost. To be acceptable, physician profiling should address clinically valid measures. They shouldn't look exclusively at cost indicators. The data should be presented at the start of a discussion about cost, quality, or productivity. Physicians and other clinicians are problem solvers. When presented with the evidence, most will have an inherent desire to want to do better. When setting up the system for creating information reports, always allow the possibility to delve further into a particular number. Examine the patient-level data to identify outliers,

FIGURE 7.6

Illustration of Executive Summary of Performance Benchmarking Findings, Indicator Status, and Trends

Executive dashboard: At a glance you can see where you are and where you are going

SAMPLE CENTER

EXECUTIVE BENCHMARK TABLE: INDICATOR STATUS AND TRENDS
Quarter 1, 1999 to Quarter 4, 1998
Table was created on 09/16/1999

	Arthroscopy, Knee	Carpal Tunnel	Cataract Removal	Hernia Repair	Laparoscopy, Gyne
Perioperative Complications (IND1)	◉ ↘	● ↘	◉ ↔	◉	◉ ↗
Delayed in Discharge (IND2)	● ↗	● ↗	● ↘	◉	○ ↘
Returns to Surgery (IND3)	◉ ↔	◉ ↔	◉ ↔	◉	◉ ↔
Admits to Hospital (IND4)	◉ ↔	◉ ↔	◉ ↔	◉	◉ ↔
Pain Episodes Not Relieved (IND5)	◉ ↔	◉ ↔	◉ ↗	◉	◉ ↔
Care Not Needed After Discharge (IND6)	◉ ↔	◉ ↘	◉ ↔	◉	◉ ↘
Pain Controlled After Discharge (IND7)	○ ↗	◉ ↗	◉ ↗	◉	◉ ↗
Satisfied Patients (IND8)	◉ ↗	◉ ↗	◉ ↗	◉	◉ ↗
Effective Discharge Instructions (IND9)	◉ ↔	◉ ↔	◉ ↔	◉	◉ ↔
Patients Prepared for Self-Care (IND10)	◉ ↔	◉ ↔	◉ ↔	◉	◉ ↔

Comparison with all centers (where you are now)
- ○ – Better than average
- ◉ – Average
- ● – Worse than average

Comparison of current results with those for the previous period (where you are going)
- ↗ – Improving
- ↔ – No change
- ↘ – Worsening

and focus on detailed data about particular patients or procedures. Physicians tend to think in terms of particular cases, so a bar chart or table that identifies a problem is immediately a candidate for further investigation about what is behind the data. They'll want to find out why the problem appeared. It could simply be data errors, and physicians will want to check for accuracy. In this regard, case-mix adjustment is often necessary for profiling physicians for most systems of benchmarking and comparing.

Pharmacy Benefits

Pharmacy benefits deserve special mention in the chapter on costs and quality because for several years they have been the fastest growing component of total costs. Table 7.10 assumes pharmacy is 9.7 percent of total costs for a fairly restrictive benefit. But pharmacy can be from 9 to 15 percent of total costs, and this figure is growing at double-digit rates. The average Medicare beneficiary has between 16 and 21 prescriptions filled per year—more than one per month. The drivers of pharmacy benefits are prescriptions per beneficiary; ingredient costs; pharmaceutical manufacturer rebates on the price of drugs; the cost of claims processing (because pharmacy generates an immense number of claims); dispensing fees to community pharmacies; and the administrative costs of single-component computerized review systems such as drug utilization review, prior authorization, and restrictive formulary.

Most plans deal successfully with rising drug costs by restructuring the drug benefit:

- maximum benefits; and
- copayments that step up as the patient is prescribed
  - generic,
  - brand on formulary, and
  - brand not on formulary.

More studies seriously question rather than support the cost effectiveness of the single-component approaches to pharmacy benefits (Soumerai et al. 1994; Horn, Sharkey, and Phillips-Harris 1998). One study found a maximum allowed number of prescriptions sent patients scrambling for inpatient hospital stays to get access to drugs, raising costs by 17 times. Computerized drug review systems seem to be evolving to more online point-of-sale claims processing. These systems have built in prospective drug utilization review to look for drug errors and adherence to the treatment regimen. The old prior authorization and restrictive formulary systems are increasingly being replaced by disease management and experimental pharmaceutical care programs. These programs carve out a greater role for the pharmacist in providing chronic care in the pharmacy or a greater role for the nurse manager. Strategically, your plan should have a clear path for addressing pharmaceutical services with an approach that views drugs as a part of the system of care. They have enormous benefits when they work effectively at reducing the use of costly inpatient and other settings. Your plan may want to see drug costs continue to go up, which they certainly will, based on scientific advances alone because it can mean the cost of some other component of care has gone down.

Screening, Wellness, and Prevention Programs

Traditional fee-for-service Medicare has expanded coverage of selected preventive services because studies indicate they are cost effective to the program or widespread screening is considered medically necessary. Medicare covers flu shots in full, mammograms subject to a schedule of frequency and copayments, prostate exams, and periodic bone-density scanning. Medicare managed care plans always have covered a wide range of preventive services as part of their add-on benefits that they offer beneficiaries to enroll in the health plan. The federal HMO Act mandates coverage for preventive services, and the culture that prevention is a good thing is characteristic of managed care plans.

In actuality, the use of preventive services varies widely by income and age. In a survey done of fee-for-service beneficiaries, 55 percent of poor beneficiaries surveyed had received a flu shot, compared with 70 percent of those with incomes above 200 percent of the poverty level. Poor and near-poor women were about 20 percent less likely to have had mammograms. Only 40 percent of poor men had undergone prostate exams versus nearly 70 percent of men at twice the poverty level. Preventive care use is disproportionately low among the under-65 disabled (Davis and Schoen et al. 1998).

The implications of these figures are twofold. First, offering and marketing extensive preventive services can tilt your plan toward enrolling people who are more likely to demand such services and appreciate the fact that they are available at little or no cost. These beneficiaries might be cost conscious or they could worry more about their health. In all the studies of the Medicare population and their attitudes and beliefs, this relationship has not been uncovered. Second, preventive services and screening cost money. They do not always pay for themselves because it could take many years to recover the costs of screening and preventive services (Scheffler and Paringer 1980; Russell 1986). In the case of markets with a large number of Medicare plans and higher than average enrollment turnover, an investment in screening, wellness, and prevention programs may backfire. If an enrollee leaves your plan, you wind up giving your competitors a prevention-conscious beneficiary. Such programs with net benefits that are far off to the managed care plan do not make economic sense (Dowd 1982).

All this is to say that preventive care is most effective and cost effective when it is targeted. Health risk assessment is the standard fare for most managed care companies. This type of assessment enables them to identify risky behaviors, determine willingness to change, and explore opportunities for improvement. Beneficiaries, while visiting the office as part of the busy practice routine, can complete them. A recent study found that patients felt their own care was improved by completing a health risk assessment with components like the one shown in Table 7.11. Compared with patients who did not have a health assessment, patients who did receive one had smaller declines in ability to perform activities of daily living, and had lower mortality rates, fewer inpatient hospital days, and lower estimated total costs. However, only 23 percent of the patients recalled that their doctor or someone else in the practice had discussed the results of the health assessment survey. As such, managed care companies did not take full advantage of the potential cost savings that the health risk assessment offers. As mechanisms for improving communication,

TABLE 7.11
Summary of
Components of
Typical Health
Assessment

*Risk assessment
is an asset: A
simple patient
survey can
reveal plenty for
follow-up and
improved
outcomes*

Component
HEALTH STATUS
Difficulty: Traveling Alone
Shopping
Doing Housework
Handling Own Money
Rating of health in general on a scale of 1 to 4
Rating of overall quality of life
Need for special support
Feeling depressed
What they think of their medical care
SERVICE USE AND COSTS
Seen any healthcare workers
Number and out-of-pocket costs of drugs
Been hospitalized recently
HEALTH RISK
Smoker
Drinks more than six alcoholic drinks per week
Unclear about who would make decisions in an emergency
Had a flu shot
Had a tetanus shot
Had a TB test [Why are these risks?]

Source: Adapted from Wasson, J. et al. 1998. "Can We Afford Comprehensive Supportive Care for the Very Old?" *Journal of the American Geriatric Society* 46 (7): 829–32.

as Wasson and colleagues suggest in Table 7.11, enhancing trust between physician and patients and lowering the number of transactions through preventive efforts fit into the transaction cost framework for improving quality and cost.

Strategic Decisions Checklist

Strategic Questions	Strategic Analyses
What kind of managed care process and culture are you building in your health plan?	A command and control approach to organizing economic transactions might work for your situation. One that relies on markets and prices is probably one you should adopt in the professional environment of a managed care plan. Each approach has its transactions costs for: • coordination; • motivation; and • transfer prices. Whatever process and culture you develop, you should recognize that it is learned, shared, and externalized.
How much control of the managed care process do you give to physicians?	As the predominant form of medical practice, the incentives and direction of the professional group is a given in Medicare managed care. You should use it, not fight against it. You need to address at least eight processes and decide whether they are working for you: 1. salary and ownership; 2. networks and joint ventures; 3. physicians in governance; 4. management services provided by physicians; 5. sharing of cost information; 6. information system integration; 7. product line integration; and 8. clinical guideline utilization. Organizational shirking must be managed with incentive systems. Self-directed groups hold much promise for managing the care process and lowering transaction costs. *continued*

Strategic Questions	Strategic Analyses
How much commitment to education do you have in your plan?	Adopt the goals of a well-run Medicare managed care plan to minimize transaction costs for delivering high-quality patient care that produces favorable outcomes and avoids the use of expensive settings such as inpatient hospital services, emergency room, and unnecessary treatments.
	Encourage professionals to accept the goals
	Invest in professional skills development
	Use Medicare databases to study and identify problem areas
	Adopt targeted clinical intervention strategies that improve health outcomes
How is your quality assurance system structured?	Process follows structure. The Quality Improvement Standards for Managed Care (QISMC) reflects the principles of total quality management (TQM). You should best be able to meet these standards by creating a TQM structure, which requires:
	• management commitment;
	• total participation;
	• continuous improvement with internal and external customers;
	• continuous improvement with internal/external suppliers; and
	• systematic analysis.
	Your QISMC projects should be easy if you have a structure for all the elements in a TQM approach.
How are you deploying management information systems and medical informatics?	Disease-structured databases from claims files should be essential for managing costs and quality.

continued

Strategic Questions	Strategic Analyses
	Use the Internet not only for e-health purposes with patients but to share clinical information and benchmark processes and outcomes across sites of care.
	Do not computerize for the sake of computerization. Ensure that people will be able to set higher performance standards with new computer resources.
Are you in compliance with fraud and abuse regulations?	You should have an ongoing mechanism for verifying compliance with fraud and abuse regulations in the following areas: • marketing materials and personnel; • anti-selective marketing and enrollment; • disenrollment; • underutilization and quality of care; • data collection and submission processes; • antikickback; and • antidumping. For a well-run Medicare+Choice plan, compliance programs are easy ro run and send a message to all customers.
What physician incentive systems does your plan use?	Your physician incentive systems are your most important tool for controlling cost and improving quality. You should have a quantifiable system for selecting physicians to serve your membership based on cost and quality. You should have clear and fair payment systems for primary care and specialist physicians. A shared-risk pool may be the best approach. You should link payments to physician performance. Measure and benchmark performance outcomes.

DISEASE MANAGEMENT:
THREE IMPERATIVE DISEASES

In the competitive environment that Medicare managed care plans face, success lies in being the best at meeting beneficiary expectations and providing necessary care. That means your health plan must be the market leader when it comes to managing the various diseases that affect enrollees in your health plan. You will find opportunities to make your plan the market leader as a progressive managed care plan by moving away from traditional medical management toward new, systematic approaches called disease management. This chapter will provide a practical explanation of how to take advantage of these opportunities when working with Medicare managed care.

Disease management is a vitally important aspect of strategic management of the managed care plan, especially as it applies to patients and their healthcare. Granted that marketing, financial management, and provider network development are critical to the success of a managed care plan. However, strategic management needs to include meeting the fundamental requirements of the patients in the health plan, and these requirements revolve around the best patient care for their **disease states**.

Disease management identifies and targets healthcare activities that are geared toward maintaining or improving the health of patients with specific diseases. Disease management takes many forms and varies by local medical practices for any health plan. Disease management must be viewed as a dynamic, responsive process used by managed care organizations to achieve long-range goals. For this reason, the discussion later in this chapter on specific diseases is not intended to be a step-by-step, how-to guideline that an organization plugs into existing management efforts. The aim is to illustrate management issues for three highly prevalent diseases: heart disease, cancer, and stroke. Disease management activities are patterns of organizational behavior that are carried out as essential strategic management activities. They are not canned, prescribed ways of doing things. The critical issue for managed care organizations is to give priority to understanding the diseases their enrollees face and to deliver care in a way that improves health outcomes for patients. Achieving this improvement often means changing the way a plan delivers care.

The purpose of this chapter is to clarify just how important it is for Medicare managed care plans to focus on three prevalent diseases as strategic imperatives for careful management. The final section presents some unique

Disease management is an approach to strategic management that uses multidisciplinary clinical teams, continuous analysis of relevant data, and cost-effective technology to improve the health outcomes of patients with specific diseases.

Disease states are different manifestations of symptoms and health status a patient with a specific disease may have at various points in time.

illustrations of outcomes assessment in managing the three imperative diseases. In the case of cancer, colon cancer is used because it is the one that occurs most frequently for both genders in the Medicare program. Woven throughout the discussion are comments about the three essential elements of disease management.

The final section of the chapter is taken from a series of studies done for HCFA from the 1980s and 1990s that examine the quality of care in Medicare HMOs across the nation. You will be able to collect more recent information than that shown in the final section of this chapter. But the measures of health outcome presented from these national studies of Medicare managed care plans illustrate what types of process of care and outcomes measures can help you implement a disease management program. Before discussing that data, we review a brief primer on disease management. Following this review is an examination of why disease management is a strategic issue for management and how crucial it is to understand the epidemiology of Medicare beneficiaries for management purposes.

A Primer on Disease Management

Disease management represents a new way of thinking about patient care—a new way of thinking that might encourage breaking down the current systems that serve patients and sharpening their focus on the need to improve health outcomes. Disease management is not a quick fix or cookbook of practice guidelines (Bodenheimer 1999). It is not a fad (Herzlinger 1999), and it is not always a way for some companies to market their drugs or devices.

In the context of patient care in a health plan, disease management contains four key activities:

1. professional communication among multidisciplinary clinical teams;
2. collection of information on health outcomes;
3. application of cost-effective technology; and
4. continuous analysis of relevant data on health outcomes.

Traditional medical practice has always involved these four activities, so adopting a disease management approach is a matter of emphasis.

Ultimately, disease management is a clinical activity. Professionally and by law, clinical activities are always subject to local medical practice and prone to change with evolving medical technology. That is why interdisciplinary teams play an important central role in a good disease management program. And that is why the discussion here cannot be too specific or clinical. The patient is at the center of the work of multidisciplinary clinical teams, and careful communication to the patient is the most important work teams do. Patients provide information about their health outcomes to the managed care plan through numerous means, including self-administered questionnaires, face-to-face interviews that might be recorded in the patient's medical record,

Traditional Medical Management	Disease Management
Case-by-case fragmented management of patients	Population-based coordinated management of patients
Individual physician as "captain of the ship"	Self-directed, multidisciplinary team of responsible health professionals
Individual pharmacist as "chemist" proffering advice	
Individual nurse as facilitating "caregiver"	
Components of care measured and controlled	Systems of care analyzed and improved
Passively treats everyone the same until they initiate care again	Identifies persons at risk and seeks them out to manage their disease
Affordable care	Appropriate care
Focus on process improvements	Focus on outcomes improvement

TABLE 8.1

Side-by-Side Comparison of Traditional Medical Management and Disease Management

Shift in thinking: Disease management as strategic management

telephone interviews, Internet web pages, or health exams. The managed care plan approves or promotes coverage for cost-effective technologies, including state-of-the-art medical procedures and pharmaceuticals, or methods of encouraging health risk behavior changes in patients. The managed care plan also provides patients with an analysis of relevant information about health outcomes information and then provides this feedback to the multidisciplinary clinical team. The impact of using cost-effective technology and analyzing relevant data should modify professional communication between providers and patients and advance the ability to measure changes in health outcomes. This process is continuous, with health professionals receiving feedback on the progress being made to improve health outcomes.

A Shift in Thinking

As a strategic management tool, disease management is a marked departure from traditional thinking regarding the medical management of the patient (see Table 8.1). Traditional medical management tends to lead one to think that there are unique aspects to treating each patient that need to be explored and understood on a case-by-case basis. To that end, this management model is personal and very much in demand in the market by patients. Unfortunately, similarities among patients are often overlooked or poorly documented under traditional medical management.

Disease management uses a population-based approach. This approach begins by gathering relevant data on process and outcomes. In evaluating these data, researchers try to find similar patterns of pathology, behavior, or outcomes that can lead to improved health outcomes, not only for the individual patient, but also for groups of patients upon remeasuring the process or outcome. Unlike traditional medical management, population-based management of patients relies more heavily on large databases that contain statistical results of caregiving. Medical decision making flows from the analysis of the databases, with intervention implications for large groups of patients.

Under the traditional medical model, the physician is referred to as "the captain of the ship" (Fuchs 1998). The physician charts the direction of patient care, gives the orders for each patient, provides the personalized attention, and is the professional the patient "chooses." The pharmacist controls the medicines or the chemicals and provides highly specialized advice, primarily to the physician, on the use of medicines. The pharmacist traditionally has almost nothing to do with population-based analysis of patient care and has little communication with the patient. The role of the nurse in the traditional model is to make it easy for patients to follow their regimen of care, taking directions from the physician and initiating little of what happens.

Disease management changes all of this by converting these three individual health professionals into a self-directed team as discussed previously in Chapter 7 (Fig. 7.1). Other professionals are added as needed. This approach elevates the roles of the pharmacist and the nurse, especially in terms of communication. Pharmacists and nurses often initiate care directly with patients, though each has only a general awareness of the patient's situation and not the physician's specific knowledge. Members of the team agree to this generalized approach to care for groups of patients identified from an analysis of the population-based data. They write down their approach and then follow it. Different approaches are adopted depending on the disease of the patient.

The disease management approach is best described as interdisciplinary. With an interdisciplinary approach, different health professionals join forces to form a team that creates a common approach to improving the health outcomes of a patient. They emerge on the other side of the caregiving process as distinct members of the team united by a common process. This approach differs from the one taken by the multidisciplinary team, in which the members of the team come into the process, make a contribution, and then leave the process unchanged, returning to the same way of doing things. The ultimate self-directed team is transdisciplinary. This approach brings together professional members of the team and fundamentally changes their former roles as members of their professional group. They are transformed into a new working group or team, and this team takes a single-minded approach to improving patient outcomes by reexamining every aspect of care and by looking for ways to improve that care.

Rather than merely requiring control over (or reduction in) separate budgets for inpatient hospital, physician office, and drugs, disease management follows the assumption that these components are interconnected. It is fruitless to attempt to control one component of care for quality or cost without understanding how it can affect other components. These subsequent effects can frequently influence the original component of care with unintended consequences. Disease management also contributes to the continual improvement of the system in the widely used vein of continuous quality improvement.

When it comes to quality of care, disease management breaks tradition. Traditional medical management passively enrolls patients into the private practice or the health plan and then waits for the patient to initiate care. By contrast, disease management uses all available data and means of identification, including screening and examining patterns of care, to uncover those people at risk for disease. Disease management then adopts specific approaches to manage diseases of patients, always with an eye to improving the health status or the health outcomes. Thus, case management, discussed further in Chapter 9, and demand management, discussed further in Chapter 10, have become staples of managed care.

These approaches also consider any and all settings for care, sometimes disrupting and replacing the regular channels for care management. Preventive care and creative health promotion are much more likely to be used in the outpatient setting to preempt more costly inpatient care. For example, homes of frail patients on Medicare managed care might be inspected for potential hazards to prevent falls and broken bones. Nurses or telephone dialing systems might be used to make phone calls to ensure adherence to drug treatment regimens. Letters might be generated to enroll target patients into an intervention that would teach them better diet, or an improved technique for using a peak flow meter, or better wound care, for example. These active and sometimes aggressive interventions to care management represent a sharp departure from the traditional approach.

Finally, and perhaps most important, disease management does not stop at only process improvement in the way care is delivered to conduct classical continuous quality improvement. Disease management clearly and doggedly focuses on improving health outcomes. As a result, measurement of outcomes and cost-effective methods of tracking outcomes through time become major issues for properly implementing disease management. The importance of this aspect warrants a separate discussion in the following section, along with illustrations for the three imperative diseases.

The Basic Steps in Disease Management

The three basic activities connected with disease management are influenced by the local environment, organization characteristics, and the willingness to change among participants. Local and organizational circumstances influence several issues: how to use professional self-directed teams aggressively, how to bear the cost of expensive data collection regarding outcomes of care, and whether to adopt the latest technology. The realities of disease management prohibit a cookbook approach. Rather, disease management must be viewed as a four-step process to be applied on a continuous basis:

Step 1: Perform feasibility study
Step 2: Select diseases to explore
Step 3: Conduct a pilot test
Step 4: Implement the program

These four steps can be followed with different degrees of intensity, which in turn could require either full-time or part-time resources. If you follow these four steps, you make disease management a strategic process in Medicare managed care.

Step 1: Perform Feasibility Study

A feasibility study should be performed before implementing any disease management program. To perform this study, you might need to form committees or conduct a series of focus groups or surveys among beneficiaries, seeking their input into the types of health outcomes they want to see. Many managed care plans already have support groups for people with certain diseases. These groups are often found in the community as well. Through this medium, you can begin to understand what enrollees with specific diseases expect and require in terms of health outcome. Are they hoping to achieve a specific level of physical functioning? Are they concerned about the site where care is provided and the type of care they receive? Or are patients with a particular disease most interested in costs? By answering these questions as they relate to a select group of enrollees with a particular disease, you are addressing the health outcomes desired by a broader group of enrollees with any particular disease.

The potential partners or professional participants in a disease management program should be oriented to the general concepts on which the approach is based. Ideally, they should have professional and perhaps financial incentives to take an interest in the process of disease management. Initial discussions with professional groups or individual practitioners should be done in a nonthreatening way to explore possibilities, and you should encourage all potential partners to express their concerns and ideas so that everyone can hear. After undertaking a general education effort about the new way of thinking, you may again ask participants to voice their concerns and ideas. Conducting the feasibility study is an important initial step, and it may take a long time. Completing this step successfully is crucial, however, if you want to achieve buy-in to the process later.

Step 2: Select Diseases to Explore

After conducting the feasibility study, or perhaps while conducting the study, you can bring together a group of representative clinicians most directly affected by the program so that they can participate in the disease-selection process. It is important that the group not tackle too many diseases at the same time.

DISEASE ATTRIBUTES

1. Presence of generally agreed-upon treatment protocols or guidelines
2. Presence of generally recognized problems in therapy, well documented in the literature
3. Potential for self-authorization of guidelines

PATIENT ATTRIBUTES

4. Prevalence of disease
5. Prevalence of drug use
6. Population is a high-risk group with measurable, common, serious health outcomes
7. Population receives other healthcare benefits (e.g., Medicare)

HEALTH OUTCOME ATTRIBUTES

8. Ability to measure health outcomes adequately: morbidity (health)
9. Ability to measure service use and costs adequately
10. Intervention has potential for high impact on health outcomes
11. Intervention has potential for high impact on service use
12. Poor health outcome should be preventable if therapy is improved

OTHER INTERVENING FACTORS

13. Therapeutic area is the target of other intervening factors in the managed care plan or in the political environment

OVERALL SCORE

Without regard to the diseases, assign a weight to each of the 13 criteria for disease selection (e.g., 5, 10, 15, 20, 25) to represent their relative importance for your situation. Assign a scoring value for each of the 13 attributes (e.g., 1–4) for each disease. Multiply the weight by the scoring value and sum for each disease to obtain an overall score.

Source: The Williamson Institute with the Degge Group, Ltd. 1995.

TABLE 8.2

Criteria for Disease Selection to Assign Relative Weights and Score for Each Disease

Where to start? A framework for selecting diseases

A good template for selecting diseases is given in Table 8.2. Identifying sources of information about the diseases and then developing standard methods for using the information can help to select disease candidates. Primary source data are usually available from claims data within the managed care plan. Information about disease treatment can be obtained from national consensus-based sources such as the National Institutes of Health or the Agency for Healthcare Research and Quality. Reviews of treatment guidelines may be sought from state and local entities to ensure applicability to community practice.

Diseases are selected on the basis of available information about the patients who have been targeted for the study. Selection criteria fall into four areas: disease attributes, population attributes, health outcomes attributes, and other intervening factors.

Disease Attributes   Before selecting a disease, you'll need to consider the existence of treatment guidelines, the range of treatment modalities, and the opinions on the appropriateness and effectiveness of treatment. The selection process also needs to include consideration of the natural progression of the disease and the various disease states patients might present to professionals. You may consider whether the guidelines for treatment are complex or simple. In other words, does implementing the guidelines require self-authorization by the health professionals involved in the managed care plan or does it call for more complex preauthorization?

Population Attributes   Selection of a disease may depend on how many patients have the disease. Under this criterion, population attributes pertain only to the group of patients that will benefit from any disease management intervention. Ideally, the targeted disease should be for a relatively homogeneous group with similar diagnoses, as well as similar socioeconomic and demographic characteristics. To determine the prevalence of a disease, the patients in question must be a stable group in terms of eligibility. They must also demonstrate a sufficient use of services or have a history of either medical or drug claims. Disease selection may also account for targeted patients who remain enrolled in the managed care plan.

Health Outcome Attributes   When selecting a disease, you should pay attention to factors that would interfere with any intervention and subsequent assessment of changes in health outcomes. Two factors that influence selection are how easy or how costly it is to measure health outcomes. For example, mortality is a health outcome, but sometimes it occurs too infrequently to be an adequate measure of health outcomes for disease management. There are an abundance of morbidity measures for most major diseases, and many have been tested for reliability. Service use and costs can also be good measures of health outcome changes. For example, costly emergency room visits can indicate poor adherence to the treatment regimen or access to care problems and, therefore, trigger the associated disease for management. Service use and costs also tell you where potential cost savings lie. Finally, you may select a disease because therapies exist to prevent it.

Other Intervening Factors   One final suggested criterion for selecting diseases is a general one that may involve local organizational priorities or politics. You may want to select a disease because other units within the managed care plan have targeted the disease or because political concerns in the community point toward the disease for management. There may be existing experts in the health plan or the community regarding the disease. There may also be local support groups or pharmaceutical companies with an interest in a disease, prompting a partnership in disease management. Such factors can be an important determinant of disease selection and can be considered explicitly.

The 13 attributes indicated in Table 8.2 can help you create an overall score for deciding which diseases to select. You can begin the selection process by assigning a weight to each criterion (e.g., 5, 10, 15, 20, 25), indicating the relative importance to the managed care plan of the attribute. Then, you can convene or survey expert clinicians who provide services to the managed care plan to rate potential disease candidates for specific attributes using the following scoring system:

4   Meets attribute easily
3   Meets attribute with some difficulty
2   Meets attribute with great difficulty
1   Unable to meet attribute

Once you compute an overall score for each disease, using the same weights for the attribute across all diseases, you can multiply the weight by the scoring value and sum across the results for each disease. The diseases with the highest overall scores are the ones best meeting the tips for selection.

Always pretest and prototype any disease management effort. It is easy to start too big and involve too many patients or professionals before possible problems are worked out of the intervention. A good pilot test or prototype program will alleviate this problem. You may want to conduct a pretest in one geographic area or in one site of care, and you could limit the test to one set of professionals and gradually expand to other professionals. All the systems for collecting data, receiving data, analyzing data, and providing any feedback to the health professionals involved or the patients should be tested carefully. *Step 3: Conduct a Pilot Test*

A six-month pilot testing period is reasonable. It might take several more months to establish the disease management program and begin to intervene with patient care. Depending on the disease, changes in outcome may not be apparent after six months of intervention.

The criterion on which to evaluate any program might be whether program goals were met, and you can assess the program by asking several questions:

• Did the health outcomes of patients improve?
• Did providers adopt the professional use of established practice guidelines and appropriate pharmacotherapy?
• Did participants—both health professionals and targeted patients—accept the program?
• Were costs affected favorably or negatively?

The purpose of a pilot is to determine the feasibility of a program and its preliminary impact on health outcomes. Thus, if a disease management program passes these criteria, it should be modified and improved upon for full implementation.

Step 4:
Implement
the Program

The program can be put in place gradually as you are sure the intervention will work properly. Ideally, you want to know that an intervention improves outcomes and lowers costs before implementing a full-blown program. But these results can take some time. Thus, it is always best to build the program gradually either by expanding geographically or by increasing the number of patients.

Figure 8.1 illustrates specific tools for disease management. Claims data are a basic beginning tool for disease management. They can be used first for selecting diseases, describing components of cost by disease, and estimating the expected effect on service use or cost. They are also useful for initially identifying patients who might be targeted for intervention. Patients identified by claims might also be screened and prioritized for intervention in several ways, including available patient surveys, instruments for risk assessment, and baseline measures of health outcomes or functional ability. Many disease management models use these screens for measuring and predicting which

FIGURE 8.1

Common Tools for Disease Management Programs

Tools from the tool box: Disease management involves some or all of the tools shown

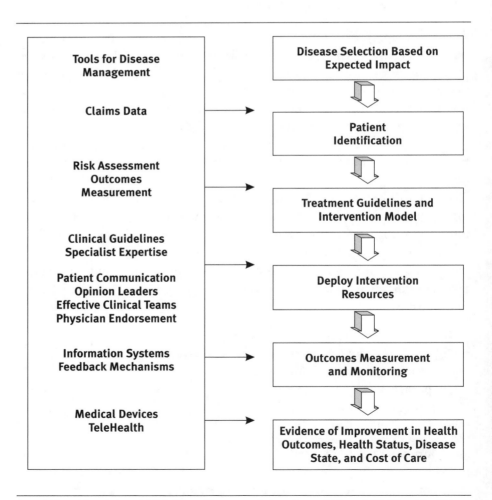

Source: Adapted from Sydnor, J. 1999. *Disease Management Industry Report*. Richmond, VA: Wheat First Union.

All Causes	Per 1,000	Percent in Age Group
65–74 Years of Age	26.1	100
75–84 Years of Age	59.5	100
85 Years of Age or Over	154.8	100
Diseases of the Heart		
65–74 Years of Age	8.5	32.6
75–84 Years of Age	21.8	36.6
85 Years of Age or Over	66.7	43.1
Malignant Neoplasm		
65–74 Years of Age	8.8	33.7
75–84 Years of Age	13.7	23.0
85 Years of Age or Over	18.1	11.7
Cerebrovascular Diseases		
65–74 Years of Age	1.4	5.4
75–84 Years of Age	4.8	8.1
85 Years of Age or Over	16.1	10.4

TABLE 8.3
Number of Deaths per 1,000 Medicare-Age Resident Population, United States

Source: Adapted from the National Center for Health Statistics. 1994. *Health, United States.*

mortality of disease. The incidence and reasons for death can also indicate the financial burden of diseases because death is a costly event to Medicare in the last year of life for a beneficiary.

In 1999, the average beneficiary cost traditional fee-for-service Medicare approximately $22,400 in the last year of life, assuming cost increases since 1996 (Medicare Payment Advisory Commission 1998). Lubitz and Prihoda (1984) found that about 28 percent of Medicare program expenditures were for the 5.9 percent in their last year of life. Within the last year of life, expenditures are further concentrated in the last months of life. About half of all Medicare costs were for service use in the last 60 days of life. About 40 percent of all costs were for service use in the last 30 days. Aside from the obvious heavy emotional burden that these final days place on beneficiaries and their families, the costs of Medicare-covered services in the last year of life clearly can create a serious financial burden.

Table 8.3 shows the death rate from all causes by age along with corresponding numbers for the three most prevalent diseases: diseases of the heart, malignant neoplasm (cancer), and cerebrovascular disease. The table shows the rate per 1,000 in each age group. A plan with 1,000 beneficiaries enrolled in the 65–74 age category could expect 26.1 deaths in a year, assuming similar rates of death as those across the country. In this age category, about one-third would be from diseases of the heart, another third from cancer, and about 5 percent from cerebrovascular diseases. The remainder would come from all other reasons. Among the older age groups, diseases of the heart become somewhat more important, malignant neoplasm declines in importance, and cerebrovascular diseases increase as a cause of death.

Unpublished research from HCFA (McMillan et al. 1990) suggests Medicare managed care plans experience lower death rates across all diseases than the national rate for Medicare beneficiaries. Enrollees tend to be somewhat healthier on average, based on self-reported health status indices. As a group, they have fewer high-cost hospitalizations before joining the managed care plan (Brown et al. 1993). This information suggests that a managed care plan probably would not experience the national average of deaths per 1,000 shown in Table 8.3.

Moreover, the figures in Table 8.3 pertain to the entire population and do not show the burden of the diseases for the typical enrollment in a Medicare managed care plan. About 60 percent of enrollment in the average Medicare managed care plan comes from the youngest age group, 65–74 years of age. Another 33 percent comes from the middle group, 75–84 years of age. The oldest group, 85 years of age and over, accounts for less than 10 percent of the average plan's enrollment (HCFA 1996). If we took into account the relatively younger enrollment in Medicare managed care plans, the relative share of deaths in a managed care plan with an enrollment of greater than 25,000 Medicare beneficiaries would closely reflect the findings shown in Figure 8.3.

Diseases of the heart would account for the bulk of deaths. The next largest single disease is malignant neoplasm, followed by cerebrovascular diseases. All other diseases would account for about one-third of the deaths.

The analysis of known incidence of death among elderly persons by disease shows that although the Medicare managed care population differs from the traditional fee-for-service population, heart disease, malignant neoplasm, and cerebrovascular disease account for more than two-thirds of deaths in a typical HMO. As such, they are a major source of risk for managed care plans in terms of expense and patient burden. Death and its high cost in the last year of life pose a major personal and financial load on patients and any

FIGURE 8.3

Distribution of Deaths in Typical Medicare Managed Care Enrollment

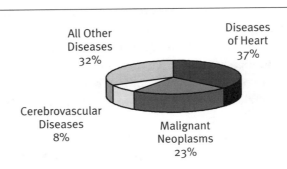

managed care plan. The burden is nearly six times the rate experienced in traditional commercial enrollment (McMillan et al. 1990), the normal source of enrollment for managed care plans. Consequently, managers of Medicare health plans must, at a minimum, carefully develop a strategy to deal with the heavy risk of these three diseases.

The Three Imperative Diseases
Heart Disease

Heart disease is the leading cause of death and is associated with more than one million heart attacks annually, making it Medicare's most frequent reason for a hospital stay. The past 30 years have seen great improvements in the efficacy and effectiveness of therapies, procedures, and interventions for heart disease. It is a remarkable number of variable treatments, including some that are controversial. Medical treatment with diet and exercise seems to help. Surgical treatment with invasive medical procedures also seems to help, as do new drug therapies. Medicines, diet, daily activities, exercise, lifestyle and health habits, and family and social supports are all elements of managing the disease. But to be effective, all these treatments require patients to adhere to a regimen. With proper management, patients can return to normal lives and avoid costly hospital episodes. Heart disease is an excellent disease management candidate based on the disease selection issues discussed above.

Heart failure is the inability of the heart to supply enough blood to meet the body's needs or, more simply, when the heart's pumping power is weaker than normal.

This is not a clinical text on the optimal treatment of heart disease. For this reason, there will be no discussion of the clinical guidelines, which change frequently and require continuous updating and interpretation. But to give an example of the critical administrative elements of disease management, the following sections discuss eligibility criteria for a disease management program and key outcome indicators that could be adopted.

Figure 8.4 shows one definition of **heart failure**. This definition is very inclusive and involves patients with related **congestive heart failure** (CHF) diagnosis. To address the patients most likely to have poor outcomes, you can either focus on the broader group or target those with a previous history of emergency room or inpatient hospital stays.

Congestive heart failure (CHF) occurs when weak heart function is accompanied by a build up of fluids in the body. This happens because blood flow slows, decreasing the amount of blood pumped from the heart. Blood returning to the heart backs up in the veins and forces fluid into surrounding tissues.

Focusing on the more complex CHF patient makes some sense because they are at relatively high risk for rehospitalization. In one national study of Medicare managed care plans, eligible CHF patients admitted to the hospital were age 75.6 on average, evenly split between males and females. In addition, 48.8 percent were single or widowed, 51.2 percent were married, 24.7 percent lived alone, 35.6 percent lived with a spouse, and 39.6 percent lived with others.

The same study on rehospitalization expected well-managed patients to experience excellent history taking and workup. Knowledge of the clinical characteristics of patients indicates good history taking, and Table 8.4 shows these

History

FIGURE 8.4
Practical
Definition of
Heart Failure

*Who is a heart
failure patient?
Eligibility
criteria for a
heart disease
management
program*

Diagnosis of congestive heart failure (ICD-9-CM 428.X) or other heart failure-related conditions (ICD-9-CM 398.1, 402.01, 402.91, 404.04).

Definition includes all claims for inpatient hospital stays, outpatient department, physician office visits, and emergency room visits. If physician office visits only (ICD-9-CM 428.X, 398.1, 402.91, 404.04), then patient was ineligible.

If not at least 65 years old, then patient was ineligible.

Source: Virginia Health Outcomes Partnership. 1998.

findings. The ability to track clinical characteristics of patients gives a health plan the ability to target patients for specific interventions that work best with that characteristic. It also allows the plan to monitor the characteristics of the population over time. Doing this helps you to tell whether the distribution of clinical characteristics changes, for example, in response to a prevention program.

Hypertension and recent weight gain were characteristics of more than half of those admitted to the hospital for CHF. Many heart failure disease management programs focus on these two markers of heart disease. These programs intervene by means of patient education, nurse phone calls, and even monitoring over the Internet, aiming to achieve good health outcomes by managing those indicators.

Medical Management

Certain types of indicators about the process of care might affect outcomes, as Table 8.5 illustrates. A health plan that does an effective job managing heart failure would know the medical management of its patients. In Medicare managed care plans, for example, about 50 percent were advised to restrict salt intake, nearly 90 percent were prescribed a diuretic, 74 percent had nitroglycerin for angina or chest pain, and nearly 50 percent were advised

TABLE 8.4
Illustrative
Outcomes

*Clinical history:
Do you know the
clinical
characteristics of
your enrollees
with congestive
heart failure?*

	Medicare Managed Care Percent of Patients (Preadmission)
Heart failure/enlargement	68.8
Hypertension	54.1
Chronic pulmonary disease	39.4
Angina/chest pain	40.2
Recent weight gain	66.9
Previous admission with acute myocardial infarction	6.5
Admission with cardiac dysrhythmias	21.2
Atrial fibrillation	35.9

Source: Williamson Institute. 1988. *National Medicare Competition Evaluation.* Baltimore, MD: HCFA. See also Retchin, S. M., and B. Brown. 1991. "Elderly Patients with CHF . . ." *American Journal of Medicine* 90 (2): 236–42.

	Medicare Managed Care Percent of Patients
Salt restriction advised	49.4
Diuretic prescribed	89.4
Nitroglycerin for angina/chest pain	73.9
Weight reduction for obese patients	48.2
Modification of medications for uncontrolled blood pressure	36.1
Referral to ophthalmologist	1.2
Follow-up visit within two weeks	75.0

Source: Williamson Institute. 1988. *National Medicare Competition Evaluation.* Baltimore, MD: HCFA.

TABLE 8.5
Illustrative Outcomes

Medical management: Do you know the medical management of your enrollees with CHF at initial evaluation?

about weight control. There are probably only a very few reasons why a CHF patient does not have a follow-up visit with two weeks of a hospital stay, but only 75 percent of patients in this study had a follow-up visit.

The items mentioned in Table 8.5 should lead to greater functioning, reduced admissions to the hospital, and better use of medications. These are all things we would like to see happen for heart failure patients.

Cancer

Patients newly diagnosed with cancer represent a significant opportunity to pursue disease management, but the numerous processes of care depend on the type and stage of cancer. With many cancers, there is not widespread agreement regarding the course of treatment, and outcomes can be poor no matter what is done for the patient. **Colon cancer** is selected here to illustrate the disease management process, however, because there is fairly wide agreement on the treatment process and successful outcomes depending on the stage of disease. Good management of this disease attempts to detect the disease as early as possible and quickly return the patient to normal activities free of the cancer.

Assuming a colon cancer prevention program is already in place, you can identify a fairly homogeneous eligible population for a colon cancer disease management program by examining records on inpatient stays and selecting patients with the disease codes shown in Figure 8.5. Approximately 22 percent of the patients are ineligible for the reasons shown. The primary reason for ineligibility is that a patient has had previous surgery for colon cancer. These patients will likely have a different course of illness, and it may be inappropriate to include them in the group defined by these criteria. They would have a separate or different disease management process.

Not all colon cancer patients are alike. Treatment regimens vary according to the personal characteristics of patients and their functional status. Eligible colon cancer patients in Medicare managed care plans are split almost

Colon cancer is malignant cells (abnormal cells that divide without control or order) found in the tissue of the colon. The colon is part of the digestive system, specifically the last portion of the large intestine.

FIGURE 8.5

Practical
Definition of
Colon Cancer

*Who is a colon
cancer patient?
Eligibility
criteria for a
colon cancer
disease
management
program*

Diagnosis of colon cancer (ICD-8-CM 143.X).

If colorectal surgery not performed during the admission (ICD-8-CM 45.X, 46.X, 48.X) then patient is ineligible. Cases with 45.0–45.41 as the ONLY procedure performed during the hospital admission are ineligible. These cases represent patients who have had only diagnostic procedures on the large intestines, or who have had only local excision of a polyp through colonoscopy.

If not at least 65 years old then patient is ineligible.

If patient did not have at least a 24-hour stay during the admission for the operative procedure then the patient is ineligible.

If previously operated on for colon cancer then patient is ineligible. Patients operated on for other cancers are included.

Source: Mathematica Policy Research. 1992. *The Quality of Care in TEFRA HMOs/CMPs*. Baltimore, MD: HCFA. See also Retchin, S. M., and B. Brown. 1990. "Management of Colorectal Cancer in Medicare Health Maintenance Organizations." *Journal of General Internal Medicine* 5 (2): 110–14.

equally between males (47.6 percent) and females (52.4 percent). Nearly 60 percent are likely to be married, 67 percent live at home with others, and about 25 percent live at home alone. More than 80 percent of patients function at the highest level and are independent in terms of activities of daily living. About 17.5 percent are Stage I cancer, 40.3 percent are Stage II cancer, 28.2 percent are Stage III, and 14.1 percent are Stage IV.

History   To achieve standardized processes of care, the history taking and workup of colon cancer patients are areas in which Medicare managed care plans can be vigilant. Taking a history of melena, taking a family history of cancer, recording examinations for fecal occult blood, and ordering endoscopies or a barium enema study are expected. Table 8.6 shows one likely profile of patient characteristics from such studies.

TABLE 8.6

Illustrative
Outcomes

*History: Do you
know the
clinical
characteristics of
your enrollees
with colon
cancer?*

	Medicare Managed Care Percent of Patients (Preadmission)
Hematocrit <30	15.5
Gastrointestinal bleeding	52.4
Recently altered bowel habits	20.4
Recent abdominal pain	29.6
Weight loss	19.4
Palpable mass	3.6
Obstipation	4.13
Bowel obstruction	4.9

Source: Mathematica Policy Research. 1992. *The Quality of Care in TEFRA HMOs/CMPs*. Baltimore, MD: HCFA. See also Retchin, S. M., and B. Brown. 1990. "Management of Colorectal Cancer in Medicare Health Maintenance Organizations." *Journal of General Internal Medicine* 5 (2): 110–14.

TABLE 8.7
Illustrative
Outcomes

*Initial
evaluation: Do
you know the
days from
presenting
symptoms to
diagnosis for
your enrollees
with colon
cancer?*

	Medicare Managed Care Average Time Lapse (Days)
Anemia	34
Gastrointestinal bleeding	40
Weight loss	40
Abdominal pain	30
All symptoms	37

Source: Mathematica Policy Research. 1992. *The Quality of Care in TEFRA HMOs/CMPs*. Baltimore, MD: HCFA. See also Retchin, S. M., and B. Brown. 1990. "Management of Colorectal Cancer in Medicare Health Maintenance Organizations." *Journal of General Internal Medicine* 5 (2): 110–14.

A majority of patients have gastrointestinal bleeding. About 30 percent have recent abdominal pain. Somewhat fewer have recently altered bowel habits or weight loss. Decreased hematocrit, a palpable mass, and bowel obstruction are likely to be observed among a minority of patients.

Initial Evaluation

Some of the clinical characteristics at the time of admission to the hospital for colon cancer could be associated with delay in treatment. Careful monitoring of the history taking of patients and tracking of the initial evaluation statistics shown in Table 8.7 should provide useful information about disease management for improving outcomes.

For Medicare managed care plans, the average time from presenting symptoms to receiving diagnosis is 37 days. This time varies depending on the symptom. When the symptoms are abdominal pain and anemia, the time lapse is less than 37 days. Gastrointestinal bleeding and weight loss are about ten days longer than other symptoms. Information such as this across sites of care and physicians responsible for first-contact care can be used to improve the time from presenting symptoms until diagnosis.

Diagnostic Studies

Most Medicare managed care plans perform colonoscopy and barium enema on almost all patients (Table 8.8). A flexible sigmoidoscopy is performed on about half of colon cancer patients. Only one-tenth receive rigid sigmoidoscopy.

Medicare managed care plans are much more likely to perform these procedures in an outpatient hospital setting or physicians office, but about 40 percent occur in the hospital, usually in association with the hospital stay for the colon cancer.

The days between the various diagnostic procedures and the operative procedure in the hospital stay vary markedly. But these statistics could be tracked on an ongoing basis to guard against delay between diagnosis and treatment, a potentially important determinant of outcome. Groups of

TABLE 8.8

Illustrative
Outcomes

*Diagnostic
studies: Do you
know the
diagnostic
procedures
performed for
your enrollees
with colon
cancer?*

	Medicare Managed Care Percent of Patients
Colonoscopy	86.4
Barium enema	88.9
Flexible sigmoidoscopy	47.1
Rigid sigmoidoscopy	9.6
Site Procedure Performed	
Inpatient hospital	43.4
Outpatient hospital	33.7
Physician office	10.3
Health plan facility	9.2
Days Between Diagnostic Procedure and Operative Procedure	**Days**
Colonoscopy	15
Barium enema	28
Rigid sigmoidoscopy	3
Flexible sigmoidoscopy	29

Source: Mathematica Policy Research. 1992. *The Quality of Care in TEFRA HMOs/CMPs*. Baltimore, MD: HCFA. See also Retchin, S. M., and B. Brown. 1990. "Management of Colorectal Cancer in Medicare Health Maintenance Organizations." *Journal of General Internal Medicine* 5 (2): 110–14.

patients, individual physicians, or hospitals could perform poorly on this indicator. Corrective action would be suggested if the delays were observed.

Other Examinations

Table 8.9 documents when special services are ordered and what those services are. Managed care plans order nutritional consultation, social work, and home health for patients with colon cancer. They take the longest to order physical therapy and are least likely to order enterostomal therapy. When enterostomal therapy is ordered, however, it is ordered quickly.

Special services such as physical therapy, enterostomal therapy, social work, home health, and nutritional consultation are useful and costly services that the clinical team will want to use effectively. Information on the use of these services can be desirable for showing when the services are most effective and whether some clinicians are overordering or underordering. More specifically, if you can relate the use of special services to improved outcomes, it can be used as evidence for clinical pathways and standard treatment guidelines on an ongoing basis to improve the ordering patterns of clinicians over time.

Staging

Stages II and III are the most common stages of cancer (Table 8.10) for patients in Medicare managed care plans. But colon cancer patients make up as much as 14 percent of Stage IV. Lymph nodes are involved in 37 percent of Medicare managed care patients with colon cancer. Less than 5 percent have evidence of tumor in margin of the resection.

	Medicare Managed Care Percent of Patients
Referrals for Special Services	
Physical Therapy	30.9
Enterostomal Therapy	17.1
Social Work	67.1
Home Health	47.8
Nutritional Consultation	75.5
	Days After Admission When Ordered
Referrals for Special Services	
Physical Therapy	9
Enterostomal Therapy	5
Social Work	7
Home Health	5
Nutritional Consultation	5

TABLE 8.9
Illustrative Outcomes

Other examinations: Do you know the referrals for special services during hospitalization for your enrollees with colon cancer?

Source: Mathematica Policy Research. 1992. *The Quality of Care in TEFRA HMOs/CMPs.* Baltimore, MD: HCFA. See also Retchin, S. M., and B. Brown. 1990. "Management of Colorectal Cancer in Medicare Health Maintenance Organizations." *Journal of General Internal Medicine* 5 (2): 110–14.

	Medicare Managed Care Percent of Patients
Stage I	17.5
Stage II	40.3
Stage III	28.2
Stage IV	14.1
Lymph node involvement	37.6
Evidence of tumor in resection margin	4.9

TABLE 8.10
Illustrative Outcomes

Staging: Do you know the staging and tumor characteristics for your enrollees with colon cancer?

Source: Mathematica Policy Research. 1992. *The Quality of Care in TEFRA HMOs/CMPs.* Baltimore, MD: HCFA. See also Retchin, S. M., and B. Brown. 1990. "Management of Colorectal Cancer in Medicare Health Maintenance Organizations." *Journal of General Internal Medicine* 5 (2): 110–14.

The stage of the cancer is the most important determinant of the approach you should take toward disease management. The clinical team will want to develop customized approaches to manage the disease within each stage of cancer. Of course, the managed care plan should strive to implement those techniques and procedures that find colon cancer as early as possible in terms of stage. Such techniques would begin at initial enrollment into the plan and continue with primary care and specialty care. Screening and preventive services according to recommended guidelines from professional societies should be used and followed in their most current form. Tracking stages of cancer data over several months, quarters, or years should produce a decline in the high stage cancers in the best managed care plans.

Treatment   As Table 8.11 shows, chest x-rays are ordered a great deal to investigate postsurgical elevated temperatures. Chemotherapy is the most likely adjuvant therapy. About one-fifth of patients require wound culture and a urine culture. A protocol for administration of presurgical antibiotics may be necessary. A minority has confusion, perhaps requiring medication or a consultation. The clinical team will want to develop carefully thought-out protocols regarding the administration of sedative-hypnotics for postsurgical confusion.

Follow-Up   Table 8.12 shows that slightly less than 70 percent of colon cancer patients in Medicare managed care have a follow-up appointment after the procedure. Very few patients have occupational therapy, but nearly half receive home health services post discharge. Wound care instructions are important for nearly one-third of colon cancer patients. About one-fourth have enterostomal therapy. Nearly all colon cancer patients are sent home, either alone or with others at home. Almost none go to the rehabilitation hospital. Nearly all plans describe diet, give medication instructions, and describe the new limitations on activities to their colon cancer patients.

Follow-up across sites of care—inpatient and outpatient—and the information technology systems to make it work are where Medicare managed care plans can excel. These plans have higher organizational structure and financial interest in avoiding costly hospital services.

This presentation of specific process of care and measures of health outcome for colon cancer shows us what needs to be done and how much needs to be done to manage information. A good disease management program for any cancer—but colon cancer specifically—should begin with identifying which patients require management. This identification process could start before patients even get the disease. It could involve primary prevention and

TABLE 8.11
Illustrative
Outcomes

*Treatment: Do
you know the
prevalence and
treatment of
postsurgical
complications
for your colon
cancer patients?*

	Medicare Managed Care Percent of Patients
Temperature >101 degrees Fahrenheit	24.4
Chest x-ray	49.5
Wound culture	18.2
Urine culture	49.4
Confusion	14.5

Source: Mathematica Policy Research. 1992. *The Quality of Care in TEFRA HMOs/CMPs*. Baltimore, MD: HCFA. See also Retchin, S. M., and B. Brown. 1990. "Management of Colorectal Cancer in Medicare Health Maintenance Organizations." *Journal of General Internal Medicine* 5 (2): 110–14.

	Medicare Managed Care Percent of Patients
Follow-up appointment scheduled	69.1
Diet described at discharge	89.7
Medication instructions given	87.8
Limitations on activities described	88.1
Occupational therapy post discharge	8.3
Home health services post discharge	48.6
Wound care instructions given	65.3
Enterostomal therapy planned	23.0
Discharge destination:	
Home alone	10.6
Home with others	72.5
Nursing home	6.4
Rehabilitation hospital	0.5
Other unspecified	10.0

TABLE 8.12

Illustrative Outcomes

Follow-up: Do you know the discharge planning services and destination for your enrollees with colon cancer?

Source: Mathematica Policy Research. 1992. *The Quality of Care in TEFRA HMOs/CMPs.* Baltimore, MD: HCFA. See also Retchin, S. M., and B. Brown. 1990. "Management of Colorectal Cancer in Medicare Health Maintenance Organizations." *Journal of General Internal Medicine* 5 (2): 110–14.

screening for various cancers and include providing patients and physicians with information about cancer in general.

Having the methods and systems for early detection and diagnosis is vital, and you should conduct a critical review of your plan to make sure these are in place. At the same time, it is meaningful to know the clinical characteristics of your patients with any cancer. Such information will permit you to adopt customized approaches to care management and adjust health outcomes data for risk, if necessary, to account for differences among patients in personal characteristics, stage of cancer, and comorbid conditions.

Another thing the colon cancer example illustrates is how information on health outcomes can be extremely valuable to an interdisciplinary team trying to change dramatically the way it provides care. Having the ongoing capability to monitor the stage of cancer, postsurgical complications (in the case of colon cancer), functional status, and destination of patients is a powerful tool for knowing what does and does not work as changes are made in the process of care. Feedback on patient outcomes can provide evidence as to whether intended strategies for disease management are realized or whether you need a new emerging strategy such as those discussed above.

Stroke

A disease management program for **stroke** should begin with several of the many available good indicators of health outcomes for patients. A workable definition of patients with stroke should be developed to track stroke outcomes. To have a fairly homogeneous mix of patients to measure changes and

Stroke, or cerebrovascular accident, is the result of a sudden reduction in blood flow to an area of the brain. When blood cannot reach the brain, cells there become deprived of oxygen and die. When this happens, abilities or functions controlled by that part of the brain become impaired or lost.

make comparisons of outcomes properly, certain patients should be included and others excluded.

For example, Figure 8.6 shows the criteria for identifying patients with stroke and the criteria for excluding certain patients. Patients with stroke are identified as those having an inpatient hospital stay that falls in the prescribed ICD-8-CM codes shown in Figure 8.6. A managed care plan using these criteria is likely to find, among all patients with the prescribed ICD-8-CM codes, that approximately 19 percent will be ineligible for the reasons shown.

Eligible cerebrovascular accident patients in Medicare managed care plans are equally likely to be male as female, and about 60 percent are married. In terms of admission to the hospital, about 70 percent come to the hospital from home where they live with others, nearly 4 percent transfer from another hospital, nearly 90 percent are admitted through the hospital emergency room, and about 8 percent are admitted through another hospital's emergency room. The admission through another hospital emergency room reflects the influence of managed care in terms of transferring patients to a network hospital from a non-network hospital after the initial hospital admission. The well-managed health plan will want to track transfers and develop enrollee education efforts to minimize transfers from non-network hospitals to network hospitals. Of course, a patient with a stroke should go to the nearest appropriate hospital to be stabilized and evaluated.

Stroke patients require urgent hospitalization to ensure proper diagnosis. A team of clinical experts should become involved with the care of the patient immediately upon admission and begin to plan for discharge. Stroke patients also require care post hospitalization. The type of care and its duration can dramatically affect outcomes and costs. Thus, the same clinical team should follow the health plan's stroke patients and build a database of ongoing outcomes to determine what works best for patients in a particular health plan.

History   From the data shown in Table 8.13, most patients with stroke in a managed care plan have hypertension. About a third of stroke patients have had a previous stroke.

Good documentation of the medical history of the patient is standard medical practice. For managed care plans, having information about the medical history of your patients helps to interpret outcome results. Well-documented medical history can account for beginning differences in the case mix of stroke patients that might explain differences in outcomes. Table 8.13 shows a workable list of clinical characteristics of patients that might be taken from a clinical history and reported in the hospital record for good patient management. This information is useful to have in a database when conducting a retrospective review and analyzing outcome results.

It would be reasonable to make a separate comparison of health outcomes, such as neurological deficit at discharge, for patients with and without hypertension. That way, you could evaluate the effect of posthospital care after each stroke on subsequent strokes and costly hospitalization.

Diagnosis of cerebrovascular accident (CVA), stroke, or cerebral thrombosis or the following ICD-8-CM codes 431, 434.X, 346.X.

If a physician noted that all of the marker CVA symptoms resolved within 24 hours then the patient is ineligible. Answer on the admission history and physical, consult, or progress reports from day 1 or 2, and the discharge summary.

If first symptoms associated with CVA had onset more than 14 days prior to the admission then the patient is ineligible. Answer should be based on the admission history and physical, consult, or progress reports from day 1 or 2, and the discharge summary.

If patient had any of the following diagnoses then the case is ineligible: subdural bleed, multiple sclerosis (MS), head trauma resulting in skull fracture, meningitis, encephalitis, brain abscess, primary or metastatic cancer involving the brain, on chronic dialysis, or history of kidney transplant.

If patient was noted to have evidence of definite, probable, or possible new myocardial infarction (MI) or heart attack on an EKG report on day 1, then the patient is ineligible.

FIGURE 8.6

Practical Definition of Stroke

Who is a stroke patient? Eligibility criteria for a stroke disease management program

---

If the patient did not have at least one of the following symptoms or signs on admission, the patient is ineligible:

Visual deficit: loss of or diminished eyesight, blurred vision, field defect, optic atrophy, hemianopsia or visual inattention.

Sensory/motor deficit or face: change in feeling, tingling, numbness or paralysis of face

Speech deficit: aphasia, dysphasia, dysarthria, difficulty talking, slurred speech

Motor deficit of limbs: compromise, paralysis, paresis, weakness of extremities (fingers, hands, arms, toes, feet, or legs), ataxia, abnormal gait

Sensory deficit of limbs: change in feeling, tingling, numbness, dysethesia, paresthesia of extremities (fingers, hands, arms, toes, feet, or legs)

Coma: comatose, unresponsive, unarousable, coma vigil, unconscious, responding only to painful stimuli

Symptoms of neurological change: somnolent, lethargic, poorly arousable, semicomatose, stuporous, obtunded (exclude seizure, syncope, restlessness, or agitation)

Exhibiting posturing: described as decerebrate or decorticate

Not responding to touch or tactile stimuli

Unable to follow commands

Confused or having a seizure

Source: Mathematica Policy Research. 1992. *The Quality of Care in TEFRA HMOs/CMPs.* Baltimore, MD: HCFA. See also Retchin, S. M., and B. Brown. 1990. "Management of Colorectal Cancer in Medicare Health Maintenance Organizations." *Journal of General Internal Medicine* 5 (2): 110–14.

TABLE 8.13
Illustrative
Outcomes

History: Do you know the clinical characteristics of your enrollees with stroke?

	Medicare Managed Care Percent of Patients (Preadmission)
Myocardial infarction within four months prior or history of CHF	22.5
Atrial fibrillation or flutter on admission	20.3
Previous CVA, stroke, or transient ischemic attack	33.3
Prior hospitalization within previous six months	15.3
Dementia	12.3
Do-not-resuscitate orders given during hospital admission	25.4
Cancer	12.4
Diabetes mellitus	21.4
Hypertension	59.5
Angina	9.2
Chronic pulmonary disease	14.7

Source: Mathematica Policy Research. 1992. *The Quality of Care in TEFRA HMOs/CMPs*. Baltimore, MD: HCFA. See also Retchin, S. M. et al. 1997. "Outcomes of Stroke Patients. . . ." *Journal of the American Medical Association* 278 (2): 119–24.

Medical Management

Most stroke patients in Medicare managed care plans have a motor deficit (86.6 percent) or speech deficit (67.7 percent) at admission. The percentage with motor deficit declines from admission to discharge (61.6 percent), and the percentage with speech deficit declines from admission to discharge as well (55.6 percent). Likewise, the percentage of patients with a visual deficit falls. Between 20 and 30 percent have a visual deficit, obtundation or stupor, an inability to follow directions, or confusion. Some of these indicators of deficit improve while others do not improve during the hospital stay (Table 8.14).

Monitoring neurological deficit at admission, discharge, and post discharge can provide constant feedback about the physician care and medications

TABLE 8.14
Illustrative
Outcomes

Medical management: Do you know the neurological deficits of your enrollees with stroke at admission and at discharge?

	Medicare Managed Care Percent of Patients	
	Admission	Discharge
Visual deficit	28.4	20.4
Speech deficit	67.7	55.6
Motor deficit	86.6	61.6
Coma or unresponsive	8.2	14.3
Obtundation/stupor	20.4	19.7
Unable to follow commands	17.4	24.0
Confusion	23.8	28.4

Source: Mathematica Policy Research. 1992. *The Quality of Care in TEFRA HMOs/CMPs*. Baltimore, MD: HCFA. See also Retchin, S. M. et al. 1997. "Outcomes of Stroke Patients. . . ." *Journal of the American Medical Association* 278 (2): 119–24.

that improve outcomes. A relatively simple assessment of a stroke patient's neurological deficits at both admission to and discharge from the hospital can provide a useful mechanism for comparing different processes of care. The assessment also allows you to compare variations in the performance of the physicians and hospitals caring for stroke patients. The assessment shown in Table 8.15 could be a start for ongoing data collection and analysis for each disease state during and after the initial hospitalization.

The health outcomes of stroke patients can also be measured in terms of functional status as shown in Table 8.15. Some of the information can be obtained from the medical record, but **activities of daily living** are perhaps best captured by the discharge planning or case management staff. With a database that contains the functional status of patients at discharge, physicians can track methods of improvement. And for patients with similar functional status, providers and case management staff can plan best practices for patients with certain posthospital care, reducing variations in the posthospital care processes.

Activities of daily living (ADL) is a patient-reported measurement of an individual's ability to cope with his or her environment. Major components can include the following: eating, getting in and out of bed, getting around, dressing, bathing, and using the toilet.

A large number of Medicare managed care patients have an indwelling catheter at discharge (36.4 percent), requiring special posthospital home care. About one-fourth are bed-bound upon discharge. Over 10 percent die while in the hospital. In terms of activities of daily living, nearly two-thirds of patients require help with transfers as they conduct their daily living. Half or more require assistance with dressing, bathing, and toileting.

The interdisciplinary clinical team, when presented with ongoing assessment of the patient with stroke, can develop approaches to improve activities of daily living. Improved outcomes in the hospital, along with intervention and patient education while an outpatient or at home, will return the patient to normal functioning and make efficient use of posthospital nursing and other services.

	Medicare Managed Care Percent of Patients (at Discharge)
Indwelling catheter	36.4
New incontinence	7.4
Bed-bound	25.3
New ducubitis ulcer	2.7
Died	12.2
Activities of Daily Living (ADL)	
Eating	39.7
Transfer	60.3
Dressing	50.1
Bathing	55.5
Toileting	51.8

TABLE 8.15

Illustrative Outcomes

Functional status: Do you know the functional status of your enrollees with stroke at discharge?

Source: Mathematica Policy Research. 1992. *The Quality of Care in TEFRA HMOs/CMPs*. Baltimore, MD: HCFA. See also Retchin, S. M. et al. 1997. "Outcomes of Stroke Patients. . . ." *Journal of the American Medical Association* 278 (2): 119–24.

Nursing Care, Respiratory therapy is applied for about 15 percent of patients on the first day.
Respiratory Speech therapy starts early on the stay at two days for about 25 percent of
Therapy, and patients. About 40 percent of patients have physician therapy by the second
Vital Signs day. Nearly half of stroke patients see the dietitian during their stay in Medicare
managed care settings. (See Table 8.16.)

Though not shown in the table, a significant number of stroke patients
have cardiac disease at discharge, as evidenced by findings of cardiomegaly
(enlarged heart), intertestinal edema, and pulmonary edema (fluid in the
lung). Approximately 20 percent of patients with stroke have a temperature
greater than 101 degrees Fahrenheit at discharge.

Medicare managed care stroke patients have shorter lengths of stay
than an otherwise similar set of traditional Medicare fee-for-service patients.
According to one study, nevertheless, mortality rates during hospitalization
are very similar. For patients in Medicare managed care, the mortality rate is
12.2 percent. In the traditional fee-for-service plan, the rate is 14.7 percent.

It is easy to skimp on these therapeutic services in the hospital and lower
the cost of hospitalization, depending on how the hospital is paid. However,
if some services are not provided and outcomes deteriorate, the risk of costly
rehospitalization and higher levels of posthospital care are obvious. It is crucial,
therefore, to balance the provision of services to achieve the best outcome that
requires the fewest resources.

How and when the therapies shown in Table 8.16 should be delivered
during and after the stay is an issue best left for the interdisciplinary clinical
team managing the care. The strategic management issue is whether you know
the answers for your patients and your clinicians have sound reasons for patterns of service use you observe. These and other vital signs might bear watching by the health plan to guard against premature discharge from the hospital.

Intensive Care In Medicare managed care settings, approximately one-fourth of Medicare
and Ethical managed care patients have do-not-resuscitate (DNR) orders in their hospital
Decisions stay. Fewer than 10 percent have ventilation withheld or withdrawn, and fewer
than 5 percent have vasopressors withheld or withdrawn. Intensive care is
provided to more than 20 percent of stroke patients, and 15 percent of all
days for the average stroke patient are spent in intensive care.

TABLE 8.16
Illustrative
Outcomes

Therapies: Do
you know the
services for your
enrollees with
stroke during
the hospital stay?

	Medicare Managed Care Percent of Patients (During Hospital Stay)
Respiratory Therapy First Day	14.8
Speech Therapy Second Day	27.7
Physical Therapy Second Day	42.8
Dietitian During Stay	47.1

Source: Mathematica Policy Research. 1992. *The Quality of Care in TEFRA HMOs/CMPs*. Baltimore, MD: HCFA.
See also Retchin, S. M. et al. 1997. "Outcomes of Stroke Patients. . . ." *Journal of the American Medical Association*
278 (2): 119–24.

	Medicare Managed Care Percent of Patients	TABLE 8.17

TABLE 8.17
Illustrative
Outcomes

	Medicare Managed Care Percent of Patients
Do Not Resuscitate (DNR) Orders	25.4
Ventilation Withheld/Withdrawn	8.5
Vasopressors Withheld/Withdrawn	4.5
Admitted Intensive Care Unit	21.6
Proportion Days in Intensive Care Unit	15.0

*Intensive care:
Do you know the
ethical decision
making and use
of resource-
intensive services
of your enrollees
with stroke?*

Source: Mathematica Policy Research. 1992. *The Quality of Care in TEFRA HMOs/CMPs.* Baltimore, MD: HCFA. See also Retchin, S. M. et al. 1997. "Outcomes of Stroke Patients. . . ." *Journal of the American Medical Association* 278 (2): 119–24.

Each of the items in Table 8.17 has important outcome and financial consequences for a Medicare managed care plan. In data not shown here, 85 percent of patients with DNR orders during their hospital stay died within 30 months post discharge.

DNR orders are not uncommon, but any good managed care plan should have a mechanism for carefully monitoring the frequency of DNR orders on its inpatients. Normally, such practices are established hospital by hospital and physician by physician in consultation with the patient and the patient's family. But managed care plans will want to avoid even the appearance of a connection between the economic incentives offered to providers and provider decision making with regard to DNR orders.

An ongoing database of such orders should be an invaluable tool to track patterns and changes in patterns of such orders by hospital, physician, and type of patient. Admission to the intensive care unit is costly but necessary. Over time, it is better to know what the trends are when it comes to patients with DNR orders rather than not know those trends and then guess at what happens to your stroke patients in the hospital.

Medicare managed care stroke patients have substantially fewer discretionary tests and procedures performed than traditional fee-for-service patients. A small number of stroke patients receive carotid angiography, about one-third receive carotid doppler, and roughly 17 to 30 percent receive an EEG or an echocardiogram. (See Table 8.18.)

**Test and
Procedure
Ordering**

The relationship between the use of discretionary tests and procedures and outcomes is not well documented. Well-managed health plans should develop protocols and pathways to achieve optimal use of tests and procedures. A multidisciplinary team of appropriate providers would be the best group to develop these protocols in accordance with local standards of medical care. If the outcome data described above are collected, gradually your own stroke patients can provide the evidence for the benefit of ordering discretionary tests and procedures. Table 8.18 provides an illustration of what can be done for Medicare managed care plans.

TABLE 8.18

Illustrative
Outcomes

*Tests: Do you
know the
number of tests
and procedures
performed on
your enrollees
with stroke?*

	Medicare Managed Care Percent of Patients
Carotid angiography	3.5
Carotid doppler	33.3
EEG	17.7
Echocardiogram	29.1

Source: Mathematica Policy Research. 1992. *The Quality of Care in TEFRA HMOs/CMPs*. Baltimore, MD: HCFA. See also Retchin, S. M. et al. 1997. "Outcomes of Stroke Patients. . . ." *Journal of the American Medical Association* 278 (2): 119–24.

**Discharge
Planning**

A follow-up appointment would seem to be a simple feature of good discharge planning, but only 54 percent of stroke patients in Medicare managed care have one (Table 8.19). Most patients have diet prescribed, medication instructions given, and their new limits on activities described. Occupational therapy or home health services continue post discharge for only about 30 percent of stroke patients.

One of the most important functions in managing this disease is discharge planning because certain destinations can be very costly with poorly documented outcomes. Rarely are stroke patients sent directly home alone. Nearly 40 percent are sent home with others. Twenty-eight percent go to the nursing home. About 20 percent are sent to a rehabilitation hospital.

Medicare managed care plans are well known for having higher use of nursing homes. In the case of stroke patients, managed care plans would appear to substitute nursing home care for rehabilitation facility use compared with traditional fee-for-service care. Whether that is judicious use of expensive

TABLE 8.19

Illustrative
Outcomes

*Discharge
planning: Do
you know the
destination for
your enrollees
with stroke?*

	Medicare Managed Care Percent of Patients
Follow-up Appointment Scheduled	54.0
Diet Described at Discharge	83.0
Medication Instructions Given	90.1
Limitations on Activities Described	80.2
Occupational Therapy Post Discharge	31.4
Home Health Services Post Discharge	30.9
Discharge Destination:	
Home Alone	3.1
Home with Others	37.1
Nursing Home	28.7
Rehabilitation Hospital	20.4

Source: Mathematica Policy Research. 1992. *The Quality of Care in TEFRA HMOs/CMPs*. Baltimore, MD: HCFA. See also Retchin, S. M. et al. 1997. "Outcomes of Stroke Patients. . . ." *Journal of the American Medical Association* 278 (2): 119–24.

care for managed care plans and excessive use on the part of traditional fee-for-service is unclear. However, in at least one study, managed care and fee-for-service patients had similar survival patterns.

Approximately two dozen outcome-assessment tools for stroke patients are available and have been used. The measures of health outcomes shown here are presented because they have been used to study Medicare managed care plans and are the most current available for such plans, rather than traditional fee-for-service Medicare. Showing precisely what measures of process and outcome can be obtained for stroke patients illustrates the potential for managing the disease. Of course, you assume that health professionals charged with the management of care at the local level are capable of using feedback on health outcomes to improve the care.

New diagnostic approaches and pharmaceuticals are brought to the market all the time for this disease, making it impossible for a book of this type to address these approaches precisely. Rather, this chapter illustrates the strategic possibilities for combining the four elements of disease management to improve health outcomes for elderly enrollees. For patients, after all, improved health outcomes is the bottom line.

WHERE TO START: *Available Guidelines for Heart Failure*

- Mayo Foundation for Medical Education and Research. 1997. "Congestive Heart Failure: What Happens When You Can't Keep Up?" *Mayo Clinic Health Letter* (July); www.mayohealth.org.
- American College of Cardiology/American Heart Association. "Guidelines for the Evaluation of Management of Heart Failure." Report of the American College of Cardiology/American Heart Association; www.americanheart.org.
- U.S. Department of Health and Human Services. 1995. "Cardiac Rehabilitation." Rockville, MD: Public Health Service, AHCRQ.
- Committee on Evaluation and Management of Heart Failure, 1995. "Task Force in Practice Guidelines." *Journal of the American College of Cardiology* 26 (5): 1376.

WHERE TO START: *Available Guidelines for Cancer*

- "ACS Guidelines for Screening and Surveillance for Early Detection of Colorectal Polyps and Cancer: Update 1997." *Cancer* 47 (3): 154–60.
- "Clinical Practice Guidelines for the Use of Tumor Markers in Breast and Colorectal Cancer." *Journal of Clinical Oncology* 16 (2): 793–95.
- Association of Community Cancer Centers. 1999. *Rectal Cancer.* Rockville, MD: ACCC.

WHERE TO START: *Available Guidelines for Stroke*

- American College of Physicians. 1994. "Guidelines for Medical Treatment for Stroke Prevention." *Annals of Internal Medicine.* 121 (1): 41–55.
- Canadian Task Force on Preventive Health Care. 1994. "Hypertension in the Elderly: Case-Finding and Treatment to Prevent Vascular Disease." Ottawa, Canada, 944–51; www.ctfphc.org.
- AHCRQ. 1995. *Post-Stroke Rehabilitation.* Clinical Guideline Number 16, publication no. 95-0062.

Strategic Decisions Checklist

Strategic Questions	Strategic Analyses
How important is strategic management in your health plan?	Know the requirements of your customers.
	Know how you know the requirements of your customers.
	Take time to plan change, even when the payoff is in the future.
Are you striving to manage diseases?	Emphasize using multidisciplinary clinical teams that encourage health professionals to plan changes in the way they treat patients.
	Collect and analyze relevant data that can help these groups plan for changes in the way they treat patients.
	Adopt cost-effective technologies for managing diseases.
Do you have managers or decision-making units who evaluate strategic management efforts?	Encourage flexibility and experimentation.
	Recognize when a disease management effort is not working and facilitate new, emerging strategies.
Do you take a manager's view of the epidemiology of your enrollees and know the incidence and prevalence of imperative diseases?	Use your data systems to analyze the types and burden of diseases among your enrollees so you can track increases or decreases over time.
	Frequently prioritize diseases for new programs and monitor outside "best practices" for inclusion in your efforts to manage disease.
Do you have an outcomes-based disease management program for patients with heart failure?	Know the clinical characteristics of your enrollees with heart failure.
	Know the medical management of your enrollees with heart failure at initial evaluation.
	Constantly improve the interventions that lower blood pressure and cause sudden weight gain.

continued

Strategic Questions	Strategic Analyses
	Know the recommendations for your patients with heart disease, and check for adherence to patients' treatment regimens.
	Monitor readmissions to the hospital for heart disease and identify the factors that are associated with costly admissions.
Do you have an outcomes-based disease-management program for patients with cancer?	Know the clinical characteristics of your enrollees with cancer.
	Know the number of days from presenting symptoms to diagnosis.
	Know the diagnostic procedures performed.
	Know the referrals for special services during hospitalization.
	Know the staging and tumor characteristics.
	Know the prevalence and treatment of postsurgical complications.
	Know the discharge planning services and their destination post hospitalization.
Do you have an outcomes-based disease management program for patients with stroke?	Know the clinical characteristics of your enrollees with stroke.
	Know their neurological deficits.
	Know their functional status at discharge.
	Know the special services during the hospital stay.
	Know the ethical decision making and use of resource-intensive services.
	Know the diagnostic test and procedures performed.
	Know the discharge-planning services and the destination post hospitalization.

continued

Strategic Questions	Strategic Analyses
How do you start a good disease management program?	Follow the basic steps: 1. Feasibility 2. Disease Selection 3. Pilot Testing 4. Implementation
Have you determined the epidemiology of diseases among the enrollees in your health plan for management purposes?	Manage diseases by managing information technology with data systems that support analysis of the types and burdens of diseases. Track changes in disease incidence and prevalence, especially to show improvement from interventions. Frequently prioritize diseases for interventions. Monitor the best practices of others for possible implementation.

BASIC CARE

The **basic care** your health plan delivers to Medicare beneficiaries has a strategic influence on how effectively your plan enrolls, retains, and satisfies your members. And it almost goes without saying that how well you enroll, retain, and satisfy members has a major effect on your bottom line.

How does one define basic care? What does it include? Basic care means delivering appropriate primary care, and it includes evaluating patients, taking medical history, conducting diagnostic tests and screenings, providing immunizations, and managing common chronic conditions found in the elderly population. Managed care plans can help their network of primary care providers deliver good basic care in a variety of ways. First, these plans can collect appropriate data on their members on an ongoing basis. They can also adopt cost-effective technologies for sharing information and communicating, and they can provide clinicians with feedback on the care they provide and the outcomes they achieve.

In addition to what good basic care means to your providers, it also represents an opportunity to educate your members. More than a way to screen and assess patients, good basic care that is fully developed can be a way to engage your enrollees in a dynamic relationship with your health plan. If you're able to communicate both to your providers and your members the value of good basic care, then enrollees will begin to have a vested interest in the managed care ethic. The evidence shows, however, that Medicare managed care plans are not achieving the best basic care that they can provide, even though they're better than traditional fee-for-service on a number of fronts. They lack the tools they need to retain members, and these tools affect enrollee satisfaction dramatically.

Naturally, all these components of care—enrollment, retention, satisfaction—influence the operation of your plan, but they also have strategic consequences. Why? Because the basic care that enrollees receive represents the experience most members will have with your health plan most of the time. The experience you create for your enrollees is the primary way you differentiate your plan from those of your rivals. Members will talk with nonmembers about the basic care your plan provides and, assuming the comments are positive, encourage new enrollment. For these members, good basic care can be low-cost care, so it's important to remember the financial side of strategic advantage.

It is well beyond the scope of this book to provide a serious clinical analysis of good basic primary care. Still, we know from our experience with

Basic care is the ambulatory care given to enrollees by physicians and other clinicians including primary (first contact) care, medical evaluation, history taking, diagnostic tests, screening, immunizations, and management of chronic conditions found in the elderly.

Medicare managed care plans what constitutes good basic care. This chapter, which is based on that experience, takes a simple, strategic management approach to evaluating good basic care for Medicare beneficiaries—an approach that relies on outcomes measurement and benchmarking. In this respect, defining good basic care is similar to evaluating disease management, which is discussed in Chapter 8.

The strategic approach on which our discussion is based also relies on feedback to the clinicians who are the first line of contact for your Medicare enrollees. That first-line contact can be nurtured and improved through good patient-physician communication, and your managed care plan can help its clinicians improve their communication skills. Your plan can also build a relationship or a physician-enrollee partnership around information sharing to enhance patient self-care and to anticipate patient problems. Thus, strengthened, physician-patient communication can build up enrollment and reduce healthcare costs.

Initial Patient Evaluation and Performance of Tests, Screenings, and Immunizations

Most successful Medicare managed care plans have well-defined expectations of the primary care physicians who serve their membership, and these expectations include prompt intake procedures for new enrollees. After perhaps years of being exposed to the unbridled fee-for-service Medicare system, Medicare patients are familiar with a system in which no one seems to mind the store. These patients are accustomed to seeing multiple physicians and being prescribed numerous drugs. So ushering new enrollees quickly under well-directed basic care is a first priority at enrollment. This initial situation is a perfect opportunity to teach new enrollees how to use your plan effectively so that they can get the care they need.

Initial Evaluation

What types of things should be done when new enrollees come into the system? What should Medicare managed care plans do at initial patient evaluation? Table 9.1 presents actual rates of compliance with indicators of standard basic primary care. The data are taken from HCFA's evaluation of the early experience with Medicare managed care and represent a large sample of patient records from more than 800 physician practices within eight large HMOs in different parts of the country. The data were collected through medical chart reviews from the early Medicare managed care experience. The results represent the only known level of compliance with initial patient evaluation and medical history taking in Medicare managed care. Of course, the goal is to have 100 percent adherence to each criterion of basic care.

Are the rates of adherence for *your* plan higher or lower than the actual rates for the average network of primary care physicians? To answer

	Percent
Post-Medical History or Hospitalization	88.5
Drug Allergies	83.0
Display of Drug Allergies	78.2
Med Listing	90.9
Gastrointestinal History	58.5
Genitourinary History	58.0
Respiratory History	59.3
Mental Status History	46.4
Musculoskeletal History	55.4
Neurological History	53.2
Implicit History	31.2
History of Tobacco Use	74.7
History of Alcohol Use	67.8
Social History	38.7
Functional Status	59.6

TABLE 9.1
Illustrative Primary Care Outcomes

Start at the beginning: Do you know initial patient evaluation and medical history taking in your health plan?

Source: Williamson Institute. 1988. *National Medicare Competition Evaluation.* Baltimore, MD: HCFA. See also Retchin, S. M., and B. Brown. 1990. "The Quality of Ambulatory Care in Medicare Health Maintenance Organization." *American Journal of Public Health* 80 (4): 411–5.

this question, you need to know the rates of adherence among your network of primary care physicians. Table 9.1 shows actual rates of adherence, which we expect to be lower than the ideal rates. If you know the rates for your health plan, you also know whether you need to improve this key component of basic care in your network. The assumption is that better rates of adherence translate into higher quality care, and higher quality care leads to healthier patients. Healthier patients have fewer costly medical problems, and the problems they do encounter are caught sooner.

When you look at the charts of primary care physicians serving Medicare beneficiaries enrolled in managed care plans, 88.5 percent indicate whether a post-medical history or previous hospitalization is in the patient's background. Likewise, 83 percent indicate drug allergies and the types of display of drug allergies, and most indicate a medication list. The medication list is very important for gaining control of the ongoing treatment regimen, and having access to this list is one of the major benefits of the coordination of care that can come from Medicare managed care. Good initial patient evaluation also means thorough history taking across all the major systems shown in Table 9.1. But detailed history taking is not noted in most charts for Medicare beneficiaries. Taking a patient's medical history for gastrointestinal, genitourinary, respiratory, mental status, musculoskeletal, and neurological problems occurs less than 60 percent of the time. An implicit history—meaning a complete and detailed history—occurs only about one-third of the time.

The rates of adherence increase when it comes to the use of tobacco and alcohol. A social history of the patient's living arrangements—alone, with one other cohabitant, familial, institutionalized—is found less than 40 percent of the time. And a simple indication of functional outcome is only noted around 60 percent of the time, suggesting that most practices don't have an ongoing mechanism for monitoring improvement in functional status.

Baseline Tests, Screening, and Immunizations

Medicare beneficiaries increasingly know the general guidelines for screening and immunization, and they demand to have these types of tests completed. The Medicare program emphasizes these benefits in a variety of communications to beneficiaries. Beyond simply responding to the demands of beneficiaries, the well-run managed care plan will want to perform baseline tests, periodic screening, and immunizations at recommended levels because it is good medical care. The direct effect on total costs in Medicare managed care is not documented, but good-quality care and early detection of disease are presumed to lead to lower healthcare costs and more satisfied beneficiaries in your plan.

Table 9.2 suggests that the rates of adherence vary for most practices in Medicare managed care. For blood pressure recording, weight recording, UA, hemoglobin, BUN/creatinine levels, and ECG readings, the data show that medical plans demonstrate a respectable, high rate of completion. Most practices should do well if they meet or exceed the levels reported here. Less often do we find that plans provide baseline tests for visual acuity, tonometry, mammography, hemoccult tests, and flu immunizations.

Basic Diabetes Care

Diabetes is a chronic illness that requires continual medical care and education to prevent acute complications and to reduce the risk of long-term

TABLE 9.2

Illustrative Diabetes Care Outcomes

It's expected: Do you know the rates of completion of baseline tests, screening, and immunizations?

	Percent
BP Recording	97.0
Weight Recording	88.4
Visual Acuity	44.2
Tonometry	73.9
Mammography	32.8
Hemoccult Test	49.7
UA	80.6
Hemoglobin	87.8
BUN/Creatinine	85.0
ECG	78.3
Flu Immunization	18.2

Source: Williamson Institute. 1988. *National Medicare Competition Evaluation.* Baltimore, MD: HCFA. See also Retchin, S. M., and J. Preston. 1991. "The Effects of Cost-Containment on the Care of Elderly Diabetics." *Archives of Internal Medicine* 151 (11) 2244–8.

complications. Type 2 diabetes mellitus affects approximately 16 million Americans, usually occurring in people over age 45 who are overweight. The prevalence of type 2 is higher in Native Americans, African Americans, Asian Americans, and Latino populations than in European Americans. However, an estimated nearly 20 percent of Americans age 65–74 have diabetes, and many of these people have not yet been diagnosed with the illness. As such, diabetes should be considered a high-priority disease by any health plan. The bottom line is this: Have a game plan for improving the quality of care and lowering the costs of treating members with diabetes.

Medical Management

Patients and clinicians can find treatment guidelines for diabetes at www. diabetes.org, and these are frequently updated. Table 9.3 illustrates the types of indicators that can help any health plan do a better job managing care for diabetes. The elements of care shown in the table come from the only large national study of patients with diabetes who received care through a Medicare managed care plan (Retchin and Preston 1991). Table 9.3 shows results for diabetic Medicare patients who were enrolled in eight early Medicare managed care plans from around the country. The percentage reflects the ratio of patients according to certain standard indicators of quality.

Approximately 20 percent of patients in Medicare managed care are likely to be treated with insulin, and nearly all (98.1 percent) had the oral

TABLE 9.3
Illustrative Diabetes Care Outcomes

Medical management: Do you know the basic diabetes care provided in your health plan?

Indicators	Percent
Oral Hypoglycemic Schedule Recorded	98.1
Oral Hypoglycemic Dose Recorded	100
Oral Hypoglycemic Type Recorded	100
Oral Hypoglycemic Agents at Any Time	66.7
Blood Sugar Recorded (Six Months)	21.2
Insulin Schedule Recorded	94.3
Insulin Dose Recorded	94.3
Insulin Type Recorded	97.1
Cases Treated with Insulin at Any Time	21.6
Change in Regimen	94.1
Referral to Ophthalmologist	44.7
Renal Function Determined	75.2
Repeat Blood Sugar	95.4
Urinalysis Performed	88.9
Blood Pressure Recorded (Annually)	95.5
Weight Recorded	95.1
Peripheral Vascular Exam	70.4
Fundoscopic Examination	47.5

Source: Williamson Institute. 1988. *National Medicare Competition Evaluation*. Baltimore, MD: HCFA. See also Retchin, S. M., and J. Preston. 1991. "The Effects of Cost-Containment on the Care of Elderly Diabetics." *Archives of Internal Medicine* 151 (11) 2244–8.

hypoglycemic schedule recorded in their chart. Two-thirds are treated with oral hypoglycemic agents. Blood sugar tests are recorded every six months only 21.2 percent of the time. Insulin schedules, dose, and type are almost always recorded. Only about 44 percent have a referral to an ophthalmologist. Referrals to subspecialists for ophthalmology lag behind recommended guidelines, which suggest frequent referrals to check the eyes. Approximately three-fourths have renal function tests at least annually following diagnosis, and most managed care providers perform urinalysis frequently.

Basic Hypertension Care

Hypertension is even more prevalent than diabetes among Medicare managed care enrollees. Approximately 60 percent of people 65 years or older have diastolic hypertension, which is associated with numerous comorbid conditions including renal dysfunction and renal disease. Hypertension can be difficult to manage because patients must adhere to the treatment regimen and continually change drugs as they become available. If patients are to adhere to recommended guidelines for treatment and receive good basic care for hypertension, they must get frequent updates on those regimens. The drug regimen for hypertension can lead to electrolyte disturbances that affect the heart, so it is imperative that patients receive careful primary care management it they're to receive optimal care and avoid expensive complications.

Initial Evaluation

According to guidelines, clinicians should order a urinalysis on all new patients every six months. However, this occurs in only 75 percent of cases identified as hypertensives in the only study of the disease in Medicare managed care plans (Preston and Retchin 1991). Pyuria is detected in nearly 8 percent of cases, but a follow-up culture was documented only 64.7 percent of the time for those cases. Other recommended tests for persons with hypertension were performed with approximately equal frequency—about two-thirds to three-fourths of the time. These tests include creatinine (73.9 percent), potassium (71.7 percent), sodium (68.5 percent), chest x-ray (68.4 percent), and electrocardiogram (77.2 percent), even in the face of a new complaint of chest pain (78.1 percent) (see Table 9.4). Two other basic tests are performed more frequently: serum glucose (90.9 percent) and hemoglobin (92.2 percent).

Medical Management

Table 9.5 shows other treatment indicators of basic care for hypertension that you may examine in your plan. Dietary counseling is standard treatment care, especially for those age 75 or younger. That said, do you know whether patients with hypertension in your plan are getting dietary counseling? The same is true of weight loss for patients exceeding high weight levels with hypertension. For the managed care plans represented in Table 9.5, the primary caregivers did

Indicators	Percent
Urinalysis Ordered	75.3
Pyuria Detected	7.7
Urine Culture for Cases with Pyuria	64.7
Creatinine	73.9
Potassium	71.7
Sodium	68.5
Glucose	90.9
Hemoglobin	92.2
Chest X-ray	68.4
ECG	77.2
ECG: New Complaints	78.1

Source: Williamson Institute. 1988. *National Medicare Competition Evaluation.* Baltimore, MD: HCFA.

TABLE 9.4
Illustrative Hypertension Care Outcomes

Initial evaluation: Do you know the lab test and radiologic procedures for patients with diastolic hypertension?

better on weight loss recommendations (78.2 percent) than dietary counseling (42.9 percent). The drug regimen recommendations change frequently and fall into beta blockers, calcium blockers, and alpha blockers. Again, do you know the pattern of drug use for hypertensives in your health plan and whether patients follow recommended guidelines?

Medications should be adjusted when there is a change in mental health status, but this is only done 42.3 percent of the time. Likewise, bradycardia should prompt an adjustment in medication, but this is done only 50 percent of the time. The cases with poor control should be driven down as low as possible, or it should at least improve as a percent of the hypertensive population. Lastly, hospitalization is always indicated with hypertensive complications.

One of the most important aspects of treating a chronic disease such as hypertension is ongoing management and follow-up care. Table 9.6 suggests some indicators of best practices for treating hypertension.

Indicators	Percent
(Cases ≥75 yrs.) Dietary Counseling	42.9
(Weight >225lbs.) Weight Loss Recommended	78.2
Diuretic Treatment	76.3
Beta Blocker Treatment	27.4
Calcium Blocker Treatment	7.3
Alpha Blocker Treatment	5.5
Mental Status Medications Adjusted with Change in Mental Status	42.3
Medications Adjusted with Bradycardia	50.0
Cases with Poor Control	59.8
Medications Adjusted with Poor Control	96.2
Hypertensive Hospitalization with Hypertensive Complications	100.0

Source: Williamson Institute. 1988. *National Medicare Competition Evaluation.* Baltimore, MD: HCFA.

TABLE 9.5
Illustrative Hypertension Care Outcomes

Medical Management: Do you know the management of patients with hypertension?

TABLE 9.6
Illustrative
Hypertension
Care Outcomes

Follow-up: Do
you know the
follow-up,
medical history,
and physical
exam of
patients with
hypertension in
your health
plan?

Indicators	Percent
Blood Pressure Checked Each Visit	71.6
Hypertensive Medications Prescribed	85.0
Monthly Blood Pressure Check	81.5
Follow-up Visit in Three Months	95.0
Hypertension History	90.9
Cardio or Cerebro History	60.3
History of Tobacco Use	72.2
Orthostatic Blood Pressure	12.3
Fundoscopic Exam or Referral to Ophthalmologist	42.0
Peripheral Vascular Exam	60.7
Elements of Cardiac Exam	
Heart Size	18.3
Auscultation	65.6
Heart Rate	75.3
Heart Rhythm	74.0

Source: Williamson Institute. 1988. *National Medicare Competition Evaluation.* Baltimore, MD: HCFA.

Follow-up

Managed care physicians and health plans are supposed to excel at following up and monitoring chronic conditions, and they appear to do well according to Table 9.6. But there is room for improvement. Elements of medical history taking, physical examination, laboratory tests, and interventions were high for patients with hypertension. For example, 72.2 percent of patients in Medicare managed care plans had a recorded history of tobacco use. In addition, orthostatic hypertension is prevalent among the elderly and can influence the choice of treatment options. Yet although this blood pressure should be taken, it seems to be done only 12 percent of the time. A fundoscopic exam or referral to an ophthalmologist occurs less than half the time. A peripheral vascular exam was more likely (60. 7 percent). Elements of a heart exam are done only about 60 percent of the time.

To help your primary care network improve on these general indicators of good hypertension care, you can invest in patient education, clinician education, feedback reports to clinicians, chart checklists, and other tools. Again, these outcome indicators only suggest a strategic approach to managing basic care, including diabetes and hypertension, and it's an approach that relies on measuring outcomes of care as a way to improve them.

Responsibility for a Defined Population

Responsibility for a
defined population
is achieving an
acceptable level of
quality for all the
care provided to a
group of health plan
enrollees subject to
a predetermined
pool of financial
resources.

Responsibility for a defined population means achieving an acceptable quality level for all the care provided to a group of health plan enrollees subject to a predetermined pool of financial resources. There is a dual responsibility to provide basic care of good quality without running out of money. The two responsibilities often clash. While there is the larger trade-off between total care provided and total dollars available, there is a micro level that is connected to the dual responsibilities. Each singular interaction between a patient and physician adds up to the sum total of care. Thus, there is an essential connection between the personal side of basic care involving many distinct patient-clinician interactions and the responsibility to manage those interactions subject to a budget constraint.

Sadly, what is sometimes lost in the daily grind of managing a large health plan and the allocation of resources is the inextricable link to each personal interaction between patient and clinician. Many health plans spend enormous resources on contracting and financial issues to meet their responsibility for a defined population. But healthcare remains, after all, a private and personal matter. At the core of the delivery system is what clinicians say and do in the privacy of an examining room. There, they discuss the most personal issues their patients face. This one-on-one interaction is vital. Great time and expense are invested in training clinicians to deliver medical care with this private, human connection. How well they deliver this personalized basic care is central to the success of a health plan. Patients place enormous value on this human element and often make enrollment decisions based on the quality of interpersonal communication with their clinicians. To manage the delivery of care for a defined population, your plan must reconcile the need to assure highly personal, private, patient-physician interaction with the fiscal management for the aggregate of care.

Resolving the dichotomy of care for *one* and care for *many* begins with each patient being supported by a number of organizational features of a progressive health plan and ends with the effective personal communication with each patient. Figure 9.1 illustrates the ideal relationship.

The Medicare managed care plan obtains relevant information from patients about the care patients want and the care they receive. The plan most often gets this information when a patient requests a visit and, in the process, reports a health problem. This information also surfaces when the patient is being evaluated and is answering medical history questions. In these instances, patients tend to give their perceptions of care and indicate their level of satisfaction with the treatment they've received. Much of this information is conveyed by the patient directly to the providers of care during a visit. That information is recorded on claims records or electronic medical records and is captured by the managed care plan. Another source for such data is through direct report to the health plan from disease management or health risk assessment programs. Increasingly, the best health plans do not wait around for patients to encounter problems, but they become assertive about finding out from individual patients or groups of patients the kinds of data needed to develop effective healthcare. The health plan that can obtain this information and summarize it for a defined population can use it to make

FIGURE 9.1

With the
Patient in
the Middle,
Managed Care
Plan and
Clinical Team
Excel

*Making basic
care work:
Information
and technology
converge to
improve patient
outcomes*

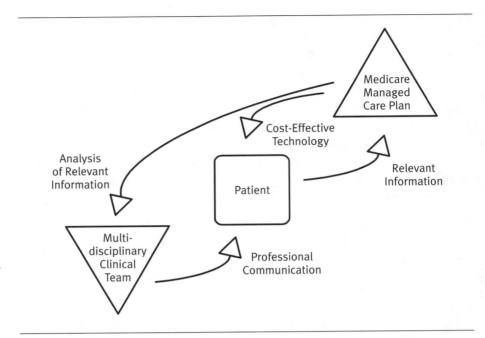

decisions about how best to use resources. That is an important first step toward becoming a successful health plan.

Once patients provide the information, the health plan can use a number of cost-effective technologies to influence the care they receive. Electronic medical records, Internet-based communication with patients, claims data processing, provider profiling of medical treatment, educational programs, and materials for patients to treat themselves—these are examples of the tools a managed care plan can apply to improve patient care. The application of some of these tools was discussed in Chapter 7, "Quality Really Can Cost Less."

The loop in the lower half of Figure 9.1 is a function that has enormous potential when it comes to caring for patients, and many managed care plans are just beginning to recognize its value. In this loop, the health plan analyzes relevant information from patients and gives that information to clinicians so that they can enhance the quality of care they provide. This information can take the form of lists of patients who should be seen for special intervention, feedback on outcomes of care, reminders for saying or doing certain things for patients, and general support of the clinicians as a team of self-directed professionals. The loop is closed when clinicians communicate with patients in a way that enhances the quality of information given to the health plan by the patient during the next round of interactions. When managed skillfully, this process encourages patients to assume greater responsibility for their health. The following sections discuss a variety of techniques for using individual physician-patient interactions to improve the sense of responsibility among patients.

Partnership, Not Paternalism

Charles Longino, M.D., describes the dominant model of medicine in the United States as the Western biomedical model, which comes with a heavy dose of paternalism. Physicians act as the "captain of the ship," expecting other disciplines and the patient to obey orders. The major doctrines seem to include, in Longino's words, "body-mind dualism, the mechanical analogy, specific etiology, and the body as the appropriate object of regimen and control" (Longino 1997). In this view, treating a patient is analogous to fixing a machine.

The paternalistic view may work fine for some patients, but Medicare managed care is different. The chief difference between commercial managed care and Medicare managed care is the type of patient each plan treats, plus the needs those patients bring to the plan. For Medicare managed care, chronic conditions abound. There are no quick fixes, and cures are elusive. Other clinical professions related to medicine may have the same or more to offer to the patient, thereby providing an alternative to the paternalistic physician. In light of the challenge facing Medicare managed care, Longino's assessment rings true. Medicine will have to change its essential self-understanding if it is to be successful in the future.

One way to change the system is to replace the paternalistic model with a partnership model. A partnership model stresses the relationship between the physician and the patient, but it also encourages a partnership among the various health professionals who make up the caregiving team. With the team approach taken in the partnership model, caregivers can begin to broaden their view, seeing the patient as a physical, social, and emotional body whose life is spent interacting with the environment. This new, broader view of patients should be communicated among the new partners, patients, and the entire multidisciplinary team.

Three driving forces are causing a shift away from the paternalistic medical model. First, there's the growth of managed care, which discourages autonomous relationships and rewards certain cooperative relationships. Second, there's a growing elderly population with chronic conditions. For these patients, caregiving is probably better handled by a multidisciplinary team rather than a sole medical practitioner. Third, the far-reaching Internet is reducing the near monopoly medicine has had on a patient's knowledge of diseases and drugs. With this knowledge, patients educate themselves about their own diseases. Physicians and clinicians in managed care plans must respond to, even anticipate, these changes by devising a creative approach for treating their enrollees. The key to success with any new approach, however, is effective communication, and the next section discusses how that works.

Communicating to a Defined Population

At the core of managing a defined population of patients is what the frontline clinicians say and do with patients. This patient-clinician interaction comprises three principal issues: communication, medical treatment, and disease

FIGURE 9.2

Common
Problems in a
Defined
Population in
Medicare
Managed Care

*Problems are
nothing new:
Communica-
tion about basic
problems can
help manage the
care of a defined
population*

- Inadequate understanding of the potential severity of the disease and the importance of medical treatment
- Need for repeated instructions
- Difficulty following suggested lifestyle changes
- Anxiety and stress from not knowing what to expect
- Variety of factors influencing successful management
- Lack of involvement by patients in developing their treatment plan
- Self-monitoring assessments and therapeutic changes
- Progressive nature of many diseases in the elderly
- Development of complications before acute symptoms appear
- Importance of overall adherence to the patient's health

Source: Whitehurst-Cook, M. et al. 1994. Virginia *Health Outcomes Partnership.* Richmond, VA: Williamson Institute for Health Studies.

management. The population of Medicare beneficiaries enrolled in your managed care plan face special challenges. Their chronic diseases require treatment in the form of visits to physicians or other clinicians, drugs, and certain behavior changes. The goal of your plan should be to communicate certain basic ideas that support the work of the clinicians directly involved in their care.

Figure 9.2 describes some of the common problems that elderly patients have across numerous diseases. Recognizing these problems as especially unique to the elderly population will help your health plan respond to them, both as a health plan and as a manager of care. This care can then be carried out by individual clinicians on the front line.

Too often, we think that if we give a health problem a name, much of the care is completed, and patients can go about their daily lives. But Medicare patients need special attention. They need to understand their health problems and the potential severity those problems present. Perhaps more than other population groups, instructions about the treatment regimen need to be repeated, along with instructions about the way the health plan operates. The health plan can suggest ways for patients to change their lifestyle or to deal with anxiety and stress. In addition, your plan can also help patients recognize the multiplicity of factors that affect the success of managing care. But this is not one-way communication. Figure 9.2 highlights the importance of two-way communication.

One area vital to improving patient-physician communication is the management of what happens during clinical contact. Too often, patients are not involved when it comes to developing their treatment plan. Patients do not get involved sufficiently in self-monitoring assessments and implementing therapeutic changes. Sometimes clinicians and patients set up unrealistic expectations about the progressive nature of many diseases, and this is especially true with elderly patients. They do not recognize complications until acute symptoms appear.

In any case, it is crucial that patients adhere to treatment regimens and the recommended lifestyle changes, and the quality of communication affects how readily patients follow through with the recommendations they receive. Feedback mechanisms that measure and report back to clinicians and patients on progress are more than helpful. They are a necessary factor for success. Education groups, advisory groups, interest groups, focus groups, patient surveys (mailed, telephone, or Internet), case managers, disease management coordinators—these and other resources are ways to obtain relevant information from patients in systematic way. These resources also reinforce one-on-one clinical contact, creating an environment of trust so that the feedback is honest and the core plan is responsive.

Responding to the common problems in Figure 9.2 can take several forms when you are managing a defined population. Figure 9.3 summarizes some basic rules to follow. First, try to use a nontechnical, straightforward means of communication. The way you communicate should be tailored to the need or the disease. Sometimes, it is necessary to use technical communication depending on the specific type of care. But generally, you cannot take a communication method for a commercial population and overlay it in Medicare. A communication expert is a vital member of the team for achieving nontechnical communication. It is often best to have someone who isn't an expert in Medicare managed care to help with the communication effort.

Responding

Second, involve your enrollees in the planning, implementation, and evaluation of communication efforts. One successful health plan had beneficiary awareness social gatherings and had members "bring a friend" to these programs. The spokespersons were actual members of the health plan, and they answered each other's questions. An advisory committee could help you achieve this goal.

Third, be sure to apply adult education techniques when you work with your enrollees. These techniques are based on participatory learning

---

1. Use nontechnical, straightforward methods to communicate
2. Involve Medicare enrollees in the communication effort
   - Planning
   - Implementation
   - Evaluation
3. Include Medicare enrollees as instructors/communicators
4. Apply adult education techniques
   - Participation
   - Self-contract process or negotiating and maintaining the treatment regimen
5. Use print, video, and Internet media to communicate

FIGURE 9.3

Five Rules for Effective Communication to a Defined Population

Keep it simple: Effective methods to reach older enrollees exist

Source: LaCroix, A. Z., and L. J. Rubenstein. 1990. "Health Promotion and the Elderly." In *Medicare. . . .* Baltimore, MD: Group Health Association of America.

and include elements of contracting or negotiating. Do not presume that a simple brochure with factual information will suffice if you're trying to promote a particular health or disease prevention issue. Develop clever ways to reach out to beneficiaries, as though you are negotiating buy-in on a particular point or trying to involve enrollees in a transaction of knowledge. Communication is a transaction. And as such, it needs systems to support it, such as requests for proposals for new ideas, discussions about options, and trial balloons or pilot programs. Promote information, based on relevant, clinical data about your beneficiaries. Use the feedback loops you've established to understand the barriers older persons may face when it comes to maintaining a treatment regimen.

Fourth, use multimedia to communicate. This approach addresses the need for repetition. Any communication should have several forms of media to carry the same message. The more the message is repeated and given a fresh look, the more receptive your enrollees become.

Listening Listen to your enrollees. Sure, it's great to provide educational information about smoking cessation, mammography, proper nutrition, physical exercise, alcohol and drug use, mental health, hip fractures, falls, immunizations, and infectious diseases. But the communication should not consist solely of brochures on these topics, nor should the communication be one way. For instance, clinicians can educate their patients about common conditions and their treatment, but then they need to check each patient's baseline knowledge as well as the overall knowledge of the plan's enrollees.

You can help in this process by encouraging clinicians to ask their patients what they know about the conditions they present during a visit. The listening should extend beyond merely determining whether patients have a factual understanding of their condition. Clinicians need to know how patients feel about their conditions and what their anxieties might be at that moment. In addition to this one-on-one listening forum, you can use surveys and focus groups as a way to listen to your entire membership. You can also provide opportunities to discuss health problems in the form of support groups and advisory groups.

To be effective listeners, clinicians need to be inquisitive. They need to encourage patients to ask questions. Most health plans now have a special toll-free line for seniors that is answered promptly by people who are experienced in answering questions from older persons. The plans capture information about the questions and follow-up. But check frequently on how well your enrollees understand their conditions and their treatment. Although it's important for clinicians to understand the variety of stressors that affect older persons, the issues they have to address are medical, not holistic.

Reporting Back Use an advisory group of Medicare enrollees to evaluate your ongoing communication efforts. Be sure to summarize the results of your communication effort and report them to the entire membership. People like to receive feedback on their efforts. By reporting how many attended a function, how many mailings were sent, or how many persons with a particular condition changed their behavior, you can reinforce your communication effort for a defined population. Health plan managers, affiliated physicians and hospitals, and the membership in general want to know how many people your communication effort reached, how it changed behavior, and what influence it had on the cost and quality of care.

Coaching for Enhanced Patienthood

In a path-breaking analysis of the relationship between physicians and patients, Roter and Hall (1992) described the ideal pattern of communication at the clinical level. Their ideas have been developed and applied by others and have resulted in the concept of enhanced patienthood. By communicating more as a coach than as a purveyor of technical information, primary care physicians and other partners on the clinical team are more persuasive when it comes to getting patients to adhere to treatment regimens. The techniques that enable clinicians to enhance patienthood include negotiating and maintaining treatment plans, probing for adherence, and achieving adherence.

Several nonverbal and verbal techniques can be used to achieve better patienthood, and Figure 9.4 summarizes those. One study of general internal medicine specialists found that the average time between a physician's addressing a patient to find out what is wrong and interrupting them was

---

- Nonverbal techniques
  - Listen actively
  - Present a receptive demeanor
  - Establish eye contact
  - Maintain a position that puts physician or other clinician at same height
  - Open sitting and office space
- Verbal techniques
  - Ask open-ended questions
  - Facilitate comments
  - Check or repeat information
  - Survey or ask, "What else is bothering you?"
- Responding to patient's emotions
  - Reflect
  - Legitimate
  - Offer personal support
  - Build partnership
  - Show respect

FIGURE 9.4

Rules for Effective Communication to a Defined Population

Enhanced patienthood: Techniques for better communication with patients exist

Source: Whitehurst-Cook, M. et al. 1994. Virginia *Health Outcomes Partnership*. Richmond, VA: Williamson Institute for Health Studies.

18 seconds. This time should be used to put patients at ease. When patients feel comfortable, they communicate more freely; and clinicians can encourage this with active listening, a receptive demeanor, and good eye contact. They can also establish trust by physically positioning themselves at the same level as their patients. Consider pharmacists. Pharmacists are frequently found behind high counters or even in caged areas in some pharmacies. To instill a sense of comfort and trust, it's important to have open sitting and office space where caregivers do not hide behind desks or tower above their patients.

Patients can set the agenda for the visit to the physician or other clinicians and feel more in control when they can ask open questions. Many experienced clinicians may feel that open-ended questioning invites wasted time and rambling about useless information. Open-ended questioning might take more time initially, but it could save time later. This is especially true for repeat visits, when certain information could have been obtained earlier, saving treatment time and improving outcomes.

Open-ended questioning can be combined with clinical interviewing to facilitate comments and to check information as the visit progresses. Using this approach, clinicians can uncover information that might be missed and make patients more involved in their care. The technique of surveying can be used to manage the visit without compromising one-on-one interaction. This approach helps physicians avoid the problem of listening to patients discuss one problem for 15 minutes and then finally getting around to the real reason for the office visit. The properly placed question "What else is bothering you?" can help patients gain confidence in their own problem identification skills. That, in turn, facilitates communication, as long as probing questions are gentle and the physician does not jump at the first problem to put the intervention in place.

Finally, it's important to empathize with the patient's feelings and emotions. Reflecting on the emotions as they are revealed, legitimizing those feelings ("I can certainly understand why you would think the pimple could be cancer"), and showing personal support are all valid techniques for enhancing patienthood.

Partnership is the crux of the relationship. Patients are more likely to be involved with their care if they feel something is being done *with* them, rather than *to* them. If the physician, the other clinicians, and the health plan think of the patient as the primary caregiver rather than anyone else, this notion can go a long way to changing the prevailing culture of seeing a patient as something that someone needs to fix.

All patients, especially elderly patients enrolled in Medicare managed care plans, deserve respect, and that has to be the prevailing attitude you and your staff take toward older adults. All the efforts by clinicians to promote a culture of communication work only if they're supported by the way the health plan operates, beginning at the first moment of contact.

Membership Retention and Member Services Operations

Providing good basic primary care is the essential ingredient to retaining your plan's membership. Member service operations and its patient representatives must be geared toward managing the primary care network and its members effectively and efficiently. In most plans, patient representatives or plan representatives handle this. These representatives are typically smart, articulate people. They take the handoff from the health plan's sales staff, help enrollees select primary care physicians, answer questions at enrollment, and schedule first visits. The plan's membership must view these people positively as facilitators rather than obstacles. But to earn this sentiment, the staff must be knowledgeable about the physicians in the network, and they must know the plan.

Patient representatives should know the basic coverage requirements including current requirements for emergency care. They should be the primary point of contact for initiating consumer grievance and appeals procedures, and they should be trained to avert such actions by helping with negotiations between patients and the providers and health plans that serve them. Granted, the key to retaining members is to offer an excellent network of primary care physicians and other clinicians. But membership operations is an indispensable support mechanism that should not be underresourced, especially when it comes to new member orientation.

Three rules seem to prevail in these new member orientation programs (Hiramatsu and Mason 1991):

1. Elderly patients will develop a satisfactory relationship with the health plan more readily in a system in which members see a personal physician for most of their healthcare needs.
2. Elderly patients should be offered a wide choice of personal physicians.
3. Elderly patients should choose a personal physician before they need medical attention.

New member orientation is the perfect place to use patient representatives to begin building relationships with new enrollees. During these orientations, new members can put a personal face on the relationship they're establishing with the health plan. But the orientation process is most efficiently carried out by a centralized department charged with seeing that each new enrollee is called or visited within days of signing up or at the beginning of enrollment. A new member orientation package should have general brochures along with a list of physicians that includes biographies of the physicians and photographs (Fig. 9.5). Internet sites with similar information should be made available for new enrollees, or their children and friends, so that new members and their families can review the available network of physicians. A brief letter could encourage new members to select a primary care physician immediately and schedule an appointment. Follow-up calls to the new member can ensure that everyone has selected a physician upon enrollment, and the process of intake can begin.

FIGURE 9.5

Contents of New Member Orientation Package

First impressions matter: The standard information sent to new members should have one goal—to choose a physician

- Welcome letter with instructions on selecting primary care physician
- Identification cards
- Guide to accessing care
- Service area map with location of network physicians and hospitals
- Physician biographies and photos
- Evidence of coverage
- Patients bill of rights
- Description of health plan organization
- Coordination of benefits information
- Frequently asked questions and answers
- Contact information and phone numbers

The other point to remember when putting together the new member package is not to overwhelm people with too many pieces of paper and too much information. You can make it clear which activities and steps are needed by the new member right away (for example, select a primary care physician). Another tactic is to send out information in stages. Information required for enrollment can go out first, followed by other mailings in a few days or weeks. This approach helps you avoid the problem of overwhelming your members.

Enrollee Satisfaction

The Consumer Assessment of Health Plans Survey (CAHPS) assesses the satisfaction of enrollees in Medicare+Choice plans annually. HCFA-approved contractors administer a customized Medicare version of the survey to 600 members of each plan and publish the enrollee satisfaction results on the Internet at www.medicarecompare.gov for each plan. That means the basic care your primary care network is delivering is being watched by HCFA, and your enrollees' perceptions of your plan's performance are being reported on the Internet annually. Figure 9.6 shows the specific items being tracked for each health plan with results posted on the Internet by plan name. We don't yet know what influence the Medicare Compare Internet Reports have on the decisions of new enrollees. Even if they play a small role, now or in future decision making, they should serve as an indicator of what is being said about your health plan in the oldest communication network around: word of mouth. Whether directly or indirectly, these Internet-reported perceptions of beneficiaries show your relative rank among your competitors, so you need to take them seriously.

Compared with fee-for-service, Medicare+Choice plans fare well on patient satisfaction. In a 1998 Medicare Payment Assessment Commission report, beneficiaries enrolled in managed care plans generally reported good access to care. As Table 9.7 reports, these beneficiaries reported few problems obtaining care, and their level of satisfaction was high. Whereas managed

FIGURE 9.6

Four
Performance
Indicators from
CAHPS

*Your primary
care is being
watched:
Medicare
Compare
annually
monitors the
performance of
Medicare+
Choice plan
performance
and publishes it
on the Internet*

1. The percentage who rated their own managed care plan as the best possible managed care plan (a rating of 1 to 10)
2. The percentage who rated their own care as the best possible care (a rating of 1 to 10)
3. The percentage who said the doctors in their own health plan always communicate well, described as:
   - Listened carefully
   - Explained things in a way they could understand
   - Showed respect for what they had to say
   - Spent enough time with them
4. The percentage who said it was not a problem to get a referral to a specialist

care beneficiaries reported statistically significant lower levels of satisfaction, the differences were slight. Whether in traditional Medicare fee-for-service or Medicare managed care, more than 90 percent of beneficiaries reported strong agreement or agreement with statements such as "physician checks everything" and "great confidence in physician." Most beneficiaries (low 90 percent) were very satisfied or satisfied with the availability of medical care on evenings and weekends, and they were also satisfied with the overall quality of care.

The findings create a real dilemma when the same physicians and hospitals serve the traditional fee-for-service market as well as other managed care plans in your market. The steps your plan takes to improve the basic primary care provided by your network of primary care physicians—especially in terms of communication—probably carry over to fee-for-service patients in competing health plans. There is really no easy solution to this dilemma. You can help address it by concentrating on enrollment, purchasing physician

TABLE 9.7

Satisfaction in
Fee-for-Service
and Managed
Care, 1996

*The basic care
dilemma: How
to differentiate
your primary
care when you
draw from the
community*

	Fee-for-Service	Managed Care
	Percent	
Strongly agree/agree with "physician checks everything"	94.2	92.3
Strongly agree/agree with "great confidence in physician"	95.3	93.2
Very satisfied/satisfied with availability of medical care, evening/weekends	94.6	93.5
Very satisfied/satisfied with overall quality of care	96.0	94.6

Source: Medicare Payment Assessment Commission. 1998. *Report to Congress.* Washington, DC: MedPAC.

practices, and setting up your own staff model practices and clinics. To the extent you can build your network with the best primary care providers and help improve their performance, the dilemma is minimized.

Your health plan's success in terms of retaining enrollment probably depends more on the good basic care you offer than your competition with Medicare fee-for-service plans. As you recall from Chapter 6, beneficiaries give relatively few reasons for joining managed care plans. But when they do, their decisions most often revolve around costs and benefits. In a 1996 survey (Medicare Payment Advisory Commission 1998), only 10 percent of beneficiaries said they joined a plan because of a recommendation or reputation. Forty percent joined because of lower costs, and 25 percent joined because of better benefits. The remaining 25 percent joined for a variety of other reasons.

So, yes, enrollment depends on costs and benefits relative to traditional fee-for-service Medicare and competing health plans. Your challenge, however, is to change the way beneficiaries perceive the core benefits of belonging to the health plan. Good basic primary care is your trump card.

Strategic Decisions Checklist

Strategic Questions	Strategic Analyses
How well do you manage initial patient evaluation and performance of tests, screens, and immunizations?	Create a well-defined, organized initial patient evaluation process for new members.
	Monitor the outcomes of patient evaluation and medical history taking in your health plan.
	Monitor the outcomes of baseline tests, period screening, and immunizations in your health plan.
	Act continuously to improve the measures of good performance by gathering relevant information, applying cost-effective technology, feeding back relevant information, and enhancing professional communication.
Do you know the outcomes of basic diabetes care provided in your health plan?	Know the number of patients with diabetes and their total annual costs in your health plan.
	Monitor the outcomes of diabetes care from the physicians and other clinicians primarily caring for your diabetic patients.

continued

Strategic Questions	Strategic Analyses
	Ensure that physicians and clinicians know the guidelines for providing good diabetic care.
	Act continuously to improve the measures of good performance by gathering relevant information, applying cost-effective technology, feeding back relevant information, and enhancing professional communication.
Do you know the outcomes of basic hypertension care in your health plan?	Know the number of patients with hypertension and how much they cost your health plan annually.
	Monitor the outcomes of hypertension care from the physicians and other clinicians primarily caring for your hypertension patients.
	Ensure that physicians and clinicians know the guidelines for providing good hypertension care.
	Act continually to improve the measures of good performance by gathering relevant information, applying cost-effective technology, feeding back relevant information, and enhancing professional communication.
How are you supporting a culture of responsibility for a defined population?	Gather relevant data on health outcomes of patients.
	Apply cost-effective technology in the form of electronic medical records, Internet-based communication with patients, claims data processing, and targeted educational programs for patients.
	Analyze relevant information and give it to multidisciplinary clinical teams to help them improve care.

continued

Strategic Questions	Strategic Analyses
How and what do you communicate with elderly patients?	Help your physicians and other clinicians improve their communication skills and convey partnership to your members, not paternalism.
	Develop effective approaches to reach older enrollees with nontechnical communication, including using enrollees in the communication, adopting adult education techniques, and incorporating multimedia.
	Listen to your enrollees. Establish beneficiary advisory groups to monitor and report back on the success of plan communication efforts.
	Monitor concerns and satisfaction levels of enrollees.
	Report back frequently to enrollees on what you are hearing and doing.
Are your Medicare managed care enrollees good patients?	Patients can be coached toward better patienthood. You should try to develop a communication plan around patienthood.
	You can teach enhanced communication and patienthood to your physicians and other clinicians.
Did you know your enrollee satisfaction is being watched? What are you doing about it?	The determinants of successful enrollment are not the same as successful member retention. Have different strategies for each.
	Have a plan for dealing with the basic care dilemma that improvements you make to your network may work to the advantage of the larger health delivery community in your area.

DEMAND MANAGEMENT

Curbing the demand for inappropriate or unnecessary health services is an essential ingredient of successful managed care. Granted, any successful managed care plan can trim expenses, unlike unbridled fee-for-service. However, that's more a byproduct of managed care than its purpose. Managed care is all about ensuring the appropriate use of care, and how well you achieve this goal largely depends on developing just the right systems and processes, not only for delivering care but especially for managing demand.

How difficult could it be to wipe out most of the inappropriate or unnecessary uses of health services? Some people might say that all one has to do is require a physician's second opinion for all services. Of course, such an approach is highly impractical. Requiring second opinions would be costly for health plans and time consuming for physicians and patients, although it might lead to more appropriate and necessary use of health services. The trick is balancing effectiveness with the cost of implementing and operating systems to manage demand.

Fortunately, you can get help creating this balance. A growing number of specially designed programs on the market are designed to manage resource consumption, and they accomplish this by focusing on the patient and how patients initiate demand for health services. These programs, known as demand management programs, are different from the cost-control systems discussed in Chapter 7. Demand management programs sometimes go around the physician or other clinicians, and sometimes they operate with the full cooperation of the clinicians involved with the ongoing care of the patient. This chapter is about these demand management programs, and our discussion will cover nurse **telephone triage**; **emergency authorization**, including emergency and urgent care procedures; and **discharge planning**.

Demand management programs are among the most prominent patient-focused efforts to curb inappropriate or unnecessary health services. Vickery (1996), an early developer of the demand management concept, describes **demand management** as "the use of decision and behavior support systems to enable individuals to use medical care appropriately." The underlying premise of demand management is that individuals are empowered by knowledge. Individuals become better consumers when they have the information they need to make informed decisions regarding the resources they consume. For healthcare specifically, demand management encourages an appropriate use of services, which has a related benefit of controlling expenses. This chapter begins with a conceptual discussion, under the heading

Telephone triage *offers easy calling (usually to licensed nurses) 24-hours a day, seven days a week to answer health questions and help patients decide whether to seek acute care before initiating such a request.*

Emergency authorization *is prior approval from the health plan of medically necessary emergency care.*

Discharge planning *means arrangements for care after leaving the hospital, including home health service, setting up durable medical equipment, or a skilled nursing facility.*

Demand management *is the use of interventional decision and behavior support systems that enable people to use medical care appropriately.*

flat-of-the-curve medicine, about why health plans should be concerned with demand management.

Telephone triage is becoming an important feature of these programs. Telephone triage can consist of several specific components: 24-hour access to registered nurses for advice and referral counseling; self-care guides; audio or video tape libraries, and Internet sites on various health topics; a process for referring identified high-risk enrollees to more intensive monitoring programs; and services that provide after-hours telephone coverage for physicians. Most physicians are not paid for handling telephone calls from patients, so many managed care plans establish these programs as a prop to their network of primary care physicians. Some even use it to replace the physician call. This chapter discusses these issues.

Emergency authorization is another important feature of demand management. Since prior authorization is not permitted by Medicare+Choice plans for emergency services, health plans must educate beneficiaries about how to use the emergency room appropriately—especially beneficiaries who are repeat offenders. Then, the plan must channel them to alternatives. Given the public concern over prior authorization and restrictive opinions regarding medical necessity, the topic is all the more relevant at this time.

Finally, one of the staples of managed care has been hospital discharge planning. This chapter also presents the basics of this important demand management technique.

Avoiding Flat-of-the-Curve Medicine

There are a number of complex reasons why enrollees demand healthcare from their insurance plan, and it's important for managed care plans to understand these reasons if they intend to manage the care they coordinate. Although the media have made much about the stringent policies that managed care plans use to regulate demand, they need to remember that regulating demand is, in fact, a key role of these plans. Traditional insurance was not concerned with the "hows" and "whys" of demand. It merely arranged to pay whatever the insured patient or the family demanded. Meanwhile, the market began to show that the public is unwilling to pay for such unbridled insurance, and cost-conscious health plans began to dominate. People and payers want plans that do a better job balancing unbridled demand with the cost of paying for covered services.

Somatization is when people experience or report physical symptoms that have no medical explanation. People may also attribute symptoms to the wrong disease and seek inappropriate services.

Thus, managed care plans must take great pains to understand how their members set the demand for services. Although most demands for medical care are appropriate and necessary, some are heavily influenced by a phenomenon known as **somatization**. This phenomenon reflects "the propensity to experience and report somatic symptoms that have no patho-physiological explanation, to misattribute them to disease, and to seek medical attention for them" (Barsky and Borus 1995).

Various reports describe the impact of somatization on the use of healthcare services. One estimates that up to 60 percent of patients treated in primary care practices report symptoms for which no serious medical condition is found (McCarthy 1997). Another report states that studies have shown that up to 55 percent of emergency room visits are unnecessary (Gemignani 1996). A third report claims that 60 percent of all ambulance transports are inappropriate (McCarthy 1997).

From an economic standpoint, the existence of unnecessary or inappropriate medical services is flat-of-the curve medicine. Whether it is derived from somatizing patients or from physicians practicing defensively in response to a presenting somatizing patient, excessive ordering of services by patients or physicians means more care for no incremental improvement in health. Figure 10.1 illustrates the idea.

Health status will increase as spending on healthcare services increases —up to a point. There comes a time at which additional spending makes no improvement to health status. This same principal holds whether applied to individual patients or to a group of enrollees from a health plan. Direct cost and utilization management techniques, as well as demand management programs, are aimed at moving back along the curve. But demand management programs add another dimension—that of helping patients alter their perceptions of what it takes to achieve good health status. Programs do this by putting information in the hands of patients so that they can address their immediate health concerns. The approach is enabling and self-supporting when compared with traditional medical care, which fosters dependency and paternalism. These programs educate enrollees, helping them to make better choices about what they can do to improve their health status.

Vickery proposes that the demand for healthcare is a function of four factors, each operating either independently or jointly with the others:

1. morbidity,
2. perceived need,
3. patient preference, and
4. nonhealth motives.

The first, morbidity, presumes that a high correlation exists between the presence of injury or disease and the demand for healthcare. Evidence suggests otherwise. As much as 94 percent of the variation in healthcare utilization is unaccounted for by morbidity alone; that is, there is considerable variation among persons with similar types and severity of illness when it comes to the way they consume healthcare resources (Lynch and Vickery 1993; Vickery 1996).

The second factor, perceived need, refers to an individual's perception of what services are required based on a self-assessment of health status. Perceived need is highly influenced by attitudes, beliefs, cultural norms, and various other sociodemographic characteristics. Vickery indicates that perceived need may be the most important predictor of healthcare utilization.

Related to perceived need is the third factor, patient preference. This refers to the decision-making process that occurs between patients and their

FIGURE 10.1

Relationship
Between
Healthcare
Services Versus
Health Status
with Flat-of-the-
Curve Medicine

*Too much of a
good thing:
Flat-of-the-
curve medicine
is when more
health services
make no
incremental
improvement to
health*

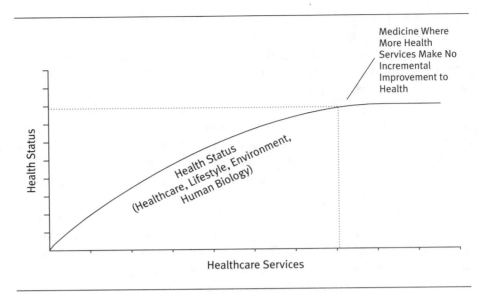

physicians regarding treatment. Physicians provide patients with information on available treatment options relevant to their specific conditions, and patients then make decisions on the basis of their understanding of those options.

The final factor is nonhealth motives. Nonhealth motives arise when healthcare services are used for purposes unrelated to individual health status. Such a motive appears when individuals use healthcare services in a malingering attempt to qualify for short-term sick benefits, long-term disability, or workers' compensation. Although the magnitude of their influence is generally unknown, various nonhealth motives seem to influence how individuals use healthcare (Vickery 1996).

Demand Management Programs

Demand management programs address somatization and flat-of-the-curve medicine (Rossiter et al. 1999). Although demand management programs have various designs, they generally embrace four primary components:

1. telephone triage to provide advice, referral counseling, or both;
2. self-care informational materials to address minor injuries and illnesses;
3. health education to focus on the self-management of chronic conditions such as asthma and diabetes; and
4. wellness initiatives to change unhealthy behaviors.

By improving access to and the availability of appropriate health information, demand management programs empower consumers to participate in decisions that affect their health. Then, by avoiding inappropriate utilization, these consumers save costs (McEachern 1995). Vickery, however, stresses that "demand management is not demand reduction, nor is it need reduction; these are among its results, but they are not its goals" (Vickery 1996).

The effectiveness of telephone triage programs is difficult to determine because much of the existing evidence assessing their value is limited to largely descriptive and anecdotal reports (Harris 1996; Sabin 1998; Gemignani 1996; McCarthy 1997; McEachern 1995; Marosits 1997). Only recently have researchers started using more sophisticated statistical methods to study telephone triage (Rossiter et al. 2000; Lattimer, George, and Thompson 1998; Delichatsios, Callahan, and Charlson 1998). But the widespread adoption of demand management programs and the early results from serious studies seem to underscore their value. Done right, they can achieve a balance between totally unfettered patient demand for services and modulated demand that, nevertheless, leaves the patient in charge.

The Role of Telephone Triage

Telephone triage is a cornerstone of many demand management programs (Lester and Breudigam 1996; Sabin 1998). Most triage lines operate 24 hours a day and are staffed by specially trained nurses. Although variously configured, telephone triage systems may encompass a variety of services.

For calls received by the triage line, nurses systematically assess the symptoms presented, determine their seriousness, and give advice. Offering advice is distinctly different from providing medical diagnoses, which nurses are legally prohibited from doing (Sullivan 1997). For most telephone triage systems, computerized algorithms guide the interaction with the caller providing a detailed step-by-step process. These algorithms are typically developed from peer-reviewed databases of treatment protocols and abstracts extracted from the medical literature (McCarthy 1997; Wolcott 1996). Callers identified as having certain chronic diseases, such as asthma and diabetes, may be referred to more intensive disease management programs for ongoing monitoring and education. Often, callers are not seeking symptom-related advice but are looking for information on specific health issues, such as what to do for pain of a certain variety or how to control an asthma episode. Nurses may assist these callers by providing the necessary information or, when available, directing them to an audiotape library.

The Available Evidence on the Cost Effectiveness of Telephone Triage

Although limited, existing descriptive and anecdotal evidence suggests that demand management programs, including telephone triage, may be effective in containing costs by controlling inappropriate utilization. A study of Medicaid claims data for Blue Cross Blue Shield of Oregon found an annual savings of $184 per member for those individuals with access to telephone triage services (McCarthy 1997). A study of 24,000 Wisconsin state school employees done by William Mercer, Inc., found a five-to-one return for those employees using the demand management program, which included a telephone triage line as a component (Gemignani 1996). Other demand management programs with telephone triage, including those for such employers as Dow Chemical, Hannaford Brothers Supermarkets, and General Motors, all report that the initiatives have helped control the inappropriate use of healthcare services (McCarthy 1997). What is unclear, however, is how effective telephone triage might be for older patients. Older people tend to have many more comorbid conditions that are not as easy to target with specific interventions. It is also more difficult for older patients to change their long-established attitudes and behaviors. Willingness to change is less likely.

Cost savings may be achieved by providing callers with interventions that are matched more appropriately to the condition for which they are calling. Findings indicate that in many cases, home care advice that comes with instructions to be seen the following day by a physician provides an appropriate intervention. Cost savings are achieved because in the absence of telephone triage, many of these callers may have otherwise sought high-cost medical care, including a visit to the emergency room (Poole et al. 1993). This finding corroborates previous research that the majority of medical-seeking behaviors is not premised on a truly emergent condition or situation (Barsky and Borus 1995). In fact, the design of most telephone triage systems anticipates that only 5 percent of the calls received will be true emergencies (Lester and Breudigam 1996).

Emergency Authorization

Emergency services are defined broadly to mean covered inpatient and outpatient services that are needed to evaluate or stabilize an emergency medical condition that is found to exist using a prudent layperson standard.

The Medicare managed care policy for the provision of **emergency services** for beneficiaries is clearly laid out in federal regulation at Title 42 Part 417.414(c)(1). A Medicare+Choice managed care plan must assume financial responsibility and provide reasonable reimbursement for emergency services and urgently needed services (as defined in 417.401) that Medicare enrollees obtain from providers and suppliers outside the health plan *even in the absence of health plan prior approval* (emphasis added).

Medicare+Choice managed care plans cannot require prior authorization for emergency services. This policy also is stated in section 2104 of the Medicare+Choice manual: "Do Not Require Prior Authorization." In addition, section 2104 of the manual states: "Do not retroactively deny a claim because a condition, which appeared to be an emergency, turns out to be non-emergency in nature." Therefore, if emergency services appeared to be needed, plans may not decide on retrospective review to refuse to cover emergency services provided.

Although the requirements from Medicare are clear and unequivocal, obviously Medicare+Choice plans cannot pay for every service provided in an emergency room. Normally, this is handled through prior authorization procedures. These procedures are designed to educate beneficiaries about when to seek emergency care and channel them to the appropriate alternatives. They also address repeat offenders who use emergency services inappropriately. Emergency services are defined broadly to mean covered inpatient and outpatient services that are needed to evaluate or stabilize an **emergency medical condition** that is found to exist using a "prudent layperson" standard. This standard encompasses clinical emergencies, and it also clearly requires health plans to base coverage decisions for emergency services on the severity of the symptoms at the time of presentation. Health plans are also required to cover examinations where the presenting symptoms are of sufficient severity to constitute an emergency medical condition in the judgment of a prudent layperson.

Emergency Room and Urgent Care Procedures

How do managed care plans educate and channel beneficiaries to the right source of healthcare? What can they do to alter the behavior of repeat offenders who obtain nonemergency or even unnecessary services in emergency settings? There are three primary mechanisms available to Medicare managed care plans: education, national coverage decisions rules, and use of objective evidence-based standards.

First, medically necessary emergency care must be available and accessible 24 hours a day, seven days a week. All information that goes to beneficiaries should include a clear definition of a medical emergency and the procedures for obtaining care in such a situation. The definition and the procedures should be prominently and repeatedly displayed in enrollment materials, newsletters, and communications that announce changes in your plan. Paperwork sent to a member following an incident of emergency services should repeat the definition and procedures. Specifically, these materials should address how to obtain care or authorization for care:

* during office hours in the service area,
* after office hours in the service area, and
* outside of the service area.

Medicare+Choice plans are required to provide their enrollees with those services that are covered under Medicare and available to other fee-for-service Medicare beneficiaries who live in the geographic area covered by the plan. That means you must view emergency services and budget for them much like fee-for-service Medicare. But that also means you can manage the demand for the services.

This leads to the second way that managed care plans can address emergency room and urgent care procedures. Any Medicare+Choice plan must abide by HCFA national coverage decisions. **National coverage decisions** are a codified group of rules for coverage representing somewhat of a consensus set of decisions made by carriers and fiscal intermediaries. These are available in HCFA's Coverage Issues Manual. Durable medical equipment is handled through regional contractors, and coverage decisions for this area may be

Emergency medical condition is a medical condition manifesting itself by acute symptoms of sufficient severity (including severe pain). Given this condition, a prudent layperson—someone who possesses an average knowledge of health and medicine—could reasonably expect the absence of immediate medical attention to place the health of the individual in serious jeopardy, serious impairment to body functions, or serious dysfunction of any bodily organ or part.

National coverage decisions are a codified set of rules that set out what services under which circumstances will be paid by Medicare. These payments are made according to the ongoing consensus set of decisions made by fee-for-service carriers and intermediaries.

found from the Durable Medical Equipment Regional Carrier serving your region. You must take care to reconcile any internal coverage policies you may have had as a health plan serving the commercial population with the national coverage decisions of Medicare, which can vary.

The bottom line for your plan is this: Emergency authorization guide-lines, nurse triage programs, and other demand management programs for the commercial population must be modified to reflect the National Coverage Decisions for Medicare managed care. Their procedures and guidelines also must abide by specific written policies made by the Medicare carrier or intermediary with jurisdiction for claims in the geographic area served by the plan. (These policies are sometimes called "local medical review determinations.") In cases where the plan overlaps the jurisdictions of more than one contractor and the contractors have different medical review policies, the plan must apply the medical review policies of the contractor in the area where the beneficiary lives.

The point is that the National Coverage Decisions represent a nucleus of opportunities for improving access to emergency care. Whereas almost any emergency service the beneficiary initiates is covered by Medicare, the managed care plan should determine whether it can appropriately channel some of that demand to urgent care settings. You can make arrangements with local hospital emergency rooms so that they can channel patients who come to the emergency room for care to an available urgent care facility or to the primary care case manager for treatment. They can do this once the patient is evaluated and stablized in the emergency room. You must develop a relationship with the local emergency facilities and personnel to achieve these improvements.

Third, you should determine coverage issues based on an objective, evidence-based process. For starters, you can develop written policies and procedures that reflect current standards of medical practice, and you can distribute these to emergency providers to help them process requests for emergency services. Statements about coverage such as "it is our policy to deny coverage for service X" are unacceptable substitutes for a careful process based on authoritative evidence.

Examples of evidence that are useful in this process include studies from government agencies such as the Agency for Health Care Research and Qual-ity, including the Center for Health Care Technology, (www.ahcrq.gov) and the Food and Drug Administration (www.fda.gov). Evaluations performed by independent technology assessment groups, such as ECRI (www.ecri.org) and the Blue Cross/Blue Shield Association (www.bcbsa.org), also can provide useful background. You are on far better ground denying payment for any ser-vice that might be claimed as an emergency if you have authoritative evidence that it is not an emergency. You may want to perform your own analysis of the issue. To do this, you can search peer review journals for literature that covers well-designed, controlled, clinical studies of the service or technology involved in the service. Case studies and anecdotal information are far less persuasive in supporting coverage decisions. If there's no authoritative evidence or medical consensus that a service is reasonable and necessary, your managed care plan is justified in denying coverage.

There is a distinction between healthcare services that must be reimbursed as covered by Medicare and services that are appropriate for a particular patient. For individual patients, coverage decisions based on appropriateness are decisions based on medical necessity. Thus, it may be true that a service that is "covered" in general is found not to be "reasonable and necessary" for an individual beneficiary because of the specific medical condition of the beneficiary or the availability of more effective alternatives for treatment. That may include treatments outside the emergency room. The judgments made regarding medical necessity do not always have to be identical to those made by providers in the fee-for-service sector and allowed by carriers and intermediaries. This is permissible as long as the judgments of the managed care plan remain within the range of high-quality medical practice and are in the best interest of the patient.

One final caution is in order. You are not allowed to have clauses in managed care plan contracts or similar restrictions that prevent physicians or other providers from fully discussing all diagnostic or treatment options with a patient. Medicare beneficiaries are entitled to a variety of benefits, and this includes getting advice from their physicians on medically necessary treatment options that may be appropriate for their condition or disease. As Figure 10.2 points out, beneficiaries in managed care plans are entitled to all the benefits of other Medicare beneficiaries, and they are entitled to get advice on appropriate diagnostic and treatment options from their physician. A gag clause would have the practical effect of prohibiting a physician from giving a patient the full range of advice and counsel that is clinically appropriate. It could result in the managed care plan not providing all covered Medicare services to its enrollees, and this violates the responsibilities of the managed care plan. Anything like a gag clause is prohibited.

Discharge Planning

The objective of discharge planning should be to estimate the length of hospitalization, prepare the patient and family for timely discharge, and identify patients at risk of long length of stay at the time of admission to minimize nonacute days at the end of the hospitalization. On a day-to-day basis, patients must be assessed with a focus on the need for continued hospitalization. Key objectives of care for that day must be communicated among the multidisciplinary team.

Recent federal data (OIG 1998) show that most Medicare discharges (60 percent from hospital inpatient settings) were to the patient's home, 15 percent were to skilled nursing facilities, 10 percent were to home with home health care needed, 3 percent to intermediate care, and the remaining 13

FIGURE 10.2

Provisions from
Federal Law
Regarding
Coverage and
Medical
Necessity
Review

*By the book:
Medicare law
clearly provides
for managed
care coverage the
same as
traditional
fee-for-service*

Section 1862(a)(1)(A) of the Social Security Act excludes payment for items that "are not reasonable and necessary for the diagnosis or treatment of illness or injury or to improve the functioning of a malformed body member."

Section 1876(c)(2)(A) requires contracting plans to provide enrollees with the services covered under Part A and Part B.

Section 1876(I)(6) states that the Secretary can terminate a contract with, or apply other remedies to an entity if that contracting entity "fails substantially to provide medically necessary items and services that are required . . . to be provided to an individual covered under the contract, if the failure has affected . . . the individual (beneficiary)."

percent to some other entity. Medicare managed care plans have been shown to *increase* the use of skilled nursing facilities, home health care, and intermediate care (Rossiter, Nelson, and Adamache 1988). They do this by pursuing more aggressive discharge planning than that followed in the fee-for-service sector of Medicare—discharge planning designed to drive down the length of hospital inpatient stay and reduce the risk of readmission. The amount that managed care companies pay in higher rates of post-acute hospital care or readmissions, they save on the cost of inpatient hospital care. Many managed care plans pay hospitals on a per-diem basis to capture the lower cost of a reduced length of stay that results from their discharge planning efforts.

Both hospitals and managed care plans operate discharge-planning processes. The contract between the two organizations should specify who is responsible for the discharge planning of the health plan's patients. Depending on the method of payment, this is normally the health plan. Patients may be discharged to a variety of settings. These include a patient's home, with or without services from a home health agency, or a nursing home. There appears to be no single model for a hospital discharge-planning process. Definitions of what discharge planning is vary widely, as do the organizational structures of the departments and professional credentials of the discharge-planning staff. There aren't any federal requirements for managed care plans to follow when it comes to discharge planning.

The social work or nursing department often has the primary responsibility for discharge planning, and the department generally receives input from other members of the healthcare team. The responsibility is sometimes in the case management or utilization review department.

According to a 1998 OIG study, effective discharge planning identifies early on what the patient's needs will be after leaving the hospital. This ensures that the patient is discharged to a safe environment with the appropriate level of services. Once a determination has been made that a patient needs discharge planning, the discharge planner conducts a psycho-social assessment and meets with utilization review staff, the patient's nurses and physicians, or other relevant interdisciplinary team members to discuss the patient's care plan. Early on, the discharge planner solicits the patient's preferences and concerns and reaches out to the family or other potential caregivers to get their input and cooperation. This much is expected of Medicare managed care plans (HCFA 1998). Studies show the presence of available relatives or friends is the primary factor that influences discharge planning for a particular patient. When family is present, 66 percent of patients go home. When absent for arthroplasty, 100 percent of patients go to a rehab facility (Kane et al. 2000).

From the Institute for Clinical Evaluative Studies (ICES 1999), an effective early discharge-planning strategy includes the following: an expected date of discharge program, a reassessment flow sheet, and criteria for identifying patients with low risk of a long length of stay (Fig. 10.3).

The first strategy of discharge planning (Fig. 10.3) is assigning the expected date of discharge so that the patient, the physician, and the rest of the healthcare team will have a goal to meet. All admissions, including elective and emergency, should receive an expected length of stay. There are numerous sources of data that discuss expected length of stay. Normally, managed care

---

FIGURE 10.3
Three Strategies for Discharge Planning

Manage the demand for hospital care: An effective early discharge planning process is a strategic issue

Implement Expected Date of Discharge Program (EDD):

An expected date of discharge is an anticipated date for discharge that is largely contingent on the admitting diagnosis and the expected clinical course of the hospital stay.

Establish the expected date of discharge either prior to admission (elective surgery), at admission, or within 48 hours of admission.

The anticipated date (hereafter referred to as the target date) is generally based on a database norm, a hospital's own norm, or another external reference.

Use Reassessment Flow Sheets:

Ensures patients are receiving an appropriate level of care when occupying acute-care beds.

Provides a mechanism to prevent delays in the care process.

The principal question to be asked on a daily basis is: "Does the patient require acute hospital services? If so, what are the plans for the day? If not, what are the plans for discharge to alternate care/home. If discharge is the choice, what is the acute care plan for the day?"

Develop Criteria for Identifying Patients at Low Risk for Long Length of Stay:

Assessment for high risk of long length of stay

Worksheets to aid in the implementation of these criteria.

Source: Institute for Clinical Evaluative Sciences. 1999. *Early Discharge Planning Strategies.* Ontario Ministry of Health, Canada.

companies rely on their own database of experience and periodically establish new stretch goals for reducing length of stay on a diagnosis-by-diagnosis basis.

Reassessment flow sheets are simple check sheets that can be generalized for all patients or created specifically for particular high-volume, high-cost hospital stays (Fig. 10.3). The advantage of these sheets is that they are concise, requiring only a few check marks. In fact, they could replace some progress notes. These flow sheets should be designed in a way that encourages hospitals to review each patient's status daily, to communicate the acute-care objectives for the day, to prompt action (acute-care plan, transfer, or discharge) if acute care is not required, and to identify reasons for delays during acute-care hospitalization. They are similar to care mapping or explicit criteria used on a concurrent basis for managing the flow of the patient's care through time. The information from reassessment flow sheets should be collected or summarized and assessed by the health plan to suggest ways to improve patient care and identify persistent problems that occur when trying to discharge patients early.

Most patients will receive care in the hospital for routine services, and they require little or no discharge planning. The costly cases are the ones that are at high risk for long length of stay. To focus attention on the high risks, you should create an explicit effort to identify patients at low risk for long length of stay. Then you can pay special attention to all of the other patients (Fig. 10.3). These criteria should be used in the emergency room to identify patients appropriate for referral to a quick-response team or urgent-care team. And these criteria can be used in preoperative assessment as a component of the nurse's assessment. The intent could be to anticipate discharge planning prior to admission. It is also appropriate to use them on the nursing unit as components of the nurse's assessment. In this case, the goal is to move toward discharge planning as soon as possible. Managed care plans that are able to concentrate their patients among a few hospital facilities are better able to integrate this type of discharge planning into the care of their patients.

Skilled Care

The same rule about discharge planning applies to skilled nursing care. To help avoid problems in discharge planning, skilled nursing facilities generally work closely with hospital discharge planners and social workers to ensure that only individuals requiring skilled services are admitted to skilled parts of the nursing home. If the skilled nursing facility determines that the person does not meet skilled standards and then admits the resident to a skilled part, it must provide the individual with a Notice of Non Coverage.

Nursing homes are required to give residents the Notice of Non Coverage when they are admitted or any time after they are admitted and skilled services are no longer required. Patients may appeal the nursing home's decision for noncoverage and should never be charged for services until they receive a formal decision on the appeal from Medicare. However, if as a result of the appeal it is determined that the managed care plan will not cover the stay, the patient is liable for the cost of care since the start of the nursing home stay. The appeal should not take an extensive period of time, and if it does, the beneficiary can report the health plan to Medicare for corrective action.

Durable Medical Equipment

Durable medical equipment can be covered in the payment to the hospital or separately after discharge. Some durable medical equipment suppliers bring items to beneficiaries residing in an institution just prior to the beneficiary's discharge in order to fit them for the equipment or train them how to use it. Having fitted or trained the beneficiary, the supplier should take the item and deliver it to the beneficiary's home on the date of discharge. The supplier should be paid for this item when it is delivered or when the beneficiary is discharged from the institution. If the supplier delivers the item to the beneficiary for use in the institution prior to the beneficiary's discharge from the hospital, the item should be the hospital's responsibility, and the supplier should not submit the claim.

Rehabilitative Services

The key to effective rehabilitative care in Medicare managed care is the identification of high-risk individuals, assessment of their health-related needs, and interventions designed both to meet those needs and to prevent further undesirable outcomes.

One of the most useful studies on rehabilitation recommends a three-pronged approach (Boult et al. 1998). You should identify high-risk seniors (also called case finding) for intervention through a combination of periodic screening, recognition of high-risk seniors by clinicians, and analysis of administrative databases. Once identified, potential high-risk enrollees should undergo an initial assessment in eight domains: cognition, medical conditions, medications, access to care, functional status, social situation, nutrition, and emotional status. A 30- to 45-minute interview can accomplish the initial assessment conducted by a skilled professional—usually one with a background in nursing. High-risk persons should then be linked with appropriate services, and others might be targeted for more detailed assessments. Interdisciplinary teams of various compositions and methods of operation, depending on local circumstances, often perform detailed assessments including geriatricians under contract with the health plan (Boult et al. 1998; Mukamel et al. 1997).

Medicare+Choice plans have a reasonable track record in conservative use of rehabilitative care. In the most comprehensive and carefully designed study of rehabilitative care done to date for HCFA, Retchin and colleagues (1997) compared discharge destinations and survival rates following stroke in Medicare HMOs with similar fee-for-service settings. The study was large, with 19 HMOs selected from 12 states. The sample included 402 HMO patients from 71 hospitals and 408 fee-for-service patients from 60 hospitals. HMO patients were more likely than fee-for-service patients to be sent to nursing homes (HMO—41.8 percent; fee-for-service—27.9 percent) and less likely to be discharged to rehabilitation hospitals or units (HMO—16.2 percent; fee-for-service—23.4 percent). At follow-up, there was no significant difference in relative risk of dying between HMO and fee-for-service groups. Patients in Medicare HMOs who experience strokes are more likely to be discharged to nursing homes and less likely to go to rehabilitation facilities following the acute event. However, they have similar survival patterns compared with similar patients in fee-for-service settings and after adjusting for other factors (Retchin et al. 1997). These results parallel the results of a study of home care after hospitalization as well. Outcomes were similar even though patients in HMOs were more likely to have home care at earlier discharge (Holtzman, Chen, and Kane 1998).

Strategic Decisions Checklist

Strategic Questions	Strategic Analyses
Do you know the unique features of your membership in terms of demand for health services?	Beyond the standard Medicare demographic cost factors, you should study the characteristics of your membership that might identify members with preventable somatization.
	Understand where somatization occurs, if at all. Select indicators that help to identify preventable somatization.
	Convey to your health plan managers, hospital, and physician network an understanding of the notion of flat-of-the-curve medicine. Make sure they believe it and act on it.
	Compare your membership to national norms or other health plans on morbidity, perceived-need patient preferences, and nonhealth motives.
	continued

Strategic Questions	Strategic Analyses
Do you have a telephone triage program?	Telephone triage programs have been shown to be cost effective. You should have one. You should provide: • 24-hour access to registered nurses for advice and referral counseling; • printed self-care guides; • audio or video tapes; • access to Internet sites on health topics; and • referral procedures to disease management programs from telephone triage.
Do you have emergency authorization?	Prior authorization cannot be required by Medicare+Choice managed care plans for emergency services. However: • You should have an aggressive program of beneficiary education about when to seek emergency care; • You should have mechanisms for channeling patients to alternatives to costly emergency care when an emergency does not exist; • You must have an intervention to modify the behavior of repeat offenders of inappropriate use of emergency services; • Your definition for emergency services and procedures for urgent care must be consistent with the prudent layperson's definition of emergency; • Ensure that your emergency and urgent-care procedures follow National Coverage Decisions and local medical review determinations; and • Emergency and urgent-care procedures must be written and based on objective, evidence-based processes. *continued*

Strategic Questions	Strategic Analyses
Do you have effective discharge planning?	You want to continuously improve your plan's ability to shorten length of stay and reduce readmissions to the hospital by substituting skilled nursing facility care, home health, and intermediate care services. • Have an Expected Date of Discharge Program • Use reassessment flow sheets effectively • Have criteria for identifying patients at low risk for long length of stay, so you can focus attention every day on the remaining patients at high risk for long length of stay • Align your relationships with skilled nursing home facilities to be in line with objectives for discharge planning • Align the state of relationships with durable medical equipment suppliers to be in line with objectives for discharge planning • Have in place a general plan for dealing with do-not-resuscitate orders • Have effective rehabilitation services

PROVIDER LIABILITY IN MEDICARE MANAGED CARE

The end of the 20th century saw the rapid adoption of managed care as a means to organize the delivery of healthcare with a special focus on both quality and costs. Today, on the morning of a new century, the continued expansion of managed care faces some chilling prospects. Chief among those are attacks on managed care by expanding managed care liability.

Spurring the attacks are anecdotal reports of inappropriate treatment decisions in health plans and a growing patient distrust of managed care in general. Many groups advocate the enactment of legislation to expose managed care plans and their providers to civil litigation and tort liability. The focal point for this legislative debate, at state and federal levels, appears in the form of a patient's bill of rights. The outcome of the policy continues to evolve, and the growing case law is heading in uncertain directions, making it difficult for this chapter to provide the most recent developments concerning provider and health plan liability.

Healthcare reform that would expose health plans to **civil litigation and tort liability** could spill over to providers (Studdert et al. 1999). In many parts of the country, one of the essential aspects of Medicare managed care is the transfer of risk to physicians and hospitals. Chapter 5 describes the Medicare-imposed limits on this risk. However, when decisions about medical necessity and coverage are delegated to provider organizations, it can lead to cases of spillover liability. This liability implicates the health plan and the at-risk physicians and hospitals, with the risk relationship creating the connection. Put differently, if a health plan shares the risk of high-cost care with physicians and that relationship can be shown to compromise decisions made by physicians, both parties might be liable. The physician is liable for making wrong medical decisions, and the health plan is wrong for setting up a payment system that encourages wrong medical decisions.

With the issue of health plan liability in flux, Chapter 11 focuses on provider liability. This chapter introduces two broad areas of provider liability with respect to Medicare managed care. The first area involves the duty of the physician and hospital to be the patient's advocate—the more positive counterpoint to the legal consequences of not doing so. The second area centers on the **antitrust** and monopoly concerns that providers should heed in Medicare managed care. Antitrust looms as a liability concern because of the undiminished pace of mergers; acquisitions; and consolidation of hospitals,

Civil litigation and tort liability are lawsuits brought by patients against physicians, hospitals, and health plans for damages from malpractice including inappropriate decisions about health plans paying for coverage.

Antitrust is the field of law protecting consumers from monopolies, attempts to monopolize, conspiracies in restraint of trade, price fixing, and mergers or acquisitions that tend to create a monopoly.

physicians, and health plans. Medicare can become involved with antitrust when services or specialties that serve predominantly Medicare patients become local monopolies for whatever reason. Local monopolies affect the contracts between Medicare+Choice plans and physicians and hospitals. The connection between medical malpractice liability and antitrust is that both expect the physician, the hospital, and the health plan to serve as the patient's advocate in both medicine and economics.

This chapter discusses the issue of patient advocacy that Medicare managed care plans should adopt as part of their strategic direction. Health plans, especially the hospitals and physicians serving Medicare beneficiaries, have a duty to patients. The managed care plans and providers following this principle should not overly expose any provider to unnecessary liability. The chapter also details guidelines for hospitals and physicians to consider as they devise their roles in the Medicare managed care market, with an emphasis on monopolies or attempts at monopoly.

These basic discussions aim to give you an introductory understanding of the issues surrounding liability. From this discussion, you'll have an overview of strategic decisions that your health plan should consider when it comes to provider liability.

Duty to Be the Patient's Advocate

Liabilities exist today for managed care companies, physicians participating in managed care, and developers of clinical practice guidelines. Patients frequently suffer physical or financial injury, and it is the source of this injury and the reasons behind it that expose providers to liability. This liability is mitigated if the parties involved carry out their duty to be the patient's advocate.

Managed care companies must be concerned about taking actions that could raise their direct institutional liability. Although they're responsible for collecting premiums and arranging and paying for care, their role in medical decision making can be a point of dispute, pulling them directly into medical care gone wrong. Negligence, "bad faith," or breach of contract on the part of the managed care company or its affiliated providers can be a point of departure for showing lack of devotion to being the patient's advocate.

Vicarious liability refers to the obligation to be responsible for the negligence of a third party. Either by looking the other way or by sympathizing, a person or organization can be drawn into a lawsuit for damages.

Another theory regarding the reasons for injury to patients has been argued in court. It accuses health plans and providers of **vicarious liability** for medical malpractice committed by affiliated physicians or their staff (*Dukes v. U.S. Healthcare* 1995; *Dunn v. Praiss* 1992; *PacifiCare of Oklahoma v. Burrage* 1995; *Prihoda v. Shpritz* 1996). Vicarious liability is the obligation that a person or organization has for the negligence of a third party. Suppose a health plan looks the other way when something goes wrong, sympathizes with known questionable behavior, or pretends not to notice. Should one of these scenarios exist, a health plan can be drawn into a lawsuit against a physician or hospital even though it's not directly involved in the caregiving.

A health plan and its providers, after all, are paid premiums and fees to be agents for the patient. Thus, any deviation from this agency principle raises liability concerns.

Finally, you need to remove financial disincentives to treat, refer, or hospitalize a particular patient. There are many anecdotes in the popular press of patients being denied coverage or going untreated, or not being referred or hospitalized. There may be sound medical reasons for these decisions. They become mixed up with the financial aspects of managed care's risk-based payments, withholds, and bonuses for meeting targets. Together, these factors give the impression that a conflict exists between quality and costs. No doubt, there are cases of excessive cost containment. However, health plans and providers must balance their financial incentives with their duty to be the patient's advocate. One way health plans and providers can protect themselves is to disclose their financial incentives to their patients. Recent court cases seem to place more emphasis on the fact that the financial incentives were not disclosed, rather than the fact that they were the cause of harm to patients (*Bast v. Prudential Insurance Co. of America* 1998).

Utilization Review and Gatekeeper Decisions

Third-party payers can be held legally accountable when medically inappropriate decisions result from defects in the design or implementation of cost-containment mechanisms. For example, when appeals made by a physician on a patient's behalf for medical or hospital care are arbitrarily ignored or unreasonably disregarded or overridden by the health plan, the plan raises its potential liability (*Wickline v. State* 1986).

Ideally, the care a patient receives should be the care that the managed care plan and hospital or physician agree is appropriate. Physicians and hospitals are expected to wrestle with the bureaucracy to see that the care they have ordered for their patient is covered and paid. The physician or hospital should exhaust all procedural rights when the utilization review process has rejected a medical recommendation. Suppose further payments are available to patients but receiving them depends on following an appeals procedure. If the provider is ignorant of the appeals procedure and some harm comes to the patient that's attributable to this ignorance, the provider might be held liable. Physicians have always had an alternative. They can order the care, and if it is not covered, they can collect payment directly from the patient. The modern system of health insurance should not be an excuse for not recommending or not delivering appropriate medical care in accordance with the community standard.

Utilization review and gatekeeper decisions are more likely to be a breach of contract or bad faith denials of care. Medicare and patient-paid premiums are for Medicare coverage plus the supplemental services spelled out in Medicare and the insurance policy. As is the case with any contract for services, a breach of contract ensues when provisions are unmet. That means utilization review and gatekeeper decisions must be considered carefully, not haphazardly. You can be accused of failing to investigate a claim properly. Nurses making medical decisions can expose the plan to scope of practice charges. Managed care plans, physicians, and hospitals at financial risk need to be especially aware of these potential liabilities.

Emphasizing Best Practices

The best way to manage this liability is to emphasize best practices. Education sessions, dissemination of medical treatment guidelines from authoritative sources, and other efforts must support the practice of improving care, not denying care. In *Wilson v. Blue Cross of Southern California*, the supporting argument for denying payment was that the health plan could not pass liability to the treating physician for a discharge decision.

What is the authoritative source for utilization review and gatekeeper decisions? What standards and whose standards were used? How much research went into examining the literature and the available medical evidence for the decision? The Agency for Health Care Research and Quality has web sites (www.guidelines.gov) with hundreds of approved **clinical practice guidelines** for most major illnesses. The agency attempts to keep them current by releasing new guidelines and medical advances. If you use these and other available published guidelines that have been approved by a professional organization that has authority, you should be able to lessen your liability.

Clinical practice guidelines are systematically developed statements to assist practitioner and patient decisions about appropriate healthcare for specific clinical circumstances.

Liability for Referrals and Second Opinion

Guidelines are not fixed protocols that must be followed. Guidelines are just that: guides for aiding physicians. They're designed for healthcare professionals to consider as they make decisions about treatments and referrals. Although they identify and describe generally recommended courses of intervention, they are not a substitute for the advice of a physician or other knowledgeable healthcare professional. Individual patients may require different treatments from those specified in a given guideline. Guidelines are not entirely inclusive or exclusive of all methods of reasonable care that can achieve the same results. Whereas guidelines can be written to account for variations in clinical settings, resources, or common patient characteristics, they cannot address the unique needs of each patient nor the combination of resources available. Deviations from clinical practice guidelines may be justified by individual circumstances. Thus, guidelines must be applied based on the needs of individual patients and using professional judgment. When in doubt, physicians should always use common sense or consult another physician.

If a provider must deviate from a guideline, the reason should be documented in the chart or in correspondence to other physicians or the health plan. Physicians are always legally and ethically responsible for an appropriate medical discharge. Denial of certain medical treatments should be considered a denial of benefits rather than a medical decision; physicians always have the duty to provide the standard of care. Guidelines do not define the standard of care, but they may be used as evidence that the physician followed or did not follow the community standard of care.

Advance Directives

Medicare managed care plans must recognize that all adults in hospitals, skilled nursing facilities, and healthcare settings have certain rights. Confidential personal and medical records, informed consent about medical treatment, and the right to prepare an **advance directive**—these three rights are inextricably linked. Advance directives can be a statement written ahead of time directing the kind of treatment patients want or don't want if they ever become mentally or physically unable to make choices or communicate their actual wishes.

In a second type of directive, a **healthcare proxy**, patients authorize another person to make those decisions for them should they become incapacitated. Federal law requires providers to give patients information about advance directives and to explain the legal choices in making decisions about medical care. This law affects hospitals, skilled nursing facilities, hospices, home health agencies, and Medicare+Choice plans serving persons covered by either Medicare or Medicaid. When it comes to these directives, state law can differ from the federal law. Medicare+Choice plans are required to give to enrollees information about the laws with respect to advance directives for the state in which they provide services.

The two most commonly prepared advance directives are a **living will** and a **durable power of attorney** for healthcare. Both can be used to ensure a patient's right to accept or refuse medical care. They can also be used to communicate with the managed care plan and the physicians and hospitals providing care on behalf of the managed care plan. These directives can indicate whether patients are saying "yes" to treatments they want, or "no" to treatment they do not want.

A living will generally states the kind of medical care patients want (or don't want) if they become unable to make their own decisions. This directive is called a living will because it takes effect while the patient is still living. Most states have their own living will forms, each somewhat different. It may be possible for your managed care plan to distribute preprinted living will forms from their state for patients to complete and sign. Your plan should support patients who want to speak to an attorney or their physician to be certain they have completed the living will in the way that ensures their wishes will be understood and followed.

In many states, a durable power of attorney for healthcare is a signed, dated, and witnessed paper that authorizes another person—a husband, wife, daughter, son, or close friend—to make medical decisions for patients who cannot make those decisions for themselves. These papers can also include instructions about any treatment that the patient wants to avoid. Some states

*An **advance directive** is generally a written document prepared by patients stating how they want medical decisions made if they lose the ability to make decisions.*

*A **healthcare proxy** allows a beneficiary to appoint someone they trust (an agent) to make their medical decisions if they are incapacitated, not only at the end of life but whenever the beneficiary cannot speak.*

*A **living will** states in writing a beneficiary's wishes about which medical treatments they do and do not want when they become incapacitated at the end of life.*

***Durable power of attorney** is a signed, dated, and witnessed paper naming another person, such as a husband, wife, daughter, son, or close friend, as your authorized spokesperson to make medical decisions for you if you should become unable to make them for yourself.*

have specific laws that allow a healthcare power of attorney, and they provide printed forms that you can use as a managed care plan for your members.

Patients are not required to have advance directives, and they may cancel them at any time. Any change or cancellation should be written, signed, and dated in accordance with state law. They should then give copies to the managed care plan, the doctor, or to others who may have received copies of the original.

In addition, some states allow the patient to change an advance directive by oral statement. If patients wish to cancel an advance directive while in the hospital, they should notify their doctor, family, and others who may need to know.

If your managed care plan serves Medicare beneficiaries, you'll deal with advance directives frequently. To avoid any misunderstandings and potentially embarrassing public charges, your plan should implement clear responsibilities and procedures for dealing with advance directives. If your members have advance directives, you should make sure that someone—the person's lawyer or family member—knows what it means and where it's located. You may even want to consider establishing procedures to ensure that contract hospitals and your own utilization review nurses check for advance directives. If a patient has a durable power of attorney, make sure a copy or the original is given to the agent or proxy. See if patients have asked their physician to make an advance directive part of the patient's permanent medical record.

Do Not Resuscitate Policy

Few studies describe the end of life for older people covered by either fee-for-service Medicare or managed care. In one available study at four teaching hospitals, the majority of Medicare 417 patients who died within one year of a serious hospitalization had measures in place to limit aggressive care (Somogyi-Zalud et al. 2000). Thus, your members are likely to have their own ideas or plans about limiting aggressive care. Do not try to change their approach to end-of-life care. You are obligated to apply only medical-necessity review criteria in the best interest of the patient.

Recognize also that attitudes about limiting aggressive care are not etched in stone for each patient, and they do change. In the same study (Somogyi-Zalud et al. 2000), before hospitalization, two out of three patients reported fair quality of life, and patients averaged 2.4 impairments in activities of daily living. During the last month of life, three of five patients interviewed in the hospital and four of five interviewed out of the hospital preferred not to be resuscitated. Yet, at the time of death, four of five patients had a do-not-resuscitate (DNR) order and two of five had an order to withhold a ventilator. In the last month of life, one out of four patients reported severe pain. Patients reported increasing functional impairments and limited quality of life. The majority preferred comfort care (Somogyi-Zalud et al. 2000).

With these characteristics of end-of-life care, there are three things to keep in mind about DNR orders:

1. Promulgation of DNR orders are not the purview of a Medicare managed care plan.
2. Beneficiaries are entitled to counsel from their physician.
3. We know very little about the impact on resources of encouraging DNR orders, and what we do know is contradictory.

DNR orders may exist for many of your patients, and you will run into them when questions of medical necessity and heroic expenditures of resources at the end of life are presented to your managed care plan for reimbursement. But your policies, procedures, and training should make it clear that DNR orders belong in the hospital, nursing home, or hospice under the direction of the physician and the patient. They are not something about which the Medicare managed care plan has an opinion.

Medicare+Choice plans must comply with advance directive requirements found in Section 1866(f). This requirement is implemented in 42 C.F.R. Part 489, Subpart I. They require your Medicare providers (including hospitals, critical access hospitals, skilled nursing facilities, nursing facilities, home health agencies, providers of home health care, and hospices) to maintain written policies and procedures concerning advance directives. This provision includes requirements that the provider document in the individual's medical record whether or not the individual has executed an advance directive that could lead to a DNR order. You can require in your contract with providers that they follow Medicare laws and conduct such documentation; but it is beyond the scope of a Medicare+Choice plan to get involved in the decision making with patients.

A physician providing care to a Medicare beneficiary enrolled in a Medicare+Choice plan may not be limited in counseling or advising the beneficiary of medically necessary treatment options that may be appropriate for the individual's condition or disease. Contractual provisions that limit a physician's ability to so counsel or advise a Medicare beneficiary are a violation of the law.

In one of the largest and most comprehensive efforts to describe patient preferences in seriously ill patients, the Study to Understand Prognoses and Preferences for Outcomes and Risks of Treatments (SUPPORT) described the communication of seriously ill patients' preferences for end-of-life care. The study looked at what patient characteristics predict patient preferences for end-of-life care. How well do physicians, nurses, and surrogates understand their patients' preferences, and what variables are correlated with this understanding? Does increasing the documentation of existing advance directives result in care more consistent with patients' preferences? (Covinsky et al. 2000).

The study found that patients who are older, have cancer, are women, believe their prognoses are poor, and are more dependent in activities-of-daily-living function are more likely to limit aggressive care in the case of heart failure. However, there are considerable variability and geographic variation in these preferences. Physician, nurse, and surrogate understanding of their patient's preferences is only moderately better than chance. Most patients do not discuss their preferences with their physicians, and only about half of patients who do not wish to receive CPR receive DNR orders. In SUPPORT patients, there was no evidence that increasing the rates of documentation of advance directives results in care that is more consistent with patients' preferences. SUPPORT documented that physicians and surrogates are often unaware of seriously ill patients' preferences. The care provided to patients is often not consistent with their preferences and is often associated with factors other than preferences or prognoses. Managed care plans are ill-positioned to assist in this situation.

In another study, hospital-based, reinforcing regulatory and educational interventions were employed to encourage physicians to discuss end-of-life (EOL) care with their patients. Specifically, the effects were measured of (1) administrative prompts to encourage discussions about EOL care and (2) a mandatory educational seminar focusing on EOL issues. Actual DNR orders were written for 28.8 percent of the time before intervention and 27.3 percent of the time after intervention. The study's authors concluded that enhanced, mutually reinforcing regulatory and educational efforts focusing on EOL care proved ineffectual at promoting either discussions about EOL issues or the use of DNR orders (Shorr et al. 2000). Managed care companies are better than most at managing health and medical care, but this is one area to leave alone.

Guidelines for the Physician's Role in Medical Management

Most physicians report that they feel they have little or no control over the practice of medicine. Yet, for antitrust purposes, they do.

For example, physicians exert significant control over the operation of hospitals. They determine the number and types of patients admitted, and they prescribe the types of services received. The laws of medical licensure provide a solitary role for physicians to diagnose diseases and prescribe medications. As such, they control the types of patients treated and what is done to them in the hospital. They also control the patient's discharge. With these influences, physicians have a great deal to say about nursing policy and what a nurse does for an individual patient. The board of directors looks to physicians for support, ideas, and approval. With so much responsibility given to the profession, so much is expected in return.

Patients demand service from physicians when they're ill. Physicians recommend visits to other physicians and inpatient hospital services. They prescribe medications and order many other services, which cannot be accessed by the patient without approval by a physician. Most physicians view the payments from patients and insurers as the only portion of the pie they are interested in. Patients, however, see themselves as usually buying much more—an entire healthcare package that runs from the initial visit to the physician to all the care that follows. As a result of these unique relationships, economics views the flow of healthcare dollars as being interconnected. In this view, the physician plays a central role. The interconnectedness raises the specter that the major players in the economics of healthcare might attempt to maximize their own income by manipulating the other pieces of the pie over which they have control or influence.

On the basis of this view, physicians switch hospitals and influence hospitals to increase physician incomes. Hospitals compete with each other, not for patients but for physicians. The not-for-profit hospitals just try to break even while trying at the same time to maintain physician satisfaction. Both hospitals and physicians do better financially if they can capture as many patients in the market as possible.

For those providers who are granted licenses to be in the market at the exclusion of others, the drive for patients and significant influence over their economic decisions can lead toward monopoly in certain markets. Monopoly can creep into the mix when patients lack realistic choices and the physicians and hospitals in the market have significant control over the price of services. Economists have shown that when monopoly power is present, prices exceed the marginal cost of providing services, patients demand fewer services, and the right mix of services is unavailable or not used in the best interest of patients. A monopoly threatens quality and restricts innovation.

These are the economic explanations for why monopoly is bad and why our federal and state antitrust laws discourage it. We have laws governing appropriate relationships, activity, and performance in the medical marketplace. Physicians and hospitals may view competitive activity as responding to managed care plans in the market or trying to protect their market share or market power; but physicians, hospitals, and health plans competing in the Medicare market, which can be viewed as its own separate marketplace, must ensure they do not run afoul of the country's antitrust laws.

Measuring Monopoly Power

This section discusses monopoly as an economic concept. Monopoly becomes a legal issue when a complaint is made in a specific situation and a judge or court decides, on the basis of the evidence presented, that an illegal monopoly exists. To see whether monopoly may be an issue for your market, you can easily compute several measures of monopoly power. Even these can only suggest monopoly power. While these measures should not be immediate cause for alarm if they indicate some level of a monopoly in your market, they may suggest the need for preliminary legal advice.

Note that the concern about monopoly revolves around the provider market, hospitals and physicians for Medicare managed care, not the health plans. Medicare+Choice plans are heavily regulated, especially their pricing for enrollment in the health plan. So you don't need to be concerned if there is a single source of enrollment in a market or only a few health plans with a large market share. But the structure of the market for these plans and the conduct of the providers in the market could be issues for monopoly behavior.

Concentration ratio offers one way to measure the potential for monopoly. This term is defined as the percent of the market (usually measured in sales) accounted for by the largest firms (for example, the top four firms). Thus, if a metropolitan statistical area (MSA) has many large primary care physician practice groups, including four large physician groups with total revenues in the fee-for-service Medicare market exceeding 60 percent of the market, there could be concerns about monopoly. This example illustrates a market with only a few large physician groups with a large market share. Normally a concentration ratio greater than 50 percent bears further examination. This same example holds true for hospitals, home health agencies, and others.

Another measure, the **Herfindahl index**, is defined as the sum of squares of market shares. Any alliance that changes the Herfindahl index a great deal could give rise to the need to challenge the alliance on the grounds of monopoly. According to federal guidelines, these alliances include any merger, acquisition, combination in the form of joint venture, provider-sponsored organization (PSO), and physician-hospital organization. For example, return to the case of four large physician group practices in the market. If the market share for each physician group practice were 15 percent, the Herfindahl index would be $(15^2) + (15^2) + (15^2) + (15^2) + n(1^2) = (225) + (225) + (225) + n(1) = 676$. This calculation illustrates four firms with the same market share adding up to 60 percent and the remainder 40 percent of the market split among many (n) sole practitioners, each with less than 1 percent of the market. If two of the groups were to decide to join together to serve a Medicare+Choice plan in the market, the Herfindahl index would change as follows: $(30^2) + (15^2) + (15^2) + (40^2) = (900) + (225) + (225) + (1) = 1,351$. The change in the Herfindahl index is 675, which would fall well below the federal threshold for concern. But if three of the larger physician groups were to combine, the Herfindahl index would change as follows: $(45^2) + (15^2) + (40^2) = (2,025) + (225) + (1) = 2,251$. This is a change of 1,575, which would put the combination in a possible area for a challenge by the Federal Trade Commission. This change is still below the area of concern, as specified in **Federal Trade Commission guidelines**, when the Herfindahl index changes by more than 1,800.

These calculations are affected by a couple of major issues: (1) what the market is like geographically and (2) what the good or service is that is being counted in the definition of market share. A related issue is what to do with attempts to calculate the power of a monopoly when patients come from outside the market or leave the market to obtain care elsewhere.

Concentration ratio is the percent of the market accounted for by the largest providers (for example, top four). The market may be defined in several ways including provider revenues, number of patients, and other measures.

Herfindahl index is the sum of squares of market share. A large change in the Herfindahl index for a market from a change in the market (merger, acquisition, joint venture, alliance) could indicate monopoly power that would be investigated by antitrust authorities.

Federal Trade Commission guidelines for Herfindahl index changes: A change in the Herfindahl index of 1,000 = no challenge; change from 1,000 to 1,800 = consider challenge; and change over 1,800 = challenge.

If these numbers are large, then the calculation of the concentration ratio or the Herfindahl index is complicated. Obviously, defendants of potential monopoly situations argue for broad definition of geographic markets, and plaintiffs argue for narrow ones.

Having laid out the basic economic principles of monopoly, the big question remains: How can providers participate successfully in the Medicare managed care market without creating a monopoly or engaging in monopolistic behavior?

Antitrust Laws

Three basic antitrust laws apply. Normally they are applied to the entire healthcare market, which covers patients of all ages and payers of all types. But it is reasonable to think that in some parts of the country, antitrust laws apply to the Medicare market as a separate market, depending on the individual circumstances. Two factors in particular would be scrutinized: (1) whether the Medicare market dominates the broader healthcare market and (2) how the Medicare market conducts itself. In other words, are beneficiaries harmed by the arrangement?

Of the three antitrust laws, the first is the Sherman Act, especially Sections 1 and 2. Section 1 states that monopolies and conspiracies in the form of trusts in restraint of trade are illegal. This can refer to contracts or collaboration among providers or among providers and health plans. They are illegal if they are designed to restrain trade or commerce among the states. Thus, it is illegal for a PSO to enter into contracts or collaborative agreements, either written or implied, overt or covert, to keep other competitors out of the market; divide up geographic areas; or engage in monopolistic pricing. Section 2 backs this up with a general prohibition to monopolize. Where Section 1 addresses the structure of the market, Section 2 addresses behavior in the market and can get you in trouble if you attempt to monopolize or conspire to monopolize. In fact, it isn't clear that you must actually gain from the monopoly. It can be enough under Section 2 of the Sherman Act to engage in the attempt without actually having achieved a monopoly. Suppose a group of physicians in the same specialty who vacation together talk about how they might work jointly to charge higher prices to a Medicare managed care plan in return for an exclusive contract with the plan to keep other plans out of the market. Although this is just talk, it's likely to be illegal.

The second important antitrust act to consider is the Clayton Act, Section 7, which covers mergers or acquisitions by one corporation of another. While the Sherman Act addresses the structure and conduct of the market and whether there is a monopoly, the Clayton Act addresses potential monopolies that arise from mergers.

Mergers are illegal if they substantially reduce competition or tend to create a monopoly. The federal or state prosecutors will apply the concentration ratios and Herfindahl index calculations described earlier and decide whether a potential merger or acquisition moves too much toward monopoly. As a rule of thumb, market share of 50 percent, defined in reasonable terms, is a cutoff for a Clayton Act violation. Merged entities that don't hold more than 50 percent market share are probably acceptable to the antitrust authorities, assuming the unmerged entity contributes to competition and the merged entity offers patients greater efficiencies.

The third antitrust law is the Robinson-Patman Act, which outlays price discrimination. Price discrimination is defined as the monopolist's ability to divide the market for exactly the same good or service and charge different prices to different purchasers. The price differences bear no relationship and cannot be justified on the basis of cost differences. Rather, these price differences are based on what the market will bear. Price discrimination is illegal if it substantially harms competition, tends to create a monopoly, or injures or prevents competition.

The Department of Justice (DOJ) and the Federal Trade Commission (FTC) collaborated to issue a joint Antitrust Enforcement statement. This statement sets out the areas of economic activity that hospitals, doctors, and other health professionals might engage in without getting in trouble. The statement sets out all the areas the two agencies agree are **antitrust safe harbors** or safe activities. The central goal in healthcare antitrust enforcement is to ensure that consumers are able to decide what they want in the marketplace instead of having providers limit their choices. Some consolidation and contracts among providers and between providers and managed care plans are intended to produce efficiencies and improve outcomes. On the contrary, sometimes these contracts and consolidations aim to gain advantage to control fees and negotiate with Medicare managed care companies on the provider's sole terms. The DOJ/FTC joint statement is not intended to support any particular aim for marketplace structure or behavior. Likewise, particular arrangements are not favored over others. It may well be that an arrangement not laid out in the joint statement is perfectly fine, in addition to the ones listed as safe harbors. Nevertheless, you should be cautious if you venture beyond the safe harbors in the joint statement. Healthcare lawyers often treat the safe harbors as the only sanctioned activities. Managers of managed care plans and providers should not accept this way of thinking. The joint statement emphasizes that there is a wide range of legal conduct outside the safety zones. There is more flexibility than might appear. Taking only one opinion from the first health lawyer you retain may close off some creative activities that are actually perfectly fine with the antitrust agencies.

Antitrust safe harbor is a description of the economic activities the antitrust agencies consider clearly acceptable under the law. Many other activities may be perfectly acceptable as well, but the agencies reserve the privilege of examining the facts of each case before deciding whether to challenge an activity outside the safe harbor.

If you believe that an arrangement with another physician group, a hospital, or a managed care company in the form of a preferred-provider organization is a better way of providing care—a way that patients and payers would prefer—you may be able to create this arrangement under the antitrust laws. As a general rule, arrangements that are not illegal *per se*, but offer the potential to create substantial efficiencies, are most likely acceptable for antitrust purposes. The overriding antitrust principle is whether a provider activity helps or harms consumers by taking away consumer choices in the form of competition. Despite this overriding principle, competitors who join together to fix their prices, even if they constitute a small percent of the market, are considered *per se* to be in violation of the antitrust acts. This means providers should never discuss prices with competitors unless they know the discussions are protected by organizational or legal arrangements with good legal counsel involved. A second corollary to the overriding principle is to get legal counsel involved early. Then you should monitor that counsel to see if it is being overly cautious.

The list of safe harbors explained in the joint statement is a minimum— not a maximum—list of acceptable activities. Anything that increases consumer choice is likely to be viewed favorably. Table 11.1 presents a very simple summary of the safe harbors in the joint statement. The joint statement first divides joint ventures of physicians networks into two broad types. The first type is an **exclusive physician network** in which participating physicians are prohibited from joining other physician networks. An exclusive network occurs, for example, when a group of general internists who mainly serve elderly patients wants to jointly purchase practice management software and retain an attorney to collectively negotiate a fee-for-service contract with a Medicare+Choice plan in the area. If part of their agreement to collaborate includes a requirement that all their Medicare+Choice is handled through the network, it would be considered an exclusive network. The physicians are agreeing to deal exclusively with this network for the Medicare+Choice market. These networks are treated differently from nonexclusive networks, which allow physicians to have multiple arrangements with several joint ventures. The exclusive network is fine if it consists of 20 percent or fewer of the physicians or specialists in the market. A nonexclusive network is fine if it consists of 30 percent or fewer of the physicians or specialists in the market. Such networks may or may not be fine beyond these threshold percentages of the market. It needs to be reviewed by antitrust authorities, or someone needs to deliver a credible opinion that, based upon other cases, exceeding the threshold under the right circumstances would be acceptable. It may be acceptable to exceed these percentages, as long as the overriding rules mentioned above are addressed.

The nonexclusive networks are further given special treatment (Table 11.1). They can be quite large in the market if there are viable competing networks, the member physicians derive substantial income from other networks, other competing networks are also nonexclusive, and there is no attempt to coordinate pricing policy.

Another type of network is a multiprovider network, which consists of competing providers and complementary or unrelated services. Physician-hospital organizations and provider-sponsored organizations make up multiprovider networks. Traditional antitrust logic applies to multiprovider networks in the form of the "Rule of Reason." This rule calls for looking

*An **exclusive physician network** is an agreement among physicians to act collaboratively in the market that includes provisions prohibiting participants from joining other networks.*

TABLE 11.1

Summary of Department of Justice and Federal Trade Commission Joint Antitrust Enforcement Statement, 1996

No bright line: The joint statement is clear because it lays out what you can and cannot do

Safe Harbor: Physician Network Joint Ventures

An exclusive network in which participants cannot join other networks is permitted if substantial risk is shared and network comprises 20 percent or less of physician/specialty in market

A nonexclusive network is permitted if substantial risk is shared and network comprises 30 percent or less of physician/specialty in market

Safe Harbor: Nonexclusive Network

Viable competing networks with adequate physician participation exist in the market

Network physicians earn substantial revenues from other networks

Absence of nonparticipation from other networks

Absence of price coordination

Safe Harbor: Multiprovider Networks

Multiprovider networks are those with competing providers or those that offer complementary or unrelated services

Rule of Reason applies, in which authorities will:

- define market
- assess network's competitive effects
- assess efficiencies created

Safe Harbor: Provider Collective Provision of Fee-Related Information to Purchasers

Collection managed by a third party

Current data collected but only three-month old data may be shared

Five providers must report, no provider's data may represent more than 25 percent of the statistic; any information disseminated must not identify the prices charged by an individual provider

Source: Federal Trade Commission and Department of Justice. 1996. Statements of Antitrust Enforcement Policy in Health Care.

at each situation on a case-by-case basis and trying to determine whether competition has been or will be harmed by a multiprovider network. The application of the Rule of Reason entails carefully defining the market, assessing known or expected competitive effects, and assessing any efficiencies created. A multiprovider network may make great sense in the Medicare market if its primary effect is to create efficiency or improve quality. For example, consider the improvements that result in both efficiency and quality when one hospital purchases another and tries to reach agreement with two surgical groups to perform heart surgery at one hospital rather than two. If this new agreement between two groups of surgeons and one hospital system leaves only one source of heart surgery for Medicare beneficiaries enrolled in Medicare+Choice plans, the data would need to be very compelling that efficiency had been achieved.

The final segment of the joint statement is the safe harbor for when providers can collect and exchange fee-related information. Generally, data on fees from competing groups of providers must never be shared directly. If they are shared—for example, to strike a contract with a managed care plan collectively—they should be given to a third party that is not involved with setting fees for any of the participants separately. A physician-hospital organization could serve this function as long as the people handling the fee-related information are not beneficiaries of the decisions over fees. Old information may be shared if it is no longer used for market negotiations. Summary statistics may be shared if five or more providers are counted in the shared statistic and no single provider represents more than 25 percent of the prices included in the calculation of the statistic. For example, a Medicare+Choice managed care plan may request fee information from the physicians in a market. It may use this information internally to strike a contract with the physicians separately. It may not disseminate or post this information for each physician so that it may be used by the physicians to set their fees, unless the information is presented so that no single provider represented more than 25 percent of the fees included in the calculation of the statistic.

Common Antitrust Claims and Remedies

The Sherman Act and the Clayton Act serve as the foundation of our antitrust laws. Together, they address provisions regarding monopoly and attempted monopoly, as well as provisions regarding mergers and acquisitions that tend to create a monopoly. Applied to healthcare, these two acts have resulted in several common types of awards from lawsuits.

In other parts of the economy, as in healthcare, the antitrust authorities do not allow firms either large or small to band together to fix prices. Even if many small firms are selling to a large firm, as in the case of physicians selling to a Medicare+Choice health plan, the small firms cannot fix prices because doing so would not benefit patients. Physicians and other providers can join together to do something that generates efficiency or improves quality. But if their only purpose is to create market power to improve their bottom line, which ultimately increases prices to consumers, that is illegal. Despite the fact that Medicare sets the payment to managed care plans with the Medicare+Choice payment rate, it would be illegal for providers to fix prices together in its dealing with the Medicare+Choice health plan.

Medicare+Choice plans are not immune from antitrust laws and can face charges of monopolistic behavior as well. One potential form of monopoly

Most-favored-nation clauses are contractual obligations that require the seller to offer the lowest price and always make the contractor receive the lowest price.

Monopsony is a single seller in the market for a product or service.

Group boycott is when members of a group combine their market power to keep another out of the market.

is the **most-favored-nation** (MFN) **clause**. MFNs are clauses managed care plans sometimes require physicians and hospitals to put in their contracts with the health plan. These clauses reflect a promise that providers will give the health plan their lowest price. In fact, these contract MFN clauses state that if the provider later agrees to a lower price with another health plan, the provider will automatically give the same price to the health plan with the MFN clause. The clauses get their name from the most-favored-nation status that countries give to one another in international trade. If the United States grants MFN status to China, then China knows it will pay the lowest taxes and tariffs the United States grants any country. When used in healthcare, these clauses are normally legal and help lower healthcare prices for consumers. But when an insurer has a **monopsony** (single-buyer) level of market share, which is 50 to 60 percent of the enrollees in a market, it could be accused of attempting to monopolize the market with its MFN clauses. Medicare+Choice plans with a large percentage of market share in a geographic area must use MFN clauses judiciously.

Another common source of antitrust complaint in healthcare is **group boycotts**. It is illegal for two or more entities to combine their market power to keep another out of the market. Thus, physicians with existing staff privileges cannot use this status with a hospital to stop another competing physician from gaining privileges. Likewise, one provider cannot convince others to deny referrals to a third because it accepts Medicare+Choice patients. Arrangements that suggest that two entities are ganging up in an economic sense to stop or impede competition from a third entity is a group boycott and can be challenged. The consequences can be grave. If the third party can show damages, the boycotting entities can be made to pay triple damages.

There are three ways providers can protect themselves against charges of antitrust. As suggested above, the most common remedy is to establish another organization that creates arm's-length decisions for providers. PSOs in the Medicare+Choice framework are a perfect example of organizations that could be created by aggressive groups of hospitals and physicians who wanted to get in the market together. PSOs eliminate some of the barriers that providers have faced in establishing risk-contracting entities. There would be concern if a large percent of providers in a market banded together in an exclusive PSO, essentially blocking competition from other managed care plans in the market. But there's a safer alternative. Rather than to try to deal directly and jointly with other providers for contracts, it's much safer to form another organization with a separate group of staff or consultants to deal with pricing issues. If there is substantial risk involved in the new organization, either in the form of initial start-up capital or risk for covered services as in the case of a PSO, the antitrust issues are significantly reduced.

From this standpoint, the ultimate way to address antitrust concerns and avoid charges of conspiracy to monopolize is to integrate under the theory that a single entity cannot conspire with itself. If physicians and hospitals are all owned by the same corporate entity, they knock out a number of antitrust issues such as conspiracy, price fixing, and boycotts. Thus, the many local hospital systems and integrated delivery systems that have grown up in the 1990s have done so in part for antitrust reasons. They must still ensure that they do not get too large in their marketplace and engage in conduct that stifles competition. But the fact that there is one ownership allows much more collaborative activity over prices, contracts, and efficient organization, than is possible almost any other way.

Strategic Decisions Checklist

Strategic Questions	Strategic Analyses
How do you create a culture that makes a health plan the patient's advocate?	Be the patient's advocate. This is good protection against liability. How do you foster patient advocacy? Review your policies and procedures explicitly to find and change items to protect against negligence, bad faith, or breach of contract. Examine your relationships with hospitals and physicians to reduce vulnerability to charges of vicarious liability. Conduct an administrative and legal review of the financial incentives you have in place for providers. Ensure they could not be viewed as financial disincentives not to treat, refer, or hospitalize a particular patient.
Are your providers well versed in the utilization review and gatekeeper systems you have developed?	Inform or educate your providers so that they know they have a duty to appeal coverage and medical-necessity decisions they disagree with. Your providers should know they have a duty to know about the coverage and medical-necessity review appeal procedures in your plan. If not, they should be told. Actively educate and disseminate quality medical-treatment guidelines to providers and encourage them to use them.

continued

Strategic Questions	Strategic Analyses
	Your utilization review and gatekeeper procedures should follow known authoritative sources that you can document as being acceptable standards.
	You should know unequivocally where your standards and medical treatment guidelines are from and who developed them.
How do you protect against liability for referrals and second opinion?	You should use medical treatment guidelines for referrals and second opinions.
	You should allow flexibility in guidelines so that they can be applied uniquely to a particular patient's situation.
	Your providers must document in the chart when they deviate from a guideline and why.
Does your plan have procedures in place for disseminating advance directives?	You should have an agreement with hospital, skilled nursing home, and other providers regarding advance directives.
	You need a mechanism for documenting advance directives for your patients and documenting cancellation of advance directives.
	Your attending physicians should know they must keep a copy of advance directives in the chart with the patient's permission.
How are your managed care plan and your providers positioned with regard to antitrust concerns?	Determine who are the major players in your health plan market and in the provider market for Medicare patients.
	Measure whether the four top health plans or provider groups in the market have more than 50 percent market share in Medicare.

continued

Strategic Questions	Strategic Analyses
	Calculate the Herfindahl index in your local health plan market and in the provider market for Medicare.
	You and your providers should refrain from engaging in marketplace activities that harm patients by taking away consumer choices.
	You and your providers should not fix prices with rivals in any way.
	Retain legal council to monitor and address antitrust concerns.
Are you exposed to common antitrust concerns?	You and your providers should not join together to gain market power to fix premium prices.
	Use MFN clauses properly.
	Do not engage in any group boycotts in Medicare managed care.

Unfolding Trends and Policy Outlook

Part I provides a primer on the Medicare program and managed care. Part II discusses strategic issues and analyzes why some Medicare+Choice health plans are successful. Part III builds on these two sections to explore where the country is progressing with its Medicare program. What does the future hold for managed care in terms of challenges and opportunities? What are the implications for strategic planning? What does all this mean to you?

This view of the future that Part III presents is for boards of directors of hospital systems, physician groups, and administrators of managed care plans, among others. The goal is to help leaders like you gain a fresh perspective and to initiate a robust dialogue. Healthcare in the United States is a competitive field for physicians, hospitals, and health plans. If the essence of strategy is doing things differently from competitive rivals for market advantage, you need to anticipate the future. You need to take the appropriate steps today to be in position to meet the future when it arrives—much as a hockey player must skate rapidly to where the puck will be.

All organizations do this. Every day, organizational leadership makes choices on the basis of alternative views of the future. Sometimes these views are clouded or dim. Too often, the alternative for some health plans simply is not to think about the future. The leadership of another Medicare managed care plan might devote time and effort to thinking about the future of Medicare and the influences it will have on their organization. If your competitors anticipate the future better than you do, that could mean trouble for your plan. History shows that missing an emerging trend or misinterpreting the implications of a new policy can lead to brutal marketplace consequences.

Part of that future vision must account for major policy issues, such as laws to "protect" patients and physicians "from" managed care. But developments in e-health commerce and biotechnology are also changing the physician-patient relationship as costs and inefficiencies are eliminated. At the same time, these developments are empowering patients and physicians by offering new treatments, thereby transforming the clinical components of care for managed care plans. Such changes in the context of "impending insolvency" for the Medicare Hospital Insurance Trust Funds raise important longer-term policy issues.

Rather than attempt to catalogue all the major policy issues, Chapter 12 is a model of what should be done for future planning. It discusses several select major policy issues and offers some preliminary conclusions. Although the precise effect of developments will be unknown for a time, this chapter speculates that Medicare *and* managed care will, as a matter of course, benefit as we move forward. The future is bright for Medicare managed care. Why? There are two obvious reasons. As Table III.1 illustrates, the population is getting older and the age distribution is tilting toward older age categories. Medicare, then, is an obvious growth market. This manifest trend might be the only thing you need to know to make Medicare the place to be in the future, but this chapter mentions several other trends as well.

Figure III.1 offers a framework for categorizing the array of issues swirling around Medicare, and it creates a visual summary of the key policy dimensions. With Medicare beneficiaries in the middle, there are four structural dimensions of policy to be considered: Medicare Benefit Structure, Medicare Payment Structure, Medicare Choice Structure, and Medicare Delivery Structure.

TABLE III.1
Selected Facts About the Epidemiology of Aging in the United States

- The population 65 years and older is 12.5 percent of the population and will rise to 16.5 percent by 2020.

- The first baby boomer will turn 65 on May 19, 2011 (9 months and 65 years after the end of WWII).

- People 85 and older represent the fastest-growing segment of the population.

Everyone knows we are getting older: Many ways to express the aging of the population, making Medicare a growth market

Medicare Benefit Structure

The first dimension, the Medicare Benefit Structure (see top of diagram), encompasses Medicare-covered services and cost-sharing provisions. One important looming issue here is expanding coverage under Medicare for pharmaceuticals (circle, Fig. III.1), and this is discussed below. Most Medicare beneficiaries (84.3 percent) are not in poverty and have wealth in the form of a house they own, pensions, annuities, dividends, or interest. With so many nonpoor beneficiaries, a recurring issue is **means testing** the Medicare premium. Means testing refers to graduating the premium paid by beneficiaries according to their income. This was attempted by Congress in the 1980s and later repealed in connection with expanded coverage for catastrophic costs. The issue could gather renewed support, especially as lawmakers launch politically popular coverage for pharmaceuticals or if the solvency of Medicare is threatened and the country looks for more money for Medicare.

Means testing is a process of making graduated increases in premiums according to level of income. The income

Medicare Payment Structure

The second dimension is the Medicare Payment Structure. In addition to the Medicare+Choice payment system for managed care plans, Medicare has at least four other major payment systems: hospitals, physicians, skilled nursing facilities, and home health agencies. These are likely to be modified and restructured to address access to care or budgetary savings. One new policy development to watch is the program for bundled payments to centers of excellence, which is represented by one of the smaller circles. With this approach, one combined payment is made for physician and hospital services for each episode of care. Because the system has long been set up to pay physicians separately from hospitals, the thorny issue becomes which party gets the single, bundled payment. But an expanded effort for bundled payment in the Medicare fee-for-service program across scores of acute procedures could serve as a basis for resolving this issue. Managed care companies could use this model to develop a new way to pay their physicians and hospitals and drive lower-cost, higher-quality arrangements.

of each beneficiary would be tested against a schedule of graduated income to determine the level of premium payments.

Medicare Choice Structure

The third dimension is Medicare Choice Structure. With the advent of the Medicare managed care program in 1985, Medicare has progressed toward greater beneficiary choice with consequences. The two major choices are between traditional fee-for-service and managed care. Medicare Compare is an effort by HCFA to provide beneficiaries with easy access to comparative information across Medicare+Choice health plans. Information is readily available regarding performance of preventive tests, access to care, disenrollment rates, member ratings of plans, and satisfaction with ease of getting referrals. Other new aspects of the new choice structure include an open-enrollment period and the new six-month lock-in period for Medicare managed care enrollees. Other efforts to help beneficiaries make a choice include providing various methods of performance measurement (Fig. III.1) and disseminating performance measurement "report cards." New efforts to protect consumers at the federal and state levels are a part of this dimension of policy issues. A well-defined process for beneficiaries to lodge complaints, grievances, and appeals against their health plan is the norm in most states, and similar rules apply at the federal level. The ability to bring suit against a health plan that has been alleged to have done harm is part of the legal protections available.

Medicare Delivery Structure

The fourth and final dimension is the Medicare delivery system structure—the types of clinical professionals and the setting for care. The delivery system

FIGURE III.1

The Four
Dimensions of
Unfolding
Trends and
Policy Issues

*Unfolding policy
issues: The
structure of
benefits,
payments,
choice, and the
delivery system
determine the
future of
Medicare*

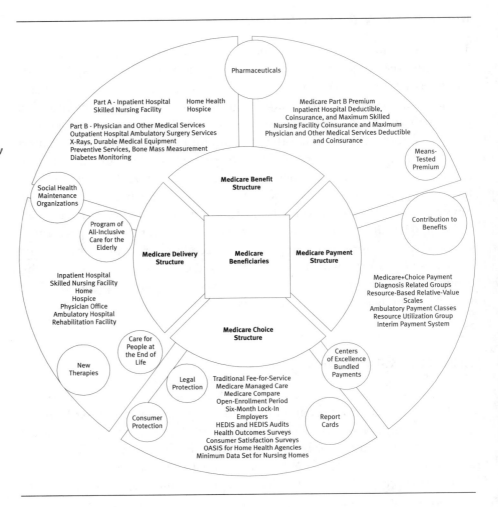

has changed over the years since Medicare was enacted, and it will continue to change given the accelerated pace of biomedical advances spurred by new information about the human genome. These developments will likely affect our ability to care for people at the end of life. Two programs already in existence and being developed, the social HMOs and the program for all include care for the elderly, could serve as the foundation for a new model of Medicare delivery.

Use the visual in Figure III.1 of unfolding trends and policy outlook to initiate a discussion with the leadership in your health plan about the future of Medicare. Add new ideas to this visual as they arise in the press or policy or professional circles. Then, use the format in the Table III.2 to chart brief comments and ideas about how various trends and policy issues could influence the structure of benefits, payments, consumer choice, and the delivery system in your health plan.

FOUR DIMENSIONS	NATIONAL TRENDS	INFLUENCE ON			
		Market Growth	Enrollment	Cost of Delivery	Competition
Medicare Benefits Structure					
Medicare Payment Structure					
Medicare Choice Structure					
Medicare Delivery Structure					

Source: Adapted from Alternative Futures Associates and Regulatory Resources, Inc. 1986. *Guidebook for Strategic Planning for Blood Service Facilities.* Washington, DC: American Blood Commission.

TABLE III.2
Environmental Analysis of the Four Dimensions to Recognize Unfolding Trends and Policy Outlook

The Medicare managed care climate: Use this simple didactic device to stimulate strategic thinking about change in your environment

The leaders of the strategic planning process working with board members, managers, or clinical leaders should present the dimensions and then have individuals take a few minutes to complete Table III.2 with their own reactions. First, the group could share ideas on national trends and what each member of the group knows about what is going on nationally. Each person can complete the column "National Trends" with his or her own perceptions. Next, complete the format in Table III.2 regarding the influence on market growth, enrollment, the cost of delivery, and competition for your situation. You do not have to be right at this point, but let your thinking and predictions "color outside the lines." Your perceptions could become reality.

Once you have some agreement on national trends, develop some scenarios or stories about what impact these might have on your health plan. Scenarios help you to reach some consensus about your view of the future, so you can make plans to meet that future when it arrives. Chapter 12 is devoted to examples of scenarios and the kinds of policy outlook you might want to explore.

THE NATURAL PROGRESSION OF MARKETS

The future of the Medicare program and its Medicare+Choice contractors will most certainly be affected by at least five major trends: the increasing attention to the protection of patients, the progress of information technology, advances in biomedical science, less in-hospital care, and the solvency of the Medicare trust fund.

The first trend is the protection of patients and providers through new legislation at the state or federal level. Highly publicized anecdotal cases of patients adversely affected by the decisions of health plan managers or clinicians have led to a demand for broadened authority to sue health plans. Physician organizations have joined the call for new laws that would curtail aggressive managed care practices and protect their autonomy as well.

The second trend, the progress of information technology, affects our ability to gather, analyze, and disseminate information that can help patients, physicians, and health plans make better decisions about healthcare. Electronic medical records and intelligent systems for supporting clinical decision making are a part of the story. **E-health**—in the form of interactive Internet web pages for patients—provides up-to-date consumer information and spurs adherence to the treatment regimen. Health information is changing the level of communication between patients and physicians, as well as what consumers expect from providers.

E-health is the use of the Internet to improve health by providing easy communication connecting patients, physicians, hospitals, and health plans.

The third trend is reflected in the advances we see in biomedical science and new therapies at the cellular level or lower.

The fourth trend is that we expect to see less hospital care combined with more of almost every other kind of care. Patients continue to pour out of hospitals, and shorter stays mean that almost half the nation's hospital beds are empty on any day. Will it end with hospital closures or continued consolidation?

Finally, there's the issue of whether the Medicare trust fund will run out of money amid the overly politicized question of when to expand Medicare benefits. This recurring issue of solvency provides pressure to lower the increase in payments to hospitals, physicians, and Medicare managed care plans. The Medicare trust funds topic continues to interject public policy issues into delivering needed care to people on Medicare and threatens the survivability of Medicare managed care plans.

This chapter discusses these trends and issues in more detail after introducing two scenarios to spark your own planning discussions. One scenario speculates on the rapid diffusion of biomedical sciences ushering in the new post-hospital era. The other scenario ponders the implications of major legal interference for the avowed protection of patients and physicians. This scenario suggests a somber period for Medicare managed care. The second half of the chapter gives example tables and charts you can use for strategic planning with your board or physicians in a managed care plan.

Possible Scenarios and the Role of Medicare Managed Care

As mentioned in previous chapters, Medicare managed care plans are required to accept prices set largely by the government and offered on a take-it-or-leave-it basis. Certainly, the process of annually fixing the price for the coming year in the form of the Medicare+Choice payment is an important economic variable in the willingness of plans to attempt to grow enrollment. The ill-advised risk adjusters that rely on actual hospital service use in the health plan and reimburse the following year based on costs is a step backward for Medicare managed care and will have its own modest contradictory effects. The policy attitude toward onerous and sometimes needless regulation of every aspect of participation in the Medicare+Choice program can influence the willingness of health plans to stay with the program. However, these are minor aspects of the passing market parade.

In the final analysis, the ultimate direction for Medicare comes down to which system—fee-for-service or managed care—is best at achieving a balance between the costs of providing care and the satisfaction beneficiaries express from the care delivered. Unbridled fee-for-service payments have inherent effects that spur excessive utilization and costs. Risk-based payments without rules give the impression that someone is skimping on care and fosters suspicion about the quality of care delivered. With approximately 80 percent of beneficiaries in one form of payment (fee-for-service) and upward of 20 percent in the other (managed care), competition among the systems for the lives of millions of beneficiaries able to make a choice leads to natural cycles. When costs seem under control, the fee-for-service sector will appear to have the upper hand. When service delivery seems wasteful and excessive, the moderating influence of managed care stands as a reasonable solution to most people. These middle cycles are affected by an overarching emerging trend: an increasing percentage of retirees with long-standing experience in the private sector with managed care organizations as their only source of healthcare.

Equilibrium is the point at which a system tends to come to rest, or toward which the system tends to move.

The concept of equilibrium applies. **Equilibrium** is a point at which a system tends to come to rest, or toward which the system tends to gravitate. To illustrate, think of any room with a thermostat as a system. The thermostat setting determines the equilibrium point. When the temperature in the room is not at the equilibrium setting, the heating or cooling devices change the temperature of the room and move it toward the equilibrium setting. Sometimes the heating or cooling devices will overshoot the equilibrium point and the room will get too hot or too cold. Then, built in mechanisms identify that the mark has been missed and the heating or cooling is shut down to gradually return the room back to equilibrium.

Markets generally work the same way. The equilibrium may be changeable or changing. Disequilibrium may dominate most of the time with equilibrium never really attained. Nevertheless, the notion of the existence of equilibrium—where the market system could come to rest—is plausible.

Operating as it does as a highly regulated market, Medicare managed care can be thought of having an equilibrium point. It might be measured in various ways. There could be equilibrium in the number of beneficiaries enrolled in traditional fee-for-service Medicare and managed care. Costs could conceivably reach a steady state of modest or no increase, essentially coming to rest. Quality could reach generally acceptable levels of excellence in both fee-for-service Medicare and managed care. However, this is unlikely because external forces cause change in Medicare and shift the theoretical equilibrium all the time. Equilibrium in the Medicare program can be upset by any number of factors: changes in the population served, variances among the physicians and hospitals providing care, and the push and pull of the general economy. The trick is identifying cycles from new trends. If overall Medicare managed care enrollment levels off, is that a transitory pause to a new rapid expansion in which Medicare costs move ahead, or is it a true long-term moderation of enrollment growth? If the number of Medicare managed care plans drops, is that because the program is doing something wrong or is it caused by the normal effects of the business cycle on health plan profits and losses to fund participation in Medicare?

The following segment discusses some of those external forces that can upset the natural progression of markets, specifically the market for Medicare managed care. Think creatively about issues that could be missing from this list of five, and don't let the setting of your organization's thermostat leave you feeling too comfortable in this dynamic, changing market.

The Coming Post-Hospital Era

Mrs. Jones enters the biomedical therapy center with the remaining pill of the three that had been delivered to her doorstep by United Parcel Service three days before. She was told to take the pills one day at a time to raise her red blood cell count for the procedure she was about to undergo. She received e-mail reminders each day to take one red-cell-stimulating pill.

Mrs. Jones is 77 and had had one hip replaced 12 years earlier at one of the local hospitals. That hospital and two others had closed and been converted to a small-business office space just last year. For her first hip replacement, she had stayed in the hospital eight days and recovered at home with great pain. Now, 12 years later, her other hip needs attention; but today she is going to stay just six hours for a procedure that would almost eliminate her symptoms of arthritis pain. She could drive herself home, and probably not notice anything initially. Nevertheless, after about eight days she would gradually improve until her pain was practically gone.

Her doctor told her the FDA had given rapid approval about 12 months ago to a new procedure developed for arthritis in the hip. The new therapy is one of the first offerings from that large pharmaceutical company she could never remember the name of but that started with a "P." She found her memory was not as good as it used to be. But she could remember this company had purchased, with great fanfare, the stock of a biotechnology company upstart that had researched the new treatment. The little biotechnology company did not have the resources to distribute the new treatment worldwide because it took careful monitoring of blood levels and specialized personnel to deliver the new procedure.

This "P" pharmaceutical company had also purchased a large chain of drugstores and converted about a third of them to biomedical therapy centers in most major cities. Moreover, they had entered into a special agreement with her Medicare managed care plan. Her doctor said he had heard about the special agreement, and her condition had deteriorated to the point this made sense. Her primary care doctor understood that the procedure was not chemically based but biologically based. He injected her with her own cells that had been treated for two weeks to modify her immune system. The doctor knew that the health plan and the pharmaceutical company were still discussing whether the payment should be made as a procedure or as a drug, and he was not sure how much he would be paid for any follow-up. The whole thing was so new.

Mrs. Jones's sister-in-law had developed a similar problem with her hip, but she had not joined a Medicare managed care plan. She is still in traditional fee-for-service Medicare, along with about 35 percent of the beneficiaries in her area who continued to select it despite higher out-of-pocket costs and heavy advertising from the Medicare managed care plan. Her sister-in-law's physician recommended the conventional hip replacement because Medicare fee-for-service had not yet recognized payment for the new procedure. But Mrs. Jones's managed care doctor said her health plan had a top-notch center at corporate headquarters for making coverage decisions about emerging technologies, and they had recommended this new procedure right away. The doctor said that while the new therapy was expensive, it would mean she would not have to undergo another costly and invasive procedure. It was thought to provide a near cure. The net effect would be to lower overall costs for Mrs. Jones and her health plan if she stayed enrolled for eight years.

The PharmD, someone with an advanced pharmacy degree, met her at the front of the biomedical center. She knew her primary care doctor would not be there because he had made the referral. A specialist was not involved because the protocol for referral and treatment was quite clear from the health plan's Internet pages. The PharmD had her take the last red blood cell activator pill and then took a blood sample. The PharmD harvested her cells that would be expanded and used in the procedure. It felt strange to Mrs. Jones to be in what was formerly a large chain drugstore. Where once she had walked past lawn furniture and Halloween candy, she found herself in a pleasant modern space for drawing blood and counseling patients privately.

The PharmD asked her if she was connected to the Internet at home, and she was. Teenage grandchildren had given her an Internet device she kept on the breakfast room table. Her son had connected it and showed her how easy it was to use in about an hour. The PharmD said she should go to a certain Web address of her health plan and report how she feels everyday for two weeks after today. If she did not do this, they would call her to see how she was doing. There would be more drugs to take and she was to be carefully monitored regarding adherence to the drug regimen.

Mrs. Jones was looking forward to a more functional and comfortable hip. She was so impressed with the biomedical center and how nice the PharmD was to explain everything that was happening to her. She hoped to remember to tell her sister-in-law to join her Medicare managed care plan—just as soon as they both had their hips replaced.

Health Plans Become Virtual Physicians and Hospitals

Mr. Brown turned 65 and enrolled in the Medicare program just six months ago. His employer had really pushed the Medicare managed care option at retirement. Not only was his former employer paying almost all the premium for retirees who joined the managed care portion of Medicare, but it was giving frequent-flyer miles to join Medicare managed care. The miles represented one dollar for every dollar in total Medicare managed care expenses, which was about $10,000 a year after the last four years of double-digit healthcare cost increases in Medicare payments.

Mr. Brown would have joined the managed care option anyway without the incentives. Of the eight plans available, he had used one of them for nearly 12 years since he started working for this employer. He could still see Dr. Irwin, his internist, without a prolonged wait or interruption.

Most physicians, including Dr. Irwin, worked for large health systems or health plans as full-time employees these days. Part of the reason healthcare costs had experienced double-digit increases was that there had been a rash of litigation against physicians, hospital systems, and health plans. That led to a major corporatization of medicine.

The way Dr. Irwin explained it to Mr. Brown, if health systems and health plans were going to be sued for malpractice for things their affiliated clinicians did, the health plans might as well employ physicians like himself to manage the entire risk better. The state legislature was even considering bills that would eliminate licensure for physicians. Institutional licensure would apply.

Licensure would be for the medical director of the health plan and all the physicians who work for the health plan as a collective. Dr. Irwin said he did not mind the arrangement because he did not have to worry about malpractice insurance, which had become nearly 40 percent of his practice expenses, and that percentage was rising.

Mr. Brown complained to Dr. Irwin that he had recently gained weight and needed to purchase new slacks because his waist had grown. Dr. Irwin told him about the new Lifestyle Center at the academic medical center, which used behavioral techniques combined with drugs to help men lose weight.

The academic medical center had started the Lifestyle Center because it had large amounts of empty space left from the period in the 1990s and early 2000s when it had overbuilt tremendously. The leadership at most academic medical centers thought society would just continue to pay for more and more specialists, so impressive structures were constructed to house all the academic departments. All of that collapsed when the rash of litigation forced clinicians into corporations and the corporations eliminated all of the artificial walls created by the specialist system. Now, interdisciplinary teams of clinicians worked closely together like a software team attacking a problem—only, the interdisciplinary clinical teams attacked specific diseases and developed the most advanced techniques to improve health outcomes for patients. They worked rapidly to redesign systems and were totally driven to improve patient outcomes because they earned substantial bonuses for doing so. Their novel techniques and processes could even be patented and licensed for even greater personal financial reward. Some of the top-paid people at the academic center were process improvement scientists who had long since replaced the procedure-based specialists as major breadwinners.

Because of all this, academic medical centers were a shadow of their former selves in terms of number of hospital beds and faculty. Medical students and other clinicians now train in the community, and health plans happily use a portion of capitation payments to support the training of students. The health plans are glad to support training because doing so helps them recruit new physicians and other clinicians to work for the health plan.

Mr. Brown knew the health plan had a lifestyle benefit because he remembered seeing it in the brochures at initial enrollment, and it was a benefit other plans did not have. Dr. Irwin told him that for a limited time, the academic medical center was encouraging physicians to send their patients so they could build awareness in the community. The academic medical center thought if it could get the beneficiaries enrolled in Mr. Brown's plan to talk about it, the other seven health plans in the community would be forced to bargain with them and add the benefit.

As Mr. Brown left Dr. Irwin's office he wondered if his health plan and the Lifestyle Center also covered hair loss from male pattern baldness.

So What?

Linear thinking is easy. Linear thinking is presuming that what happened in the past will continue to happen in the future. For example, if a Medicare managed care plan had two competitors in the local market, and each experienced enrollment growth of 5 percent last year while the Medicare+Choice payment went up 3.4 percent, a linear thinker would take for granted that the same thing would happen again next year. Sometimes linear thinking can be quite accurate about planning for the future. Sometimes, it can be useless.

The scenarios with Mrs. Jones and Mr. Brown illustrate the pitfalls of linear thinking. A managed care plan that always thought hospitals would be there and the components of care would remain the same would place itself at risk in Mrs. Jones's world. Mr. Brown represents a new kind of enrollee, well versed in managed care and ready to consume the nonessentials. But he would walk away if the health plan did not offer nonessentials, such as flat-stomach treatments and baldness reversal. The academic medical center in Mr. Brown's scenario illustrates the payoff, or lack thereof, from linear thinking.

Nonlinear thinking is modular. Pieces from the past cannot be taken apart and put back together in the same way to predict the future. With nonlinear thinking, the ideas are more intuitive, visual, and creative. Rather than strict numerical plans, there are emerging themes, issues, trends, connections and opportunities (Sanders 1998). Unlike predicting whether night will follow day (linear), it is more like predicting how the path of bright, large clouds might move across the sky (nonlinear). Although both linear and nonlinear thinking can be accurate in helping to plan, nonlinear thinking has distinct advantages. It keeps new ideas and opportunities flowing. Many ideas may not work out or they may be far too distant in the future—even a three-year horizon is considered lengthy in many business circles. But some of the ideas from nonlinear thinking will be winners that add to your success.

Scenario planning is a form of nonlinear thinking. It is one of a number of strategic planning tools that allows you to ask "what if?" Developing scenarios forces you to gather new data from outside the organization. That process and information can challenge your assumptions and cause ongoing reevaluation of your strategic direction.

The two scenarios above illustrate how it can work. When you retreat with your board, physician members, or health plan management, try to develop stories like the ones about Mrs. Jones and Mr. Brown. By doing that, you can get people out of the regular mode of linear thinking and consider alternative futures. Offbeat and futuristic scenarios are fine. In fact, sometimes they uncover major trends. They also force members of the strategy team to develop similar assumptions about the future. Shared assumptions are essential if you intend to develop the best response to whatever future you conjure up. The following discussion and associated charts and tables illustrate different perspectives on the future and describe the potential environment for

Medicare managed care. Use these as templates for developing the trends you see unfolding and the outlook on policy you take.

Five Trends That Will Change Medicare Managed Care

The scenarios in the previous section aim to help you think strategically. They offer examples of a resource for systematically exploring the uncertainty facing Medicare managed care plans. You should develop your own scenarios as you delve further into possible trends and the policy outlook from your vantage point. To explore this type of strategic process further, this section develops five proposed trends that will change Medicare managed care. They are intended as examples, and they extend some of the points brought out in the scenarios. At least one might contain the future that is in store for all of us.

Protection of Patients and Providers

Many of the rights and responsibilities that would be established in various forms of patient bill of rights legislation found at federal or state levels are already assured for Medicare beneficiaries enrolled in traditional fee-for-service or managed care plans. Table 12.1 examines several of the most prominent provisions.

The Medicare Compare effort, the extensive regulation of marketing and evidence of coverage overseen by HCFA Regional Offices, and other efforts give Medicare beneficiaries the kind of information envisioned in patient-bill-of-rights legislation. Federal law already requires distribution of information about living wills and durable power of attorney to Medicare beneficiaries. The rules for obtaining a Medicare+Choice contract govern access and choice in physicians and hospitals to Medicare managed care enrollees. The rule for prudent layperson definition is taken right from the Balanced Budget Act of 1997 covering the right to emergency services. Medicare beneficiaries are also guaranteed nondiscrimination, dispute resolution, and confidentiality from their Medicare contractors.

Several important provisions of patient bill of rights legislation are not now extended to Medicare beneficiaries. One important provision is the right to sue a health plan for medical malpractice. Some proposals recommend that consumers be involved in the governance of health plans and quality oversight organizations. Others expand the use of legal remedies for inappropriate care including coverage denials and substandard care. They consider the tort liability system the final arbitrator of and enforcement effort of quality care. Finally, Medicare carries no particular expectations about patients and their responsibility to try to remain healthy.

Managed care plans resist expanding the legal remedies available to consumers on the basis of two arguments. First, they maintain that treatment decisions and payment decisions are separate decisions. The recommendations of a licensed health professional (for example, physician, nurse, pharmacist)

Information—Consumers have the right to receive accurate, easily understood information and assistance when making informed healthcare decisions about their health plan, professionals, and facilities.

Participation in Treatment Decisions—Consumers have the right and responsibility to participate fully in all decisions related to their healthcare.

Access and Choice—Consumers have the right to a choice of healthcare providers that is sufficient to ensure access to appropriate high-quality healthcare.

Emergency Services—Consumers have the right to access emergency healthcare services when and where the need arises, such that a prudent layperson could reasonably expect the absence of medical attention to result in placing health in serious jeopardy, serious impairment to bodily functions, or serious dysfunction of any bodily organ or part.

Nondiscrimination—Consumers have the right to nondiscriminatory treatment in marketing, enrollment, and delivery of healthcare services.

Dispute Resolution—All consumers have the right to a fair and efficient process for resolving differences with their health plan, healthcare providers, and the institutions that serve them.

Confidentiality—Consumers have the right to communicate with healthcare providers in confidence and to have the confidentiality of their individual healthcare information protected. Consumers also have the right to review and copy their own medical records and request amendments to their records.

Consumer Responsibility—It is reasonable to expect and encourage consumers to assume responsibilities to help increase best outcomes and support a quality-improvement-conscious environment.

TABLE 12.1
Summary of Common Rights and Responsibilities in Proposals for Protection of Patients and Providers

Medicare already does most of this: Rights and responsibilities in most legislative proposals are common practice in many states

are subject to well-known tort liability in the case of malpractice. Nevertheless, health plans by law cannot diagnose diseases or prescribe medications, so they cannot and are not held to medical malpractice tort liability. If a health plan decides against coverage for a treatment, that is a financial decision that can be subject to normal contract law regarding breach of contract. Second, managed care plans should not be held responsible for things over which they do not have control. The decisions made or the errors committed in a licensed, accredited hospital or by a physician in the office are the responsibility of the paid health professionals involved. The managed care company normally is deciding whether to pay for something, and it is not directing the way the care is delivered. The physician or hospital and the managed care plan may differ over whether something is medically necessary and should be paid. But that can be decided later after the care is delivered.

If these long-standing views of managed care liability are replaced with tort liability for medical malpractice, it portends a world in which many consumers would sue their managed care plan under federal law. First, evidence-based coverage decisions would be even more prevalent than they are now.

Managed care plans will be forced to implement more rigorous treatment guidelines and expect adherence to the latest evidence-based approaches to care. If the value of a certain service is clearly documented in the scientific literature and can be reduced to a rule or requirement for treatment, medicine would become much more of a cookbook approach. To protect their "deep pockets," managed care plans would implement highly restrictive formularies and prior authorization procedures for physicians to follow. Ironically, the quality of care could improve as a result, but physicians who thought tort liability would protect their autonomy could see their decision making even more seriously directed by health plans trying to protect their own liability.

In the final analysis, extreme consumer protections through the tort system could lead to institutional licensure of a managed care plan's network of physicians and hospitals. Today, to become a network provider for a managed care plan, a contract must be agreed to by both parties. In a future with tort liability for managed care plans, hospitals and physicians would have to agree to follow strict protocol and authorization procedures. It would be tantamount to being licensed by the managed care plan, rather than the state to deliver care, since the health plan would have dual authority over the payment and delivery of any care to patients.

The Congressional Budget Office (CBO) estimates that patient bill of rights legislation could raise private sector premium costs by 1.3 percent to 4.1 percent, depending on the specifics of the bill. Such estimates are made with great uncertainty because so little is known about how many patients might bring suit, whether they would be class-action suits, and whether they would lead to mega-damage awards. Still, simply passing the bill could lead to immense changes in provider and health plan behavior, increasing the use of services and costs to insulate against lawsuits. Therefore, cost estimates are subject to more than the usual amount of uncertainty. The ultimate costs could be substantially larger or smaller. If the change in price of tobacco products from the large awards granted under lawsuits and settlements in the late 1990s is any indication, the cost estimates could be as much as four times higher than CBO estimates. That would mean the range is more like an increase in costs of 5.2 percent to 16.4 percent, with more of the impact in the early years. Similarly, the right to sue health plans provisions could pass and little or nothing could happen in the courts, which means the impact could be as much as one-fourth the current CBO estimates.

At this writing, no one has ventured a guess regarding what will happen to Medicare managed care plans. Threats of lawsuits or actual awards would raise Medicare managed care plan costs. Are these costs to be factored into the Medicare+Choice payment rate, just as physicians receive payment adjustments for differences in practice costs of medical liability insurance? Moreover, and perhaps even more significantly, if the ability to sue is the last straw for the participation of managed care plans in Medicare, there could be a return to double-digit rates of increase for traditional fee-for-service

Medicare costs. That conclusion is based on recent studies that find those areas of the country with greater market penetration by HMOs experiencing lower fee-for-service expenditures under Medicare. These results suggest a spillover effect from Medicare managed care. Physicians who participate in managed care plans change their practice styles for all their patients, not just for those enrolled in Medicare+Choice health plans. Managed care plans that modify their restrictions, consequently, could lead to higher costs in fee-for-service plans as well. CBO has not estimated the magnitude of such an effect for either Medicare or private insurance.

Progression of Technology

A second trend that is certain to have a significant and growing influence on Medicare and Medicare managed care is technology, especially information technology. As noted earlier, the falling cost of data collection and data management will lead to an even more robust use of medical guidelines, disease management, and continuous monitoring of outcomes by top-flight managed care organizations. The challenge for health plans is committing to technology and demonstrating a willingness to pay for hits and misses on the technology front (Peterson 1999).

There are four approaches to tackling the data needs of health plans: integrated data warehouse, dual databases, hub-and-spoke model, and outsourcing.

A massive integrated data warehouse gives a platform to a health plan for having all sorts of data at the fingertips of managers and clinicians. If all the data you collect on a patient is in one place in one accessible data system, it should be easy to analyze trends over time and across components of care. The downside is inflexibility and high cost.

The second approach is what Peterson calls dual databases. Huge quantities of claims data might be warehoused, but a decision support component splits off the most relevant bits of data for management and clinical purposes. This information might be put on a server or desktop computer for further analysis. This approach makes it easier to use data—and provides faster access—but you must be sure that the information you take from the larger database is really the information you need.

The third approach is the hub-and-spoke model. Remote, and sometimes diverse, data systems are put together through an interfacing program that finds commonalities and uses them to combine diverse sources of data. Each of the different spokes remains the same and contributes to the hub when there are common data elements. The hub can be used to process data for reports about all the spokes.

The final approach is outsourcing. With this, a vendor's approach to data processing that has been successful somewhere else can be used at your plan. This approach offers a great deal to small and midsize health plans that lack the resources to build their own systems.

Any of these approaches to information technology and data management will support any number of activities in the future. Practice management, electronic data interchange, document management, electronic medical records, reporting and analysis, and clinical reference software including intelligent systems are only a few areas of technology improvement. There should be no doubt that technology in its many forms will play a major role in the future direction of healthcare and managed care.

Biomedical Science and New Therapies

More than two decades ago, Lewis Thomas (1979) said many of the things we do in modern medicine are nothing more than fix-up technologies, not curative technologies. The rapid advances of biotechnology and pharmaceuticals are changing how medicine will be practiced in the future, offering the prospect of shifting from fix-up to cure.

Today, as in the past, physicians often use fix-up technologies to mollify the effects of a disease. Metal joints are inserted in knees and hips. Blood vessels are removed from one part of the body and stitched onto the heart to improve blood flow. Poisons are beamed or injected into the body to reduce or eliminate tumors. In the future, we can hope to prevent the disease or condition from occurring in the first place.

The Human Genome Project and related genetic/DNA research already have yielded a multitude of diagnostic tests that pinpoint the exact locations in the body and identities of genetic mutations that predispose people to certain diseases. The thinking goes that science should be able to use this information to prevent, halt, or treat diseases and conditions, if not cure them. Thus, parts of the body with immunology problems might be targeted and adverse effects regulated. New blood vessels could be grown without surgery just by subjecting the body to certain biological substances. Sending cellular messages to stop them from multiplying or causing them to die off altogether might alter the behavior of cancerous cells.

These are not theoretical propositions. In the past ten years, there have been more than 320 ongoing clinical trials in humans approved by the Research Advisory Committee of the National Institutes of Health with the label gene therapy. The vast majority is in the area of cancer (Fig. 12.1), followed by coronary artery disease, peripheral artery diseases, cystic fibrosis, and HIV/AIDS. A large collection of other diseases also have reached the stage of human clinical trials. Although some of these programs have come under public scrutiny for highly publicized failures, there is no apparent waning of appetite to pursue these trials by scientists or patients.

The overarching goal should be to target those physical and mental conditions that tend to deprive people of a meaningful life with social significance, and many of these diseases affect the older person. The major ones are listed in Table 12.2. However, this begs the questions What is aging?" and "How long can we realistically expect to live?" Genetics certainly has an influence

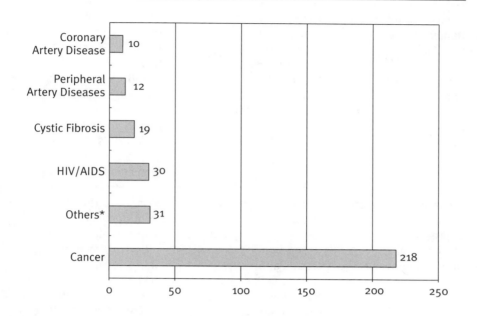

FIGURE 12.1
Total Gene Therapy Clinical Trials Approved by National Institutes of Health Research Advisory Committee in Last Ten Years

Gene studies are spiraling upward: Serious diseases are under serious investigation

Source: Adams, C. 1999. "Committee Pushes to Regain Authority Over Experiments in Gene Therapy." *The Wall Street Journal.*

* Includes 21 different diseases or disorders, most having one of two experiments each.

on aging, as do environmental factors and the aging of our cells. The body changes with aging, and body defenses are modified along with our ability to engage in physical activity. The so-called compression of morbidity, or the way in which sickness is postponed to later life, creates a paradoxical situation in which the result is longer periods of both health and sickness among the elderly (Moody 1994). Although chronic illness is postponed thanks to technological advances, we are all living much longer on average, making the period of morbidity later and longer. The fastest growing segment of the population is the age group 85 years and older, and the numbers of people in this group will more than double in the lifetime of most Americans. Advances in the biomedical sciences will vastly accelerate the compression of morbidity. With increased longevity and new medical technology, old age will no longer carry a fixed, constant meaning (Collins 1999). Instead, terms such as quality of life, successful aging, and collective acceptance of limits will increasingly come to shape the acceptable allocation of scarce resources.

Add to this mix the prospect of gene-based population screenings, diagnostic tests, and therapies becoming commonplace as soon as the next decade. Ethical debates have arisen over the subject of genetic screening and our ability to identify people predisposed or prone to certain diseases that have no cure. With the proper oversight, new genetic information can be used for the greater good. Although this is not the subject of this segment, it is important to realize that screening is a necessary step in the process.

TABLE 12.2
Conditions that
Affect Older
People

*Which will
biomedicine
cure? The next
discoveries could
be on this list
and at what
cost?*

**Memory and Thinking:
Dementia, Delirium,
and Amnesia**
Delirium (Sudden
   Confusion)
Amnesia

**Head, Neck, and
Sensory Concerns**
Hearing Difficulty
Vision Problems
Dry Mouth
Difficulty Chewing
Oral and Dental Problems
Thyroid Disease

Neurologic Disorders
Dizziness
Fainting (Syncope)
Seizures
Tremors
Speaking Difficulty
   (Aphasia)
Huntington's Disease
Parkinson's Disease
Stroke
Meningitis

Psychologic Concerns
Anxiety
Depression
Alcohol Abuse
Drug Dependency

**Joints, Muscles, and
Bones**
Causes of Joint, Muscle,
   and Bone Problems
Neck Pain
Shoulder Pain
Back Pain
Hip Problems
Knee Problems
Foot Problems
Gout
Pseudogout
Osteoarthritis
Rheumatoid Arthritis
Osteoporosis and
   Osteomalacia
Paget's Disease of Bone
Bone Fractures

Skin Conditions
Skin Dryness
Skin Discoloration in
   Body Folds (Intertrigo)
Skin Growths
Itching
Allergic Skin Rash
   (Contact Dermatitis)
Fungal Skin Infections
Infestations
Pressure Ulcers
Psoriasis
Shingles
Skin Cancers
Skin Changes Due
   to Poor Circulation
   (Statis Dermatitis)
Skin Infections

**Heart and Circulation
Conditions**
Chest Pain
Swollen Ankles
High Blood Pressure
Coronary Artery
   Disease
Diseases of the
   Heart Valves
Congestive Heart
   Failure
Abdominal Aortic
   Aneurysm
Poor Circulation
Varicose Veins
   and Other Venous
   Disorders

Digestive Disorders
Abdominal Pain
Loss of Appetite
Swallowing Difficulties
Heartburn
Constipation
Diarrhea
Excess Gas
Gastrointestinal Bleeding
Loss of Bowel Control
Peptic Ulcer Disease

Blood Disorders
Anemia
Bleeding and Clotting
   Disorders
Blood Poisoning
Leukemia
Lymphoma
Multiple Myeloma
Reduced White Blood Cells

continued

TABLE 12.2
Continued

**Lung and
Breathing Problems**
Cough
Wheezing and
   Breathing Difficulty
Chronic Lung Disease
Aspiration
Lung Cancer
Pneumonia
Tuberculosis

Gallbladder Disease
Diverticulitis
Appendicitis
Colon and Rectal Cancers
Hemorrhoids and Other
   Rectal Problems

Nutrition Concerns
Nutritional Requirements
Malnutrition
Loss of Weight
Obesity

**Bladder, Urinary, and
Kidney Conditions**
Blood in the Urine
   (Hematuria)
Loss of Bladder
   Control (Urinary
   Incontinence)
Urinary Tract Infection
Bladder Cancer
Kidney Problems
   Caused by Blood
   Vessel Disease
Problems with Kidneys'
   Filtering Apparatus
(Glomerulo-nephritis)
Sudden Kidney Failure

**Other Important
Conditions**
Cancer (General)
Disorders of Salt
   and Water
Diabetes Mellitus
Heat Stroke
Hypothermia
Infections (General)
Loss of Vitality
Medication Problems
   (Polypharmacy)
Pain
Sleep Problems
Walking Problems,
   Immobility, and Falls

**Sexuality and
Sexual Concerns**
Sexuality in Relation
   to Coexisting Illness
Counseling
Gynecologic Disorders
Vaginal Bleeding
Breast Cancer
Cervical Cancer
Uterine or Endometrial
   Cancer
Ovarian Cancer
Impotence
Prostate Problems

Source: American Geriatrics Society. 1995. *Complete Guide to Aging and Health.* New York: American Geriatrics Society.

Historically, pharmaceutical drugs have addressed populationwide diseases. But the curative drugs of the future will be more tailored to the individual. Before cures can be developed, it is only natural that genetic mutations must be identified, prevalence and incidence rates must be quantified, and serious investments of time and money must be allocated to discover cures that work.

While such cures may be several years away, today's breakthrough drugs, biologic therapies, information systems, and increased public awareness are changing the way healthcare is delivered. For example, vaccines are in development for a wide variety of conditions like cancers and coronary artery disease. A number of genetic mechanisms of cancer development and progression have been discovered, leading to genetic approaches to treatment or supports to current treatments. Bioinformatics companies identify patterns in gene variation with high-speed computers and develop graphical views of how new drugs might attack suspect genes and proteins. The companies are frequently free agents, so they can sell their systems for discovering new drugs to many established pharmaceutical companies and share in the profits. If even a fraction of the current advances under development comes to pass, we will have a biomedical revolution.

Medicare is not ready for that. Medicare covers principally hospital services and physician services. In the very near future, the population of Medicare beneficiaries will be requesting and participating in these new developments in cell and gene therapy. At the moment, Medicare simply says "No" to new coverage unless it is approved by the Food and Drug Administration. Medicare managed care plans have the flexibility to pay for new technologies if they are part of a clinical trial and the beneficiary has informed consent and agrees to participate. If new biotechnologies are cost effective, it will be in the interest of the managed care plan to cover promising treatments. It will be in the interest of us all to pay for valid, promising studies of new technologies as well. Traditional fee-for-service Medicare does not do this, and Medicare managed care rarely does it. Medicare is out of date and ill prepared for what is happening.

The accompanying diagram suggests an answer. Medicare must restructure benefits from two broad categories of coverage organized by type of service to four broad categories of coverage organized by purpose. In the first category, the traditional Part A and Part B of Medicare established nearly 40 years ago would be combined and only medically necessary services would be covered: inpatient hospital services and physician services along with uniform cost-sharing provisions (e.g., common deductible and 20 percent coinsurance with an annual maximum, rather than a lifetime maximum, based on hospital days). Medically necessary prescription drugs used in conjunction with an ongoing disease management program that tracks health outcomes over time and manages contraindications and adherence to the treatment regimen also would be a part of this category (Table 12.3).

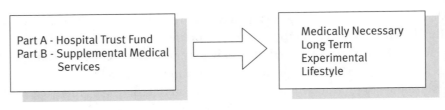

In the second category, skilled nursing facility care and hospice would be placed under a new coverage called long-term care. Some forms of cost-effective home and community-based health services, including professional all-inclusive care for the elderly (PACE), also would be captured under this coverage. Again, different cost-sharing provisions would apply, but these would have a common deductible and coinsurance where appropriate.

Experimental and lifestyle coverage under this proposal would make up the new categories. Experimental coverage would pay for promising new treatments in approved clinical trials on a cost-sharing basis of 50 percent with

OLD PART A AND PART B COVERAGE	MODERN COVERAGE	**TABLE 12.3** Reconfiguration of Medicare Benefits from Part A and Part B to Modern Categories of Coverage

Part A (Separate Inpatient Hospital and Skilled Nursing Facility Deductibles, per Day Coinsurance After Minimum Days, and No Maximum)

Inpatient hospital
Skilled nursing facility
Home health care
Hospice

Part B (Deductible, 20 Percent Coinsurance, and No Maximum)

Physician and other medical services

Outpatient hospital care

Ambulatory surgical services
X-rays, durable medical equipment

Physical, speech, and occupational therapy
Clinical diagnostic laboratory services
Home health care

Outpatient mental health services
Preventive services
Bone mass measurement and diabetes monitoring

Medically Necessary Care (Common: Deductible, 20 Percent Coinsurance, and Maximum)

Inpatient hospital
Home health care
Physician and other medical services
Outpatient hospital care
Ambulatory surgical services
X-rays, durable medical equipment

Physical, speech, and occupational therapy
Clinical diagnostic laboratory services
Outpatient mental health services
Bone mass measurement and diabetes monitoring
Medically necessary prescription drugs

Long-Term Care (Common: Deductible, Copay, and Maximum)

Skilled nursing facility
Home health care
Hospice

PACE

Experimental Care (50 Percent Coinsurance with Sponsors)

Schedule C cancer drugs
New cell and gene therapies

Lifestyle Care (20 Percent Coinsurance with Rebate for Preventive Services)

Preventive services
Lifestyle drugs

Medicare reform requires a new concept of benefits: It worked for the first 35 years but not for the next century the sponsors of trials. The trials would require FDA approval and meet new rigorous standards for producing scientific findings regarding quality of life and cost effectiveness.

The final category would emphasize the importance of personal responsibility in good health and help pay for lifestyle services and drugs, such as assistance for weight loss, smoking cessation, and other types of conditions. The cost sharing would be 20 percent Medicare and 80 percent beneficiary to highlight patients' responsibility to take care of themselves. Beneficiaries meeting prescribed preventive care guidelines would receive an annual rebate on their out-of-pocket costs for preventive services.

Shifting Clinical Sites of Care

The mix of components of Medicare services has been changing and will probably continue to change. Recent trends in the mix of components of care are affected by regulations such as certificate of need, but they will be influenced in the future by the demographics of the boomers and the compression of morbidity. We can expect even stronger pressure to change the mix of components of care as the system gives way under the pressure for those more responsible sites to the obvious needs.

Predicting the future of healthcare is risky, but the recent past can offer some insight. Figure 12.2 shows the percent distribution of spending on different types of care. Medicare expenditures are used as a proxy for indicating the clinical components of care. If more money is being spent in that area, we are counting it as a more important component of care. The early period from 1980 to 1996 is from actual spending data, and the later period 2004 to 2012 is projected on the basis of the trends established earlier. The second part of Figure 12.2 shows the distributions if Medicare drug coverage started in 2004 and were to grow through 2012.

From 1980 to 1996, the share of spending going to hospitals in Medicare fell from 67.6 percent to 49.6 percent. Physician spending increased modestly from 23.6 percent to 26.3 percent. Skilled nursing facility spending increased modestly from 5.3 percent to 8.4 percent. Home health agency spending increased nearly fivefold from 1.1 percent to 5.6 percent of spending, obviously substituting for costly inpatient hospital care. Hospice came on line as a covered service in Medicare during the period and held 1 percent of spending by 1996.

Inpatient Hospital: With or without drug coverage, inpatient hospital spending will continue to take a smaller share of Medicare, although even in 2012 it is still projected to be the largest single item. Spending on inpatient hospital care falls from 67.6 percent in 1980 (actual) to 49.6 percent (actual) in 1996 to 40.6 percent in 2004 to 31.6 percent in 2012. With drug coverage, inpatient care is projected to drop to 29.4 percent of Medicare spending in 2012.

Physician: Spending on physician services hovers in the range of 23.8 percent in 1980 to 29.4 percent in 2012. This spending is projected to take

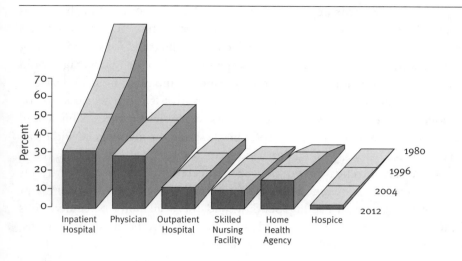

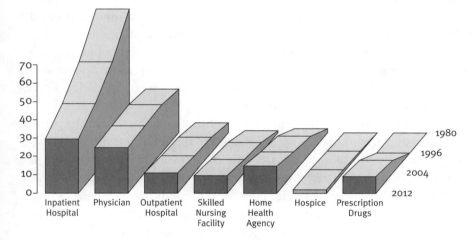

FIGURE 12.2
Percent
Distribution by
Type of Service
1980–1996
(Actual),
2004–2012
(Projected)

*Dramatic
changes in the
components of
care in the
future: Hospital
settings will
decline further
while the others
grow*

a slightly lower share if drugs are covered, allowing for some substitution of prescription drugs for physician services under Medicare coverage.

   Outpatient Hospital: Spending here increases modestly from the actual 1996 levels of 8.4 percent of spending to 10.8 percent of spending projected for 2012. With drug coverage, the trend is little changed.

   Skilled Nursing Care, Home Health Agency, and Hospice: Because of the increasing distribution of frail Medicare beneficiaries, skilled nursing care continues to grow markedly from the 1996 levels of 5.6 percent to 10.1 percent in 2012. Home health agency spending grows from 9.1 percent in 1980 to 15.6 percent in 2012. Hospice is expected to grow modestly to 2.1 percent of Medicare spending by 2012.

   Prescription Drugs: If prescription drugs come on line for Medicare, they are projected to be 7 percent of spending in 2004 and rise to 9 percent in 2012.

Some wild cards in this summary are whether the trend in the 1990s for a leveling of skilled nursing care demand will continue. Increased demand for home and community-based care will dampen the trend for skilled nursing care and accelerate home health agency spending. Also, drug coverage could have a major dampening effect on the demand for inpatient hospital services. The hospital projections could be too conservative if more services can be provided in outpatient hospital departments or physician offices. This would occur due to advances in pain control, blood salvage during surgery, and more powerful medications for infections and viruses with fewer side effects.

The actual trends shown have been affected, and the projected trends will be affected, by state regulation of sites of care. One of the most prominent forms of regulation of capital spending and the availability of clinical sites of care are state certificate-of-need laws. These require hospitals, physicians, or anyone wishing to build a facility requiring a healthcare license to obtain state approval warranting the capital spending as "needed." About half of all states have certificate-of-need laws, which restrict rapid innovation in the field and affect Medicare spending. If Medicare drug coverage is passed and the biomedical revolution discussed in the previous section happens, federal law should preempt these state laws. Competition that is more open and the opportunity for rapid adoption of new and possibly lower-cost clinical sites of care should be in the interest of Medicare.

Another way to examine the components of care is to look at the percent of beneficiaries and what they use. This helps to highlight one more comment on the prospects for long-term care. The compression of morbidity and the looming transformation in the age distribution of the baby boomer population will bring millions more older and possibly frail Medicare beneficiaries under the program. The trend on the components of care is illustrated in Table 12.3.

The columns show three categories of beneficiaries according to frailty and their components of care. Most beneficiaries see a physician during the year, and a large percentage go on to receive outpatient hospital services. Although the frail elderly are more likely to have these two services than all other beneficiaries, the pattern is close. But for durable medical equipment, home health care, rehabilitation, hospital, and skilled nursing care, the percentages are markedly different. Two to three times the use of durable medical equipment is found among the frail beneficiaries. The frail elderly in the community use five times the home health services, twice the average rate of hospitalization, and three to five times the average rate of skilled nursing home use. Unless new technologies are developed to address the needs of the frail beneficiary, the shift toward supportive services shown in this table along the magnitudes shown is in the cards for the future.

When Will the Trust Funds Be Empty?

The Medicare Hospital Trust Funds will never be empty. The question of empty trust funds is a political icon. Both sides use the prospect of depleted

Type of Service	Beneficiaries in Traditional Medicare	Frail Beneficiaries in the Community	Frail Beneficiaries in Nursing Homes
Durable Medical Equipment	18.0	53.0	33.1
Home Health Agency	9.5	50.0	8.9
Rehabilitation Facility	0.9	5.0	0.5
Inpatient Hospital	18.4	43.1	33.8
Outpatient Hospital	62.5	72.3	85.3
Physician	92.8	97.1	99.5
Skilled Nursing Facility	2.9	9.6	16.4

Source: Medicare Payment Advisory Commission. 1999.

TABLE 12.3
Percent Distribution of Beneficiaries Using Medicare Services, 1995

Frail beneficiaries drive components of care: More frail beneficiaries in the future means more durable medical equipment, home health care, rehabilitation, hospital services, and skilled nursing care

trust funds to their advantage. Sometimes the prospect of Medicare's insolvency is used to frighten elderly beneficiaries to gain their allegiance that something will be done. At other times, an empty bucket is used to intimidate physicians and hospitals that payments must be cut to keep the program solvent. Balancing the trust funds is a simple matter of either cutting benefits or raising taxes or premiums to ward off a deficit. What politicians mean when they talk about barren funds is that they and the public are unwilling to adjust spending or revenues. Depleted trust funds can be seen years ahead. Still, they can be addressed with only one year's notice. No one wants to point out that it is a game of assumptions. If you are willing to assume that spending can be cut or revenues raised, balancing the Medicare trust funds is nothing more than normal, everyday budgeting (Fig. 12.3).

The continued strong performance of the U.S. economy in the 1990s and prospects for future positive performance have improved the financial status of the Medicare Hospital Insurance Trust Fund. The dates are quite far off for when the fund is projected, under current law, to run short of money to pay full benefits. At the beginning of 2000, the Hospital Insurance (HI) Trust Fund, which pays inpatient hospital expenses, was projected to be able to pay full benefits until 2015. Low increases in healthcare costs generally and continuing efforts to combat fraud and abuse have been cited as reasons for the lengthy period of positive inflows to the funds. The Supplementary Medical Insurance (SMI) Trust Fund, which pays doctor's bills and other outpatient expenses, is expected to remain adequately financed into the indefinite future. However, this is only because current law sets financing each year to meet the expected costs next year. Although the rate of growth of SMI costs moderated in the 1990s, outlays have still increased 41 percent over the period 1994–1999 or about 9 percent faster than the economy as a whole.

The real drivers of Medicare trust funds are the share of the Gross Domestic Product (GDP) that goes to Medicare and the number of workers

FIGURE 12.3

Historical and Estimated Workers per Beneficiary, 1970–2075

Dwindling support: Fewer workers per Medicare beneficiary will mean higher contributions in revenues or forgone benefits as well as rising wages for caregivers

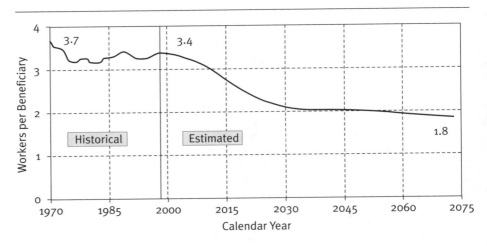

contributing to the funds versus the beneficiaries supported by the funds. As for the GDP, about 1.56 of the value of all the economy's goods and services was devoted to the HI Trust Fund in 1998. That is expected to rise to 2.2 percent (96 percent) in 25 years. The SMI Trust Fund is projected to rise from 0.98 percent to 2.23 (170 percent) in 2000–2025. The two together are to rise from 2.54 percent to 4.43 percent of GDP. Although they seem like small, single-digit percentage shares, the shift represents billions of dollars and a massive quantity of goods and services including skilled workers. Nonetheless, it is still a small fraction of all that goes on in our economy. We will probably be able to weather the impact in terms of the share of the economy devoted to Medicare.

What may be more problematic for the very long run is the number of workers needed to support one beneficiary. This will mean fewer people being productive and earning wages as the basis for revenues for the Medicare Trust Funds. More importantly, perhaps, is that the number of people to care for frail elderly beneficiaries will be lower than it is today. Wages for these caregivers should rise if they become more scarce, but we will have to change our expectations about who provides care under Medicare. If not, costs will go up to attract a sufficient number of caregivers for future home health agencies, skilled nursing facilities, and rehabilitation services.

The Role of Competition in the Financing and Delivery of Healthcare

There are millions of older Americans who reveal every day their desires for a private health plan supported with public dollars. Opting out of the predominantly government-operated system is a choice they are willing to make. The current system is set up correctly—offer competing choices for people to select a form of healthcare financing and delivery that best meets their needs. The competing choices are free to enter the market and try to do better than traditional fee-for-service Medicare. What are *you* doing?

First, with an aging population, you are competing in a growing market. Second, it is a solvent market, despite the myths about impending insolvency promulgated through the political process. The money is there. Medicare is funded. Third, because the market is growing and the money is there, it is an intensely competitive market that only the best prepared are able to participate in. Fourth, it is a market with intensive buying and selling (transactions), which means the focus must be on the beneficiary as a customer and lowering transaction costs in the system.

In 2008, when we examine the successful Medicare managed care plan, what will the best plans have done to become leaders in the field? What business practices will serve as common ground for successful health plans? What managed care cultures will flourish? What types of plans will be acquired, and what types will do the acquiring?

As much as beneficiaries can choose between fee-for-service and managed care in most parts of the country, managers of Medicare managed care plans, healthcare executives, and physicians have a choice also. The choice you make today will determine where you will be in the near term and the future.

Strategic Decisions Checklist

Strategic Questions	Strategic Analyses
How does your health plan identify unfolding trends and develop its policy outlook?	You should have formal sessions where key people in the organization can share viewpoints about the future. Try to develop a consensus about future assumptions. Use the framework examining Medicare benefit, payment, choice, and delivery structure to organize your thoughts. Scan the news and industry literature to identify emerging trends.
How do you select the key drivers of change?	You can begin with the major drivers of change presented in this chapter and then develop your own list of drivers for your own market. Try to figure out which drivers are merely swirling distractions and which are real drivers of ultimate, equilibrium change.
Do you do scenario planning?	Use the top management team and the physicians and other clinicians in your health plan to develop scenarios. Be open-minded about what might happen in the future. Even the most distant possible event could contain the seeds of a new important emerging trend. Use the scenarios to overcome linear thinking. Consider the implications for your health plan if the scenarios were to come true. Take actions now to anticipate the future you are envisioning.

continued

Strategic Questions	Strategic Analyses
What kinds of projections and simulations do you make?	Gather charts and tables illustrating the past and projecting the future of the trends you think are important. Simulate the influence of changes in future enrollment, cost, profitability. Examine the organization critically to see if resources should be deployed to address emerging trends.
Does your business strategy get adjusted?	Revisit the planning assumptions about the drivers of change in the Medicare market, the scenarios, and the emerging trends. This should be done annually. The results should be used to inform the key decision makers in your plan about the role they can play to create change to meet the future.

REFERENCES

Adamache, K., and L. F. Rossiter. 1986. "The Entry of HMOs in the Medicare Market: Implications for TEFRA's Mandate." *Inquiry* 23(4): 349–64.

Adler, G. S. 1994. "A Profile of the Medicare Current Beneficiary Survey." *Health Care Financing Review* 4: 153–63.

Alternative Futures Associates and Regulatory Resources, Inc. 1986. *Guidebook for Strategic Planning for Blood Service Facilities.* Washington, DC: American Blood Commission.

AMCRA Foundation. 1994. *1994–1995 Managed Health Care Directory,* vii–ix. Washington, DC: AMCRA Foundation.

American Geriatrics Society. 1995. *Complete Guide to Aging and Health.* New York: American Geriatrics Society.

Barrett, D. E. 1996A. "Marketing the Medicare Managed Care Product." In *Implementing a Successful Medicare Managed Care Product,* edited by D. Mlawsky, 35–44. Washington, DC: Atlantic Information Services, Inc.

———. 1996B. "Selling the Medicare Managed Care Product." In *Implementing a Successful Medicare Managed Care Product,* edited by D. Mlawsky, 45–48. Washington, DC: Atlantic Information Services, Inc.

Barsky, A., and J. Borus. 1995. "Somatization and Medication in the Era of Managed Care." *Journal of the American Medical Association* 274: 1931–34.

Begun, J., and K. B. Heatwole. 1999. "Strategic Cycling: Shaking Complacency in Healthcare Strategic Planning." *Journal of Healthcare Management* 44(5): 339–51.

Berger, M., and I. Muhlhauser. 1999. "Diabetes Care and Patient-Oriented Outcomes." *Journal of the American Medical Association* 282(18): 1676–78.

Berkowitz, E. N. 1996. *Essentials of Health Care Marketing.* Gaithersburg, MD: Aspen Publishers, Inc.

Berkowitz, K., and J. J. Martingale. 1996. "Medicare Managed Care Plans and the Employer Market." In *Implementing a Successful Medicare Managed Care Product*, edited by D. Mlawsky, 49–59. Washington, DC: Atlantic Information Services, Inc.

Bernstein, A. B., and A. K. Gauthier. 1998. "Defining Competition in Markets: Why and How? (Examining the Role of Regulation in an Evolving Healthcare Marketplace)." *Health Services Research* 33(5): 1421–29.

Bierman, A. S., E. S. Magari, A. M. Jette, M. Splaine, and J. H. Wasson. 1998. "Assessing Access as a First Step Toward Improving the Quality of Care for Very Old Adults." *Journal of Ambulatory Care Management* 21(3): 17–26.

Blendon, R. J., J. M. Benson, M. Brodie, M. Brossard, D. E. Altman, and R. Morin. 1997. "Disenrollment of Medicare Beneficiaries from HMOs." *Health Affairs* 16(5): 111–16.

Board of Trustees. 1998. *Medicare Trustee's Report.* Washington, DC: Office of the President.

Bodenheimer, T. 1999. "Disease Management: Promises and Pitfalls." *The New England Journal of Medicine* 340(15): 1202–5.

Bodenheimer, T., and L. Casalino. 1999A. "Executives with White Coats. . . ." First Part. *New England Journal of Medicine* 341(25): 1945–8.

———. 1999B. "Executives with White Coats. . . ." Second Part. *New England Journal of Medicine* 341(26): 2029–32.

Bodenheimer, T., B. Lo, and L. Casalino. 1999. "Primary Care Physicians Should Be Coordinators, Not Gatekeepers." *Journal of the American Medical Association* 281(21): 2045–9.

Boling, P. A. 1999. "The Value of Targeted Case Management During Transitional Care." *Journal of the American Medical Association* 281(7): 656–67.

Boult, C., T. F. Pualwan, P. D. Fox, and J. T. Pacala. 1998. "Identification and Assessment of High-Risk Seniors: HMO Workgroup on Care Management." *American Journal of Managed Care* 4(8): 1137–46.

Brown, R. S. 1993. *The Medicare Risk Program for HMOs: Final Summary Report on Findings from the Evaluation.* Princeton, NJ: Mathematica Policy Research.

Brown, R. S., and K. Langwell. 1988. "Enrollment Patterns in Medicare HMOs: Implications for Access to Care." *Advances in Health Economics Health Services Research* 9: 69–96.

Brown, B., and S. M. Retchin. 1990. "Quality of Ambulatory Care in Medicare Health Maintenance Organizations." *American Journal of Public Health* 80(4): 411–15.

———. 1991. "Elderly Patients with Congestive Heart Failure Under Pre-Paid Care." *American Journal of Medicine* 90(2): 236–42.

Brown, R. S., D. G. Clement, S. M. Retchin, J. Hill, and J. Bergeron. 1993. "Do Health Maintenance Organizations Work for Medicare?" *Health Care Financing Review* 15(1): 7–23.

Brown, R. S., D. G. Clement, and S. M. Retchin. 1994. "Care of Patients Hospitalized with Strokes under the Medicare Risk Program." In *HMOs and the Elderly*, edited by H. Luft, 167–94. Chicago: Health Administration Press.

Brown, R. S., and M. Gold. 1999. "What Drives Medicare Managed Care Growth?" *Health Affairs* 18(6): 140–49.

Browne, M. J., and H. Doerpinghaus. 1994. "Asymmetric Information and the Demand for Medigap Insurance." *Inquiry* 31(4): 445–50.

Burns, L. R., M. A. Morrisey, J. A. Alexander, and V. Johnson. 1998. "Managed Care and Processes to Integrate Physicians/Hospitals." *Health Care Management Review* 23(4): 70–80.

Butler, R. N. 1997. "Economic and Political Implications of Immunology and Aging on Tomorrow's Society." *Geriatrics* 93(1–3): 7–13.

Cafferata, G. L. 1984. "Knowledge of Their Health Insurance Coverage by the Elderly." *Medical Care* 22(9): 835–47.

Capitman, J. A. 1988. "A Descriptive Framework For New Hospital Roles in Geriatric

Care." *Health Care Financing Review Annual Supplement* (December): 17–25.

Cartin, T. J., and D. J. Jacoby. 1997. *A Review of Managing Quality. . . .* Milwaukee, WI: ASQ Quality Press.

Cave, D. G. 1995. "Vertical Integration Models to Prepare Health Systems for Capitation." *Health Care Management Review* 20(1): 26–39.

Chamber, L. W., D. L. Sackett, C. H. Goldsmith, A. S. MacPherson, and R. G. McAuley. 1976. "Development and Application of an Index of Social Function." *Health Services Research* 11(4): 430–41.

Christensen, S. 1998. "Medicare+Choice Provisions in the Balanced Budget Act of 1997." *Health Affairs* 17(4): 224–31.

Christensen, S., S. H. Long, and J. Rodgers. 1987. "Acute Health Care Costs for the Aged Medicare Population: Overview and Policy Options." *The Milbank Quarterly* 65(3): 397–425.

Christianson, J. B., B. Dowd, and R. Feldman. 1995. "Open-Ended Options in Medicare Risk Contracts with HMOs." *Managed Care Quarterly* 3(1): 47–55.

Clement, D. G., S. M. Retchin, M. Stegall, R. Cohen, and R. S. Brown. 1992. *Impacts of Medicare HMOs on the Quality of Medical Care.* Princeton, NJ: Mathematica Policy Research.

Clement, D. G., R. S. Brown, S. M. Retchin, and M. Stegall. 1994. "Elderly Access and Outcomes Under Managed Care." *Journal of the American Medical Association* 27(19): 1487–92.

Clement, D. G., S. M. Retchin, and R. Brown. 1994. "Satisfaction with Access and Quality of Care in Medicare Risk Contract HMOs." In *Health Maintenance Organizations and the Elderly,* edited by H. S. Luft, 95–110. Chicago: Health Administration Press.

Collins, F. S. 1999. "Genetics: An Explosion of Knowledge Is Transforming Clinical Practice." *Geriatrics* 54(1): 41–7.

Congress of the United States Congressional Budget Office. 1988. "Including Capital Expenses in the Prospective Payment System." August.

———. 1997. "Predicting How Changes in Medicare's Payment Rates Would Affect Risk-Sector Enrollment and Costs." March.

Conrad, D., R. Bonney, M. Sachs, and R. Smith. 1996. *Managed Care Contracting.* Chicago: Health Administration Press.

Covinsky, K. E., J. D. Fuller, K. Yaffe et al. 2000. "Communication and Decision Making in Seriously Ill Patients: Findings of the SUPPORT Project. The Study to Understand Prognoses and Preferences for Outcomes and Risks of Treatments." *Journal of the American Geriatric Society* 48(5 suppl.): S187–93.

Dansky, K. H., L. D. Gamm, J. J. Vasey, and C. K. Barsukiewicz. 1999. "Electronic Medical Records: Are Physicians Ready?" *Journal of Healthcare Management* 44(6): 440–55.

D'Aveni, R. A. 1994. *Hypercompetition.* New York: The Free Press.

Davidson, B. N. 1998. "Designing Health Insurance Information for the Medicare Beneficiary." *Health Services Research* 33(5): 712–13.

Davidson, B. N., S. Sofaer, and P. Gertler. 1992. "Consumer Information and Biased Selection in the Demand for Coverage Supplementing Medicare." *Social Sciences and Medicine* 34(9): 1023–34.

Davis, K., and C. Schoen. 1998. "Assuring Quality, Information, and Choice in Managed Care." *Inquiry* 35(2): 104–14.

Davis, D., M. Thompson-O'Brien, N. Freemantle et al. 1999. "Impact of Formal Continuing Medical Education: Do Conferences, Workshops, Rounds, and Other Traditional Continuing Education Activities Change Physician Behavior or Health Care Outcomes?" *Journal of the American Medical Association* 282(9): 867–75.

DeBusk, R. F., N. H. Miller, R. Superko et al. 1994. "A Case Management System for Coronary Risk Factor Modification After Acute Myocardial Infarction." *Annals of Internal Medicine* 120(9): 721–29.

Deevy, E. 1995. *Creating the Resilient Organization*. Upper Saddle River, NJ: Prentice Hall.

Delichatsios, H., M. Callahan, and M. Charlson. 1998. "Outcomes of Telephone Medical Care." *Journal of General Internal Medicine* 13(9): 579–85.

Deming, W. E. 1986. *Out of the Crisis*. Cambridge, MA: MIT, Center for Advanced Engineering Study.

DHHS Bureau of Data Management and Strategy. 1983. "Medicare Statistical Files Manual, Appendix A: Glossary." Washington, DC: U.S. Government Printing Office.

"DM Nurse Line Creates 'Win-Win' Scenario for Point-of-Service Product." 1997. *Healthcare Demand and Disease Management* 3(4): 57–59.

Dowd, B. E. 1982. "Financing Preventive Care in HMOs: A Theoretical Analysis." *Inquiry* 19(1): 68–78.

Dowd, B., R. Coulam, and R. Feldman. 2000. "A Tale of Four Cities: Medicare Reform and Competitive Pricing." *Health Affairs* 19(5): 9–29.

Draft, R. L., and R. H. Lengel. 1998. *Fusion Leadership*. San Francisco: Berrett-Koehler.

Duncan, P. W., L. B. Goldstein, D. Matchar, G. W. Divine, and J. Feussner. 1992. "Measurement of Motor Recovery After Stroke." *Stroke* 23(8): 1084–9.

EBRI. 1991. "Databook on Employee Benefits." Washington, DC: Employee Benefit Research Institute.

Ellis, R. P. 1985. *The Effect of Prior-Year Health Expenditures on Health Coverage Plan Choice*, 149–70. Greenwich, CT: JAI Press, Inc.

Ellis, R. P., G. C. Pope, L. I. Iezzoni et al. 1996. "Diagnosis-Based Risk Adjustment for Medicare Capitation Payments." *Health Care Financing Review* 17(3): 101–28.

Ettner, S. L. 1997. "Adverse Selection and the Purchase of Medigap Insurance by the Elderly." *Journal of Health Economics* 16(5): 543–62.

The Euroqol Group. 1990. "A New Facility for the Measurement of Health Related Quality of Life." *Health Policy* 16(3): 199–208.

Evans, A., and L. J. Blumberg. 1998. "Reform of the Medicare AAPCC: Learning from Previous Proposals." *Inquiry* 35(1): 62–77.

Every, N., C. P. Cannon, C. Granger et al. 1998. "Influence of Insurance Type on the Use of Procedures. . . ." *Journal of the American College of Cardiology* 32(2): 387–92.

Feldman, R., H. C. Chan, J. Kralewski, B. Dowd, and J. Shapiro. 1990. "Effects of HMOs on the Creation of Competitive Markets for Hospital Services." *Journal of Health Economics* 9(2): 207–22.

Fox, P. D. 1997. "Applying Managed Care Techniques in Traditional Medicare." *Health Affairs* 16(5): 44–57.

Fox, P. D., and T. Fama (eds). 1996. *Managed Care and Chronic Illness: Challenges and Opportunities.* Gaithersburg, MD: Aspen Publishers, Inc.

Fox, P. D., R. Snyder, G. Dallek, and T. Rice. 1999. "Should Medicare HMO Benefits Be Standardized?" *Health Affairs* 18(4): 40–52.

Freeborn, D. K., C. R. Pope, J. P. Mullooly, and B. H. McFarland. 1990. "Consistently High Users of Medical Care Among the Elderly." *Medical Care* 28(6): 527–40.

Fuchs, V. 1998. *Who Shall Live?* River Edge, NJ: World Scientific.

Gabel, J. 1997. "Ten Ways HMOs Have Changed During the 1990s." *Health Affairs* 16(3): 134–45.

Gabel, J., H. Whitmore, C. Bergston, and L. Grim. 1997. "Growing Diversification in HMOs 1988–1994." *Medical Care Research and Review* 54(1 March): 101–17.

Gemignani, J. 1996. "Demand Management: Dial-a-Nurse." *Business and Health* 14(7): 50.

———. 1997. "What's Holding Back MSAs?" *Business and Health* 15(11): 34–9.

Gold M., K. Chu, S. Felt, M. Harrington, and T. Lake. 1993. "Effects of Selected Cost Containment Efforts: 1971–1993." *Health Care Financing Review* 14(3): 193–225.

Gold, M., R. Hurley, T. Lake, T. Ensor, R. Berenson. 1995. *Arrangements Between Managed Care Plans and Physicians.* Washington, DC: Physician Payment Review Commission.

Gold, M., L. Nelson, R. S. Brown, A. Ciemnecki, A. Aizer, and E. Docteur. 1997. "Disabled Medicare Beneficiaries in HMOs." *Health Affairs* 16(5): 149–62.

Gold, M., A. Smith, A. Cook, and P. Defilippes. 1999. *Medicare Managed Care: Preliminary Analysis of Trends in Benefits and Premiums, 1997–1999.* Princeton, NJ: Mathematica Policy Research.

Goodlin, S. J., E. Fisher, J. A. Patterson, and J. H. Wasson. 1998. "End-of-Life Care for Persons Age 80 Years or Older." *Journal of Ambulatory Care Management* 21(3): 34–39.

Greenlick, M. R. 1985. *Comments on Medicare Capitation Payments to HMOs,* 97–100. Greenwich, CT: JAI Press, Inc.

Gruenberg, L., E. Kaganova, and M. C. Hornbrook. 1996. "Improving the AAPCC with Health-Status Measures from the MCBS." *Health Care Financing Review* 17(3): 59–75.

Hall, M. A. 1997. *Making Medical Spending Decisions: The Law, Ethics, and Economics of Rationing Mechanisms.* New York: Oxford University Press.

Hamel, G., and C. K. Prahalad. 1994. *Competing for the Future.* Boston: Harvard Business School Press.

Harris, J. 1996. "Disease Management: New Wine in Old Bottles?" *Annals of Internal Medicine* 124(9): 838–42.

Havlicek, P. L. 1999. *Medical Groups in the U.S.* Chicago: AMA, Division of Survey and Data Resources.

Health Care Financing Administration. 1982. *Prospective Reimbursement for Hospitals: A Glossary of Technical Terms.* Washington, DC: U.S. Government Printing Office.

————. 1996. *1996 Guide to Health Insurance for People with Medicare*. Washington, DC: U.S. Government Printing Office.

————. 1997A. *A Profile of Dually-Eligible Medicare Beneficiaries*. Washington, DC: U.S. Government Printing Office.

————. 1997B. http://www.hcfa.gov/medicare/intro.htm. December 30, 1997.

————. 1998. *1998 Data Compendium*. Washington, DC: U.S. Government Printing Office.

Heinen, L., P. D. Fox, and M. D. Anderson. 1990. "Findings from the Medicaid Competition Demonstrations: A Guide for States." *Health Care Financing Review* 11(4): 55–67.

Herzlinger, R. 1999. "Disease Management." *New England Journal of Medicine* 341(10): 767–8.

Hicks B., H. Raisz, J. Segal, and N. Doherty. 1981. "The Triage Experiment in Coordinated Care for the Elderly." *American Journal of Public Health* 71(9): 991–1002.

Hiramatsu, S., and M. J. Mason. 1991. *New Member Orientation: Its Role and Refinement*. New York: Group Health Association of America.

HMO Workgroup on Care Management. 1996. *Identifying High-Risk Medicare HMO Members*. Washington, DC: AAHP Foundation.

————. 1998. "Essential Components of Geriatric Care Provided Through Health Maintenance Organizations." *Journal of the American Geriatric Society* 46(3): 303–8.

Holtzman, J., Q. Chen, and R. Kane. 1998. "The Effect of HMO Status on the Outcomes of Home-Care After Hospitalization in a Medicare Population." *Journal of American Geriatrics* 46(5): 629–34.

Horn, S. D., P. D. Sharkey, and C. Phillips-Harris. 1998. "Formulary Limitations and the Elderly." *American Journal of Managed Care* 4(8): 1105–13.

Hornbrook, M. C., V. J. Stevens, D. J. Wingfield et al. 1994. "Preventing Falls Among Community-Dwelling Older Persons." *Gerontologist* 34(1): 16–23.

Hunt, S. M., S. P. McKenna, J. McEwen, E. M. Backett, J. Williams, and E. Papp. 1980. "A Quantitative Approach to Perceived Health Status: A Validation Study." *Journal of Epidemiological Community Health* 34(4): 281–86.

Hurd, M. D., and K. McGarry. 1997. "Medical Insurance and the Use of Health Care Services by the Elderly." *Journal of Health Economics* 16(2): 129–54.

Hurley, R. E., and R. R. Bannick. 1993. "Utilization Managers in Medicare Risk Contract HMOs." *Quality Review Bulletin* 19(4): 131–7.

Iglehart, J. K. 1998. "The Federal Trade Commission in Action: The FTC's Robert F. Leibenluft." *Health Affairs* 17(5): 65–74.

Institute for Clinical Evaluative Sciences. 1999. *Early Discharge Planning Strategies*. Ontario Ministry of Health, Canada.

Institute of Medicine. 1994. *Health Data in the Information Age: Use, Disclosure, and Privacy*, 239–246. Washington, DC: National Academy Press.

Jensen, G. A., and M. A. Morrisey. 1992. "Employer-Sponsored Postretirement Health Insurance: Not Your Mother's Medigap Plan." *Gerontologist* 32(5): 693–703.

Joch, A. 2000. "Can the Web Save Disease Management?" *Healthcare Informatics* 15(3): 59–70.

Johnson, R. E., M. J. Goodman, M. C. Hornbrook, and M. B. Eldredge. 1997. "The Effect of Increased Prescription Drug Cost-Sharing. . . ." *Medical Care* 35(11): 1119–31.

Kaiser Family Foundation, Medicare Policy Project. 1998. *Fact Sheet: Medicare Managed Care*. Washington, DC: Henry J. Kaiser Family Foundation.

Kane, R. L., Q. Chen, M. Finch, L. Blewett, R. Burns, and M. Moskowitz. 2000. "The Optimal Outcomes of Post-Hospital Care Under Medicare." *Health Services Research* 35(3): 615–61.

Kaplan, R. M., J. W. Bush, and C. C. Berry. 1976. "Health Status: Types of Validity and the Index of Well-Being." *Health Services Research* 11(4): 478–507.

Kaplan, S. H., S. Greenfield, and J. E. Ware. 1989. "Impact of the Doctor-Patient Relationship on the Outcome of Chronic Disease." In *Communicating with Medical Patients*, 228–45. Newbury Park, CA: Sage.

Kletke, P. R., D. W. Emmons, and K. D. Gillis. 1996. "Current Trends in Physicians' Practice Arrangements." *Journal of the American Medical Association* 276(7): 555–60.

Knowles, P., and R. Cummins. 1984. "ED Department Medical Advice Telephone Calls: Who Calls and Why." *Journal of Emergency Nursing* 10(6): 283–86.

Komisar, H. L., J. M. Lambrew, and P. D. Fox. 1996. *Long-Term Care for the Elderly: A Chart Book*. New York: The Commonwealth Fund.

Kotin, A. M. 1996. "Medically Managing the Medicare Population." In *Implementing a Successful Medicare Managed Care Product*, edited by D. Mlawsky, 67–79. Washington, DC: Atlantic Information Services, Inc.

Kotler, P. 1994. *Marketing Management, 8th ed.* Englewood Cliffs, NJ: Prentice Hall.

Kramer, A. M., P. D. Fox, and N. Morgenstern. 1992. "Geriatric Care Approaches in Health Maintenance Organizations." *Journal of the American Geriatrics Society* 40(10): 1055–67.

Kramer, A. M., J. F. Steiner, R. E. Schlenker et al. 1997. "Outcomes and Costs After Hip Fracture and Stroke: A Comparison of Rehabilitation Settings." *Journal of the American Medical Association* 277(5): 396–404.

Kunkel, S. R., and R. A. Applebaum. 1992. "Estimating the Prevalence of Long-Term Disability for an Aging Society." *Journal of Gerontology Social Sciences* 47(5): S253–60.

LaCroix, A. Z., and L. J. Rubenstein. 1990. "Health Promotion and the Elderly." In *Medicare, Medicaid and the HMO Experience*. Baltimore, MD: Group Health Association of America.

Lamphere, J. A., P. Neuman, K. Langwell, and D. Sherman. 1997. "The Surge in Medicare Managed Care: An Update." *Health Affairs* 16(3): 127–33.

Langwell, K. M., and J. P. Hadley. 1986. "Capitation and the Medicare Program." *Health Care Financing Review* (Special): 9–20.

———. 1989. Evaluation of the Medicare Competition Demonstrations. *Health Care Financing Review* 11(2): 65–80.

———. 1990. Insights from the Medicare HMO Demonstrations. *Health Affairs* 9(1): 74–84.

Langwell, K., L. Rossiter, R. Brown, L. Nelson, S. Nelson, and K. Berman. 1987. Early Experience of Health Maintenance Organizations Under Medicare Competition Demonstrations. *Health Care Financing Review* 8(3): 37–55.

Laschober, M. A., P. Neuman, M. S. Kitchman, L. Meyer, and K. M. Langwell. 1999. "Medicare HMO Withdrawals: What Happens to Beneficiaries?" *Health Affairs* 18(6): 150–7.

Lattimer, V., S. George, F. Thompson et al. 1998. "Safety and Effectiveness of Nurse Telephone Consultation in Out of Hours Primary Care: Randomised Controlled Trial. The South Wittshire Out of Hours Project (Swoop) Group." *British Medical Journal* 317(7165): 1026–27.

Lee, L. F. 1978. "Unionism and Wage Rates: A Simultaneous Equations Model with Qualitative and Limited Dependent Variables." *International Economic Review* (2): 415–33.

LeMasurier, J. D., G. Bailey. 1999. *Medicare+Choice Monitoring Guide*. Washington, DC: Health Care Financing Administration.

Lester, J., and M. Breudigam. 1996. "Nurse Triage Telephone Centers Key to Demand Management Strategy." *The NAHAM Management Journal* 22(4): 13–4, 34.

Levenstein, J. H. 1989. "Patient-Centered Clinical Interviewing." In *Communicating with Medical Patients*, 107–20. Newbury Park, CA: Sage.

Link, C. R., S. H. Long, and R. F. Settle. 1980. "Cost Sharing, Supplementary Insurance, and Health Services Utilization Among the Medicare Elderly." *Health Care Financing Review* 2(2): 25–31.

Long, S. H. 1994. "Prescription Drugs and the Elderly: Issues and Options." *Health Affairs* 14(2): 157–74.

Longino, C. F., Jr. 1997. "Pressure from Our Aging Population Will Broaden Our Understanding of Medicine." *Academic Medicine* 72(10): 841–7.

Lorig, K. R., P. D. Mazonson, and H. R. Holman. 1993. "Evidence Suggesting that Health Education for Self-Management in Patients with Chronic Arthritis Has Sustained Health Benefits While Reducing Health Care Costs." *Arthritis Rheum* 36(4): 439–46.

Lubitz, J., and R. Prihoda. 1984. "The Use and Costs of Medicare Services in the Last Two Years of Life." *Health Care Financing Administration* 5(3):117–31.

Lubitz, J., J. Beebe, and G. Riley. 1985. *Improving the Medicare HMO Payment Formula to Deal with Biased Selection*, 101–22. Greenwich, CT: JAI Press, Inc.

Luft, H. S. 1981. *Health Maintenance Organizations: Dimensions of Performance*. New York: Wiley.

Luke, R., and J. Begun. 1994. "Strategy Making in Health Care Organizations." In *Health Care Management, 3rd ed.*, 355–91. Albany, NY: Delmar.

Lynch, W., and D. Vickery. 1993. "The Potential Impact of Health Promotion on Health Care Utilization: An Introduction to Demand Management." *American Journal of Health Promotion* 8(2): 87–92.

Magari, E. S., M. B. Hamel, and J. H. Wasson. 1998. "An Easy Way to Measure Quality of Physician-Patient Interactions." *Journal of Ambulatory Care Management* 21(3): 27–33.

Manning, W. G., A. Leibowitz, G. A. Goldberg, W. H. Rogers, and J. P. Newhouse. 1984. "A Controlled Trial of the Effect of a Prepaid Group Practice on Use of Services." *The New England Journal of Medicine* 310(23): 1505–11.

Marosits, M. 1997. "Improving Financial and Patient Outcomes: The Future of Demand Management." *Healthcare Financial Management* 51(8): 43–44.

Marquis, M. S., and J. A. Rogowski. 1991. *Participation in Alternative Health Plans.* Santa Monica, CA: RAND.

Marshall, B. S., M. J. Long, J. Voss, K. Demma, and K. Skerl. 1999. "Case Management of the Elderly in a Health Maintenance Organization: The Implications for Program Administration Under Managed Care." *Journal of Healthcare Management* 44(6): 477–93.

Mathematica Policy Research, Inc. 1992. *The Quality of Care in TEFRA HMOs/CMPs.* Baltimore, MD: Health Care Financing Administration.

———. 1999. *Health Plans' Selection and Payment of Health Care Providers.* Washington, DC: MedPAC.

McBride, T. D., J. Penrod, and K. Mueller. 1997. "Volatility in Medicare AAPCC Rates: 1990–1997." *Health Affairs* 16(5): 172–80.

McCall, N., T. Rice, and J. Sangl. 1986. "Consumer Knowledge of Medicare and Supplemental Health Insurance Benefits." *Health Services Research* 21(6): 633–57.

McCall, N., T. Rice, J. Boismier, and R. West. 1991. "Private Health Insurance and Medical Care Utilization: Evidence from the Medicare Population." *Inquiry* 28(3): 276–87.

McCarthy, R. 1997. "It Takes More than a Phone Call to Manage Demand." *Business and Health* 15(5): 36–41.

McCormack, L., P. D. Fox, T. Rice, and M. L. Graham. 1996. "Medigap Reform Legislation of 1990: Have the Objectives Been Met?" *Health Care Financing Review* 18(1): 157–74.

McEachern, S. 1995. "Demand Management Will Be a Necessity, A Baked-in Utility." *Health Care Strategic Management* 13(10): 20–23.

McMillan, A., R. M. Mentnech, J. Lubitz, A. M. McBean, and D. Russell. 1990. "Trends and Patterns on Place of Death for Medicare Enrollees." *Health Care Financing Review* 12(1): 1–7.

Medicare Payment Advisory Commission. 1998. *Report to Congress: Context for a Changing Medicare Program.* Washington, DC: MedPAC.

———. 1999. *Report to Congress: Selected Medicare Issues.* Washington, DC: MedPAC.

Menkin, H. 1999. *Handbook of Managed Care Terminology.* New York: Healthcare Trustees of New York State.

Milgrom, R., and J. Roberts. 1992. *Economics, Organization, and Management.* Englewood Cliffs, NJ: Prentice Hall.

Miller, R. H., and H. S. Luft. 1994. "Managed Care Performance Since 1980: A Literature Synthesis." *Journal of the American Medical Association* 271(19): 1512–19.

———. 1997. "Does Managed Care Lead to Better or Worse Quality of Care?" *Health Affairs* 16(5): 7–25.

Mintzberg, H. 1994. *The Rise and Fall of Strategic Planning.* New York: The Free Press.

Monahan, M. L. 1988. "Quality of Life of Adults Receiving Chemotherapy: A Comparison of Instruments." *Oncology Nurse Forum* 15(6): 795–98.

Moody, H. R. 1994. "Four Scenarios for an Aging Society." *Hastings Center Report* 24(5): 32–5.

Mukamel, D. B., C. C. Chou, J. G. Zimmer, and B. M. Rothenberg. 1997. "The Effect of Accurate Patient Screening on the Cost-Effectiveness of Case Management Programs." *Gerontologist* 37(6): 777–84.

Mullooly, J. P., and D. K. Freeborn. 1979. "The Effect of Length of Membership upon the Utilization of Ambulatory Care Services." *Medical Care* 17(9): 922–36.

Murray, J. P. 1988. "Physician Satisfaction with Capitation Patients. . . ." *Journal of Family Practice* 27(1): 108–13.

"National Health Information, Physician Compensation, and Incentives Under Capitation." 1999. Capitation Management Report Newsletter. Atlanta, GA.

Nathan, A., L. Goodyer, A. Lovejoy, and A. Rashid. 1999. " 'Brown Bag' Medication Reviews as a Means of Optimizing Patients' Use of Medication and of Identifying Potential Clinical Problems." *Family Practitioner* 16(3): 278–82.

Naylor, M. D., D. Brooten, R. Campbell et al. 1999. "Comprehensive Discharge Planning and Home Follow-Up of Hospitalized Elders." *Journal of the American Medical Association* 281(7): 613–20.

NCHSR. 1979. "Insurance Terms." Unpublished list of insurance terms from the National Medical Care Expenditures Survey.

Nelson, E., J. Wasson, J. Kirt et al. 1987. "Assessment of Function in Routine Clinical Practice: Description of the COOP Chart Method and Preliminary Findings." *Journal of Chronic Diseases* 40: 55S–63S.

———. 1996. *Access to Care in Medicare Managed Care: Results from a 1996 Survey of Enrollees and Disenrollees*. Washington, DC: Physician Payment Review Commission.

Nelson, L. M., K. M. Langwell, and R. S. Brown. 1988. "Comparison of 'Rollovers' and 'Switchers' Among Enrollees of Medicare HMOs." *GHAA* 8(2): 63–78.

Nelson, S., K. Langwell, and R. Brown. 1990. *Organizational and Operational Characteristics of TEFRA HMOs/CMPs*. Princeton, NJ: Mathematica Policy Research.

Nelson, L., R. Brown, M. Gold, A. Ciemnecki, and E. Docteur. 1997. "Access to Care in Medicare HMOs, 1996." *Health Affairs* 16(2): 148–56.

Neuman, P., and K. M. Langwell. 1999. "Medicare's Choice Explosion? Implications for Beneficiaries." *Health Affairs* 18(1): 150–60.

Newhouse, J., M. B. Buntin, and J. D. Chapman. 1997. "Risk Adjustment and Medicare: Taking a Closer Look." *Health Affairs* 16(5): 26–43.

Ni, H., D. Nauman, D. Burgess, K. Wise, R. Crispell, and R. E. Hershberger. 1998. "Factors Influencing Knowledge of and Adherence to Self-Care Among Patients with Heart Failure." *Archives of Internal Medicine* 159(14): 1613–9.

O'Sullivan, J., C. Franco, B. Fuchs, B. Lyke, R. Price, and K. Swendiman. 1997. *Medicare Provisions in the Balanced Budget Act of 1997*, 105–33. Washington, DC: Congressional Research Service.

Office of Inspector General. 1995. *Beneficiary Perspectives of Medicare Risk HMOs*. Washington DC: OIG.

———. 1998. *Medicare Hospital Discharge Planning*. Washington, DC: OIG.

———. 1999. *Medicare Beneficiary Access to Home Health Agencies*. Washington, DC: OIG.

Pacala, J. T., and C. Boult. 1996. "Factors Influencing the Effectiveness of Case Management in Managed Care Organizations: A Qualitative Analysis." *Journal of Healthcare Management* 41(3): 29–35.

Pacala, J. T., C. Boult, K. W. Hepburn et al. 1995. "Case Management of Older Adults in Health Maintenance Organizations." *Journal of the American Geriatric Society* 43(5): 538–42.

Pacala, J. T., C. Boult, R. L. Reed, and E. Aliberti. 1997. "Predictive Validity of the Pra Instrument Among Older Recipients of Managed Care." *Journal of the American Geriatric Society* 45(5): 614–17.

Pai, C. W., and D. G. Clement. 1999. "Recent Determinants of New Entry of HMOs Into a Medicare Risk Contract." *Inquiry* 36(1): 78–89.

Palsbo, S. J. 1997. *The AAPCC Explained and Updated*. Washington, DC: American Association of Health Plans.

Paone, D., R. Levy, and R. Bringewatt. 1999. *Integrating Pharmaceutical Care: A Vision and Framework*. Reston, VA: National Chronic Care Consortium and the National Pharmaceutical Council.

Patterson, J. A., A. S. Bierman, M. Splaine et al. 1998. "The Population of People Age 80 and Older: A Sentinel Group for Understanding the Future of Health Care in the United States." *Journal of Ambulatory Care Management* 21(3): 10–16.

Pauly, M., W. Kissick, and L. Roper. 1988. *Lessons from the First Twenty Years of Medicare*. Philadelphia, PA: University of Pennsylvania Press.

Pauly, M., J. Eisenberg, M. H. Radany, M. H. Erder, R. Feldman, and J. S. Schwartz. 1992. *Paying Physicians*. Chicago: Health Administration Press.

Peterson, C. 1999. "The Technology of Disease Management." *HealthPlan* 40(2): 77–81.

Physician Payment Review Commission. 1996A. *Medicare Risk Plan Participation and Enrollment: A Chart Book*. Washington, DC: Physician Payment Review Commission.

———. 1996B. *Annual Report to Congress, 1996*. Washington, DC: Physician Payment Review Commission.

———. 1997. *Annual Report to Congress, 1997*. Washington, DC: Physician Payment Review Commission.

Poole, S., B. Schmitt, T. Carruth, A. Peterson-Smith, and M. Slusarski. 1993. "After Hours Telephone Coverage: The Application of an Area-Wide Telephone Triage and Advice System for Pediatric Practices." *Pediatrics* 92(5): 670–79.

Porter, M. E. 1998. *On Competition*. Boston: Harvard Business School.

Preston, J., and S. M. Retchin. 1991. "The Management of Geriatric Hypertension in Health Maintenance Organizations." *Journal of the American Geriatric Society* 39(7): 683–90.

Price, J. R., and J. W. Mays. 1985. *Selection and the Competitive Standing of Health Plans in a Multiple Choice, Multiple Insurer Market*, 127–48. Greenwich, CT: JAI Press, Inc.

Prince, T. R. 1998. *Strategic Management for Health Care Entities*. Chicago: AHA Press.

Read, J. L., R. J. Quinn, and M. A. Hoefer. 1987. "Measuring Overall Health: An Evaluation of Three Important Approaches." *Journal of Chronic Diseases* (40 suppl. 1): 7S–21S.

Reed, J. 1999. *MEDICARE+CHOICE: New Standards Could Improve Accuracy and Usefulness of Plan Literature*. Washington, DC: U.S. GAO.

Reinhardt, U. E. 1979. "Medicare: Its Financing and Future." *American Economic Review* 69(2): 279–83.

Remler, D., K. Donelan, R. Blendon et al. 1997. "What Do Managed Care Plans Do to Affect Care? Results from a Survey of Physicians." *Inquiry* 34(3): 196–204.

Retchin, S. M., and B. Brown. 1990A. "Management of Colorectal Cancer in Medicare Health Maintenance Organizations." *Journal of General Internal Medicine* 5(2): 110–14.

———. 1990B. "The Quality of Ambulatory Care in Medicare Health Maintenance Organizations." *American Journal of Public Health* 80(4): 411–5.

———. 1991. "Elderly Patients With Congestive Heart Failure Under Prepaid Care." *American Journal of Medicine.* 90(2): 236–42.

Retchin, S. M., and J. Preston. 1991. "The Effects of Cost Containment on the Care of Elderly Diabetics." *Archives of Internal Medicine* 151(11): 2244–48.

Retchin, S. M., L. F. Rossiter, B. Brown, R. S. Brown, L. Nelson, and D. G. Clement. 1991. "How the Elderly Fare in Health Maintenance Organizations: Outcomes from the Medicare Competition Demonstrations." *Health Services Research* 26(5): 651–69.

Retchin, S. M., S. Brown, S. J. Yeh, D. Chu, and L. Moreno. 1997. "Outcomes of Stroke Patients in Medicare Fee for Service and Managed Care." *Journal of the American Medical Association* 278(2): 119–24.

Retchin, S. M., L. Penberthy, C. Desch et al. 1997. "Perioperative Management of Colon Cancer Under Medicare Risk Programs." *Archives of Internal Medicine* 157(16): 1878–84.

Rice, T. 1987. "An Economic Assessment of Health Care Coverage for the Elderly." *The Milbank Quarterly* 65(4): 488–520.

Rice, T., and N. McCall. 1985. "The Extent of Ownership and the Characteristics of Medicare Supplement Policies." *Inquiry* 22(2): 188–200.

Rice, T., N. McCall, and J. M. Boismier. 1991. "The Effectiveness of Consumer Choice in the Medicare Supplemental Insurance Market." *Health Services Research* 26(2): 223–46.

Rice, T., and K. Thomas. 1992. "Evaluating the New Medigap Standardization Regulations." *Health Affairs* 11(1): 194–207.

Rice, T., M. L. Graham, and P. D. Fox. 1997. "The Impact of Policy Standardization on the Medigap Market." *Inquiry* 34(2): 106–16.

Rich, M. W., V. Beckham, C. Wittenberg, C. L. Leven, K. E. Freedland, and R. M. Carney. 1995. "A Multidisciplinary Intervention to Prevent the Readmission of Elderly Patients with Congestive Heart Failure." *New England Journal of Medicine* 333(18): 1190–95.

Riley, G. F., A. L. Petosky, J. D. Lubitz, and L. G. Kessler. 1995. "Medicare Payments From Diagnosis to Death. . . ." *Medical Care* 33(8): 828–41.

Riley, G., C. Tudor, Y. P. Chiang, and M. Ingber. 1996. "Health Status of Medicare Enrolles in HMOs and the Fee-for-Service Sector in 1994." *Health Care Financing Review* 17(4): 65–76.

Riley, G. F., M. J. Ingber, and C. G. Tudor. 1997. "Disenrollment of Medicine Beneficiaries from HMOs." *Health Affairs* 16(5): 117–24.

Robinson, J. 1997. "Physician-Hospital Integration and the Economic Theory of the Firm." *Medical Care Research and Review* 54: 3–24.

Rossiter, L. F. 1986. "Operational Issues for HMOs and CMPs Entering the Medicare Market." In *New Health Care Systems: HMOs and Beyond*. Washington, DC: Group Health Association of America, Inc.

Rossiter, L. F. and K. Adamache. 1990. "A Blended Sector Rate Adjustment for the Medicare AAPCC." *Journal of Risk and Insurance* 2.

Rossiter, L. F., K. Langwell, and A. Friedlob. 1985A. "Risk-Based Contracting Under Medicare: Implementing TEFRA's New Mandate." *Healthcare Financial Management* 39(5): 42–5, 48–58.

———. 1985B. "Exploring Benefits of Risk-Based Contracting Under Medicare." *Healthcare Financial Management* 39(5): 42–5, 48–58.

Rossiter, L. F., K. M. Langwell, J. P. Hadley et al. 1986. "HMOs in the Medicare Market: Part 1." *Medical Group Management* 33(6): 32–7, 44–5.

———. 1987. "HMOs in the Medicare Market: Part 2." *Medical Group Management* 34(1): 37–44.

Rossiter, L. F., R. Brown, L. Nelson, S. Nelson, and K. Berman. 1987. "Early Experience of HMOs Under Medicare Competition Demonstrations." *Health Care Financing Review* 8(3): 37–55.

Rossiter, L. F., L. Nelson, and K. Adamache. 1988. "Service Use and Costs for Medicare Beneficiary in Risk-Based HMOs and CMPs." *American Journal of Public Health* 78(8): 937–43.

Rossiter, L. F., and K. Langwell. 1988. "Medicare's Two Systems for Paying Providers." *Health Affairs* 7(3): 120–32.

Rossiter, L. F., K. M. Langwell, L. Nelson, K. W. Adamache, and R. S. Brown. 1989A. "Medicare's Expanded Choices Program: Issues and Evidence from the HMO Experience." *Advances in Health Economics and Health Services Research* 10: 3–40.

Rossiter, L. F., K. Langwell, T. Wan, and M. Rivnyak. 1989B. "Patient Satisfaction Among Elderly Enrollees and Disenrollees in Medicare HMOs and CMPs." *Journal of the American Medical Association* 262(1): 57–63.

Rossiter, L. F., H-C. Chiu, and S-H. Chen. 1994. "Strengths and Weaknesses of the AAPCC: When Does Risk Adjustment Become Cost Reimbursement?" In *HMOs and the Elderly*, edited by H.S. Luft, 251–270. Chicago: Health Administration Press.

Rossiter, L. F., D. A. Draper, S. Carswell, and M. Ely. 1999. *Demand Management: The Impact of Telephone Triage on the Use and Cost of Health Care Services*. Richmond, VA: Williamson Institute for Health Studies.

Rossiter, L., V. E. Bovbjerg, V. Olchanski, S. E. Zimberg, and J. S. Green. 2000. "Internet-Based Monitoring and Benchmarking in Ambulatory Surgery Centers." *Joint Commission Journal on Quality Improvement* 26(8): 450–65.

Rossiter, L., M. Y. Whitehurst-Cook, and R. E. Small. 2000. "The Impact of Disease Management on Outcomes and Cost of Care." *Inquiry* 42(3).

Roter, D. L., and J. A. Hall. 1992. *Doctors Talking with Patients/Patients Talking with Doctors: Improving Communication in Medical Visits, 12th edition*. Westport, CT: Auburn House.

Russell, L. B. 1986. *Is Prevention Better than Cure?* Washington, DC: Brookings Institute.

Sabin, M. 1998. "Telephone Triage Improves Demand Management Effectiveness" *Healthcare Financial Management* 52(8): 49–51.

Sanders, T. I. 1998. *Strategic Thinking and the New Science.* New York: The Free Press.

Scanlon, W. J. 1999. *MEDICARE+CHOICE: Impact of the 1997 Balanced Budget Act Payment Reforms on Beneficiaries and Plans.* Washington, DC: U.S. Government Printing Office.

Schag, C. C., R. L. Heinrich, and P. A. Ganz. 1984. "Karnofsky Performance Status Revisited: Reliability, Validity, and Guidelines." *Journal of Clinical Oncology* 2(3): 187–93.

Scheffler, R. M., and L. Paringer. 1980. "A Review of the Economic Evidence on Prevention." *Medical Care* 18(5): 473–84.

Schlenker, R. E., P. W. Shaughnessy, and D. F. Hittle. 1995. "Patient-Level Cost of Home Health Care Under Capitated and Fee-for-Service Payment." *Inquiry* 32(3): 252–70.

Seidman, J., E. P. Bass, and H. R. Rubin. 1998. "Review of Studies that Compare the Quality of Cardiovascular Care in HMO vs. Non-HMO Settings." *Medical Care* 36(12): 1607–25.

Senge, P. 1990. *The Fifth Discipline.* New York: Currency Doubleday.

Shaughnessy, P. W., R. E. Schlenker, and D. F. Hittle. 1994. "Home Health Care Outcomes Under Capitated and Fee-for-Service Payment." *Health Care Financing Review* 16(1): 187–221.

Shorr, A. F., A. S. Niven, D. E. Katz, J. M. Parker, and A. H. Eliasson. 2000. "Regulatory and Educational Initiatives Fail to Promote Discussions Regarding End-of-Life Care." *Journal of Pain and Symptom Management* 19(3): 168–73.

Short, P. F., and J. P. Vistnes. 1992. "Multiple Sources of Medicare Supplementary Insurance." *Inquiry* 29(1): 33–43.

Sobel, D. S. 1995. "Rethinking Medicine: Improving Health Outcomes with Cost-Effective Psychosocial Interventions." *Psychosomatic Medicine* 57(3): 234–44.

Somogyi-Zalud, E., Z. Zhong, J. Lynn, and M. B. Hamel. 2000. "Elderly Persons' Last Six Months of Life: Findings from the Hospitalized Elderly Longitudinal Project." *Journal of the American Geriatrics Society* 48(5 suppl.): S131–39.

Soumerai, S. B., T. J. McLaughlin, D. Ross-Regnan, C. S. Casteris, and P. Bollini. 1994. "Effects of a Limit on Medicaid Drug-Reimbursement Benefits. . . ." *The New England Journal of Medicine* 331(10): 650–5.

Splaine, M., P. Batalden, E. Nelson, S. K. Plume, and J. H. Wasson. 1998. "Looking at Care from the Inside Out: A Conceptual Approach to Geriatric Care." *Journal of Ambulatory Care Management* 21(3): 1–9.

Splaine, M., A. S. Bierman, and J. H. Wasson. 1998. "Implementing a Strategy for Improving Care: Lessons from Studying Those Age 80 and Older in a Health System." *Journal of Ambulatory Care Management* 21(3): 56–59.

Splaine, M., W. B. Brooks, J. A. Patterson, L. Von Reyn, and J. H. Wasson. 1998. "Geriatric Education: A System Approach." *Journal of Ambulatory Care Management* 21(3): 40–48.

Stacey, R. 1992. *Managing the Unknowable.* San Francisco: Jossey-Bass.

Stegall, M., D. G. Clement, S. M. Retchin, R. S. Brown, and R. Cohen. 1992. *Quality of Care, Satisfaction with Care and Access to Care in the TEFRA HMO/CMP Program Evaluation.* Richmond, VA: Williamson Institute for Health Studies.

Stewart, A. L., R. D. Hays, and J. E. Ware. 1988. "The MOS Short-form General Health Survey: Reliability and Validity in a Patient Population." *Medical Care* 26(7): 724–35.

Stewart, A. L., A. Napoles-Springer, and E. J. Perez-Stable. 1999. "Interpersonal Processes of Care in Diverse Populations." *Milbank Quarterly* 77(3): 305–39.

Studdert, D. M., W. M. Sage, C. R. Gresenz, and D. R. Hensler. 1999. "Expanded Managed Care Liability: What Impact on Employer Coverage?" *Health Affairs* 18(6): 7–25.

Sullivan, G. 1997. "Advice or Diagnosis? A Legal Perspective." *Business and Health* 5: 40–42.

Sydnor, J. 1999. *Disease Management Industry Report.* Richmond, VA: Wheat First Union.

Taylor, A. K., P. J. Farley, and C. M. Horgan. 1988. "Medigap Insurance: Friend or Foe in Reducing Medicare Deficits?" In *Health Insurance: Public or Private.* San Francisco: Pacific Institute for Public Policy Research.

Thomas, L. 1979. *The Medusa and the Snail.* Toronto, Canada: Bantam Books.

Thomas, S., and J. Jones. 1996. Report 2: Implementation Manual Medicaid Health Outcomes Partnership. Richmond, VA: Williamson Institute for Health Studies.

Timmerman, G. M. 1999. "Using Self-Care Strategies to Make Lifestyle Changes." *Journal of Holistic Nursing* 17(2): 169–83.

Tompkins, J. 1995. *The Genesis Enterprise.* New York: McGraw-Hill.

Tucker, A. M., and K. Langwell. 1988. "Disenrollment Patterns in Medicare HMOs: A Preliminary Analysis." *GHAA* 9(1): 22–41.

United HealthCare Corporation. 1994. *The Managed Care Resource: A Glossary of Terms.* Minneapolis, MN: United HealthCare Corporation.

United States General Accounting Office. 1985. *Problems in Administering Medicare's HMO Demonstration Projects in Florida.* Washington, DC: U.S. GAO/HRD-85-48.

———. 1986. *Medicare: Issues Raised by Florida HMO Demonstrations.* Washington, DC: U.S. GAO/HRD-86-32.

———. 1995. *Medicare: Opportunities Are Available to Apply Managed Care Strategies.* Washington, DC: U.S. GAO.

———. 1996A. *Medicare: HCFA Should Release Data to Aid Consumers, Prompt Better HMO Performance.* Washington, DC: U.S. GAO.

———. 1996B. *Medicare HMOs: Rapid Enrollment Growth Concentrated in Selected States.* Washington, DC: U.S. GAO.

———. 1998. *Medicare: Many HMOs Experience High Rates of Beneficiary Disenrollment.* Washington, DC: GAO/HEHS-98-142.

———. 1999. *Medicare Managed Care Plans: Many Factors Contribute to Recent Withdrawals, Plan Interest Continues.* Washington, DC: U.S. GAO.

United States House of Representatives, Committee on Ways and Means. 1994. *Overview of Entitlement Programs: 1994 Green Book,* 791–95. Washington, DC: U.S. Government Printing Office.

United States House of Representatives, Committee on Interstate and Foreign Commerce. 1976. *A Discursive Dictionary of Health Care.* Washington, DC: U.S. Government Printing Office.

University of Pittsburgh Medical Center. 1995. *Healthcare Economics: The New Tool for Clinical Decision Making*, 20–21. University of Pittsburgh.

Vickery, D. 1996. "Demand Management. Toward Appropriate Use of Medical Care." *Healthcare Forum Journal* 39(1): 14–19.

Vickery, D., and W. Lynch. 1995. "Demand Management: Enabling Patients to Use Medical Care Appropriately." *Journal of Occupational and Environmental Medicine* 39(1): 14–19.

Vistnes, J. P., and J. S. Banthin. 1997–1998. "The Demand for Medicare Supplemental Insurance Benefits." *Inquiry* 34(4): 311–24.

Wachter, D., J. Brillman, J. Lewis, and R. Sapien. 1999. "Pediatric Telephone Triage Protocols: Standardized Decision Making or a False Sense of Security?" *Annals of Emergency Medicine* 33(4): 388–94.

Wade, D. T., H. R. Langton, C. E. Skilbeck, and R. M. David. 1998. *Stroke: A Critical Approach to Diagnosis, Treatment and Management*, 171. London: Chapman and Hall.

Wagner, E. H., A. Z. LaCroix, L. C. Grothaus et al. 1994. "Preventing Disability and Falls in Older Adults: A Population-Based Randomized Trial." *American Journal of Public Health* 84(11): 1182–96.

Wagner, E. H., B. T. Austin, and M. Von Korff. 1996. "Organizing Care for Patients with Chronic Illness." *Milbank Quarterly* 74(4): 511–44.

Ware, J. E., M. S. Bayliss, W. H. Rogers, M. Kosinski, and A. R. Tarlov. 1996. "Differences in Four-Year Health Outcomes for Elderly and Poor Chronically Ill Patients Treated in HMOs and Fee-for-Service Systems." *Journal of the American Medical Association* 276(13): 1039–47.

Wasson, J., C. Gaudette, F. Whaley et al. 1992. "Telephone Care as a Substitute for Routine Clinic Follow-up." *Journal of the American Medical Association* 267(13): 1788–93.

Wasson, J., T. A. Bubolz, J. Lynn, and J. Teno. 1998. "Can We Afford Comprehensive Supportive Care for the Very Old?" *Journal of the American Geriatric Society* 46(7): 829–32.

Wasson, J. H., T. A. Stukel, J. E. Weiss et al. 1999. "A Randomized Trial of the Use of Patient Self-Assessment Data to Improve Community Practices." *Effective Clinical Practice* 2(1): 1–10.

Webster, J. and J. Feinglass. 1997. "Stroke Patients, 'Managed Care,' and Distributive Justice." *Journal of the American Medical Association* 278(2): 161–62.

Weeks, W. B. 1998. "Improving Patient Care in a Changing Environment: A Teaching Case." *Journal of Ambulatory Care Management* 21(3): 49–55.

Weiner, J. P., A. Dobson, S. L. Maxwell, K. Coleman, B. H. Starfield, and G. F. Anderson. 1996. "Risk-Adjusted Medicare Capitation Rates Using Ambulatory and Inpatient Diagnoses." *Health Care Financing Review* 17(3): 77–99.

Welch, W. P. 1985. "Medicare Capitation Payments to HMOs in Light of Regression Toward the Mean in Health Care Costs." In *Advances in Health Economics and Health Services Research*, 75–96. Greenwich, CT: JAI Press, Inc.

———. 1996. "Growth in HMO Share of the Medicare Market, 1998–1994." *Health Affairs* 15(3): 201–14.

Welch, W. P., and H. G. Welch. 1995. "Fee-for-Data: A Strategy to Open the HMO Black Box." *Health Affairs* 14(4): 104–116.

White, J. 1997. "Which Managed Care for Medicare?" *Health Affairs* 16(5): 73–82.

Whitehurst-Cook, M., M. Roberts, and M. Nelson. 1994. *Virginia Health Outcomes Partnership: Educational Planning Design Report*. Richmond, VA: Williamson Institute for Health Studies.

Wholey, D. R., L. R. Burns, and R. Lavizzo-Mourey. 1998. "Managed Care and the Delivery of Primary Care to the Elderly and the Chronically Ill." *Health Services Research* 33(2, Part II): 322–53.

Wilensky, G., and L. F. Rossiter. 1991. "Coordinated Care and Public Programs." *Health Affairs* 10(4): 62–77.

Wilensky, G. R. 1999. "A Model for Medicare's Future." *Healthplans* 40(5): 17–8, 20–1.

Williamson Institute. 1988. *National Medicare Competition Evaluation: An Evaluation of the Quality of the Process of Care*. Baltimore, MD: Health Care Financing Administration.

Windham-Bannister, S. R., and D. D. Mount. 1991. *Building a Market Management Information System for an HMO*. New York.

Wolcott, B. 1996. "Managed Care's Driving Force: Demand Management." *Infocare* (January/February): 12–15.

Wolfe, J. R., and J. H. Goddeeris. 1991. "Adverse Selection, Moral Hazard, and Wealth Effects in the Medigap Insurance Market." *Journal of Health Economics* 10(4): 433–59.

Wood, S. P. 1996. *Implementing a Successful Medicare Managed Care Product*, edited by D. Mlawsky. Washington, DC: Atlantic Information Services, Inc.

Zawadski, R. T., and C. Eng. 1988. "Case Management in Capitated Long-Term Care." *Health Care Financing Review Annual Supplement* (December): 75–81.

Zuckerman, A. M. 1998. *Healthcare Strategic Planning*. Chicago: Health Administration Press.

Legal Cases

Bast v. Prudential Insurance Co. of America. No. 97–35429, U.S. Ct. of Appeals for the Ninth Court, 150 F.3d 1003; 1998 U.S. App. LEXIS 11358; 98 Cal. Daily Op. Service 4155; 98 Daily Journal DAR 5767; 22 E.B.C. 1268, May 7, 1998.

Dukes v. U.S. Healthcare. US S. Ct. U.S. Supreme Court. 1995. 1009.

Dunn v. Praiss. A.2d: N.J. Super. Ct. App. Div. 1992. 862.

PacifiCare of Oklahoma v. Burrage. F.3d: 10th Cir. 1995. 151.

Prihoda v. Shpritz. F.Supp. D.Md. 1996. 133.

Wickline v. State. Supreme Court of California 727 P.2d 753; 1986 Cal. LEXIS 276; 231. Cal. Rptr. 560, November 20, 1986, Filed.

Wilson v. Blue Cross of Southern California 271 Cal.Rptr.876.

COMMON MEDICARE MANAGED CARE TERMS

ACTIVITIES OF DAILY LIVING (ADLs)–Activities performed as part of a person's daily routine of self-care such as bathing, dressing, toileting, transferring, continence, and eating (United HealthCare Corporation 1994).

ACTUARY–In insurance, a person trained in statistics, accounting, and mathematics who determines policy rates, reserves, and dividends by deciding what assumptions should be made with respect to each of the risk factors involved, and who endeavors to secure as valid statistics as possible on which to base these assumptions (U.S. House of Representatives 1976).

ADJUSTED-AVERAGE PER CAPITA COST (AAPCC)–A county-level estimate of the average cost incurred by Medicare for each beneficiary in the fee-for-service system. The expected cost per person–year that the Medicare program pays for hospital (Part A) and physicians' (Part B) services. The AAPCC is based on fee-for-service costs of Medicare beneficiaries in each county in the United States. From 1985 to 1999, the AAPCC was used to set the payment rate to Medicare HMOs. See U.S. Per Capita Cost (PPRC 1996B).

ADJUSTED COMMUNITY RATE–Estimated payment rates that a health plan with a Medicare risk contract would have received for its Medicare enrollees if paid its private market premiums, adjusted for differences in benefit packages and service use. Health plans estimate their ACRs annually and adjust subsequent year supplemental benefits or premiums to return any excess Medicare revenue above the ACR to enrollees (PPRC 1996B).

ADMINISTRATIVE COSTS–the costs incurred by a carrier, such as an insurance company or HMO, for administrative services such as claims processing, billing and enrollment, and overhead costs. Administrative costs can be expressed as a percentage of premiums or on a per-member-per-month (PMPM) basis (United HealthCare Corporation 1994).

ADMINISTRATIVE SERVICES ONLY (ASO)–A contract whereby an independent agent, such as an insurance company or third-party administrator (TPA), performs administrative services for a self-funded plan in exchange for a fee without assuming any financial risk. ASO services may include claims processing, actuarial support, benefit plan design, financial advice, medical management, preparation of data for reports to government units, and other administrative functions (Menkin 1999).

ADVERSE SELECTION–The enrollment in numbers higher than expected of high risk or unhealthy members into a managed care organization. Adverse selection causes costs that are higher than expected. Opposite of favorable selection.

AMBULATORY PATIENT CLASSIFICATIONS (APC)–A system for classifying outpatient services and procedures for purposes of payment. The APC system classifies some 7,000 services and procedures into about 300 procedure groups.

ASSIGNMENT OF BENEFITS–A method under which a claimant requests that his or her benefits under a claim be paid to some designated person or institution, usually a physician or hospital (United HealthCare Corporation 1994).

AVERAGE LENGTH OF STAY (ALOS)–The average number of days in a given time period that each patient remains in the hospital. Calculated by dividing the total number of bed days by the number of discharges for a specified period (Menkin 1999).

BALANCE BILLING–In Medicare and private fee-for-service health insurance, the practice of billing patients in excess of the amount approved by the health plan (PPRC 1996B).

BED DAYS–The total number of days of hospital care (excluding the day of discharge) provided to a plan member. Generally reported in "days per 1000 plan members per year" (Menkin 1999).

BENCHMARKING–A process that identifies best practices and performance standards to create normative or comparative standards (a benchmark) as a measurement tool. By comparing against a benchmark, an organization can establish measurable goals as a part of the strategic planning or total quality management process (Menkin 1999).

BENEFICIARY–Someone who is eligible for or receiving benefits under an insurance policy or plan. The term is commonly applied to people receiving benefits under the Medicare program or covered under a private health insurance plan (PPRC 1996B).

BENEFIT–The amount payable by Medicare for a covered service on behalf of a beneficiary.

BENEFIT PERIOD (SPELL OF ILLNESS)–A period of time for measuring use of Hospital Insurance (HI) benefits. For Medicare, it begins on the entitled beneficiary's admission to a qualifying hospital or other facility and ends after the 60 consecutive days during which the individual was not an inpatient of any hospital or other facility primarily providing skilled nursing or rehabilitation services. Although there are limits to covered benefits per benefit period, there is no limit to the number of benefit periods a beneficiary can have. The beneficiary must pay the HI deductible for each new benefit period (DHHS 1983).

BEST PRACTICES–Organizations that have demonstrated superior performance in both their operational and clinical processes. They are identified as such not only because of highly successful clinical performance, but also for contributions made by outstanding management practices (Menkin 1999).

BLUE CROSS AND BLUE SHIELD ASSOCIATION (BCBSA)–The national non-profit organization to which the independent Blue Cross and Blue Shield member plans make up the Blue Cross and Blue Shield Association; however, all member plans function as independent, locally operated companies. BCBSA administers programs of licensure and approval for Blue Cross plans and provides specific services related to the writing and administering of healthcare benefits across the country (U.S. House of Representatives 1976).

BOARD CERTIFIED–Describes a physician who is certified as a specialist in his or her area of practice. Usually, that means completion of a supervised program of certified clinical residency and the physician passing both an oral and a written exam given by a medical specialty group (Menkin 1999).

BOARD ELIGIBLE–Describes a physician who has graduated from a board-approved medical school, completed an accredited training program, practiced for a specified length of time, and is eligible to take a specialty board exam within a specific amount of time (Menkin 1999).

BONUS–A payment a physician or entity receives beyond any salary, fee-for-service payments, capitation, or returned withhold. Bonuses and other compensation that are not based on referral levels (such as bonuses based solely on quality of care, patient satisfaction, or physician participation on a committee) are not considered in the calculation of substantial financial risk.

BUDGET NEUTRALITY–For the Medicare program, adjustment of payment rates when policies change so that total spending under the new rules is expected to be the same as it would have been under the previous payment rules (PPRC 1996B).

BUNDLED BILLING–The practice of charging a comprehensive package price for all medical services associated with a specific procedure. Frequently used for high-cost procedures such as organ transplants, heart surgery, and maternity care. Also called global fees or package price (Menkin 1999).

BUNDLED PAYMENT–A single comprehensive payment for a group of related services or episode of care (PPRC 1996B).

CAPITATION–A set dollar payment per patient per unit of time (usually per month) that is paid to cover a specified set of services and administrative costs without regard to the actual number of services provided. The services covered may include a physician's own services, referral services, or all medical services.

CARRIER–A private or public organization with which HCFA enters into agreement to help administer the Part B benefits under Medicare. Also referred to as "contractors," the carriers determine coverage and benefit amounts payable and make payment to physician/suppliers or beneficiaries (DHHS 1983).

CARVE-OUT COVERAGE–Method of integrating payment for health benefits provided by two different policies for the same or different covered services. Most often seen with mental health, dental, and disease management (PPRC 1996B).

CASE MANAGEMENT–A process whereby covered persons with specific health-care needs are identified, and a plan that efficiently utilizes healthcare resources is formulated and implemented to achieve the optimum patient outcome in the most cost-effective manner (United HealthCare Corporation 1994).

CASE MANAGER (CM)–A professional (usually a nurse, physician, or social worker) who handles specific catastrophic or high-cost cases as a member of a utilization management team. CMs may also prevent hospital admissions or initiate early discharges by coordinating alternative care services (e.g., home care and outpatient services), thereby lowering costs (Menkin 1999).

CASE MIX–the diagnosis-specific makeup of a hospital's workload. Each hospital has a Medicare Case Mix Index under the Medicare prospective payment system for hospitals (NCHSR 1979).

CATASTROPHIC HEALTH INSURANCE–Health insurance that provides protection against the high cost of treating severe or lengthy illnesses or disabilities. Generally such policies cover all or a specified amount or percentage of medical expenses above an amount that is the responsibility of the insured himself (U.S. House of Representatives 1976).

CENTERS OF EXCELLENCE–A network of healthcare facilities selected for specific services on the basis of criteria such as experience, outcomes, efficiency, and effectiveness. For example, an organ transplant managed care program wherein employees access select types of benefits through a specific network of medical centers (United HealthCare Corporation 1994).

CHURNING–The unethical practice in a fee-for-service reimbursement environment of a provider seeing a patient more often than is medically necessary in order to increase revenue (Menkin 1999).

CLOSED PANEL–A managed care plan that contracts with or employs physicians on an exclusive basis for services and does not allow those physicians to see patients from other managed care organizations. Staff model HMOs are examples of closed-panel managed care plans (Menkin 1999).

COINSURANCE–A policy provision, frequently found in Major Medical insurance, by which both the insured person and the insurer share in a specified ratio the covered losses under a policy. The most common coinsurance is 20 percent patient, 80 percent insurance (NCHSR 1979).

COMMUNITY RATING–The HMO Act [section 1302 (United HealthCare Corporation 1994) of the PHS Act] defines community rating as a system of defining rates of payments for health services that may be determined on a per-person or per-family basis "and may vary with the number of persons in a family, but must be equivalent for all individuals and for all families with similar composition." The intent of community rating is to spread the cost of illness evenly over all subscribers (the whole community) rather than charging the sick more than the healthy for health insurance (U.S. House of Representatives 1976).

COMPETITIVE BIDDING–A pricing method that elicits information on costs through a bidding process to establish payment rates that reflect the costs of an efficient health plan or healthcare provider (PPRC 1996B).

COMPETITIVE MEDICAL PLAN (CMP)–From 1985 to 1999, recognized by Medicare as a prepaid health plan, not federally qualified as an HMO, which entered into a risk-based contract with HCFA under Medicare. Replaced with Medicare+Choice program.

CONCURRENT REVIEW–Review of the medical necessity of hospital or other health facility admissions upon or within a short period following an admission and the periodic review of services provided during the course of treatment. The initial review usually assigns an appropriate length of stay to the admission (using diagnosis-specific criteria), which may also be reassessed periodically. Where concurrent review is required, payment for unneeded hospitalizations or services is usually denied (U.S. House of Representatives 1976).

CONSUMER ASSESSMENT OF HEALTH PLANS (CAHP)–A survey and report tool that provides reliable and valid information to help consumers and purchasers assess and choose among health plans. Survey questions ask consumers about their experience with their health plans. See www.ahqr.gov.

CONSUMER PRICE INDEX (CPI)–An economic index prepared by the Bureau of Labor Statistics of the U.S. Department of Labor. It measures the change in average prices of the goods and services purchased by urban wage earners and clerical workers and their families. It is widely used as an indicator of changes in the cost of living, as a measure of inflation (and deflation, if any) in the economy, and as a means for studying trends in prices of various goods and services. The CPI is made up of several components including the medical care component (U.S. House of Representatives 1976).

CONTINUOUS QUALITY IMPROVEMENT (CQI)–The management process whereby ongoing systematic evaluation and modification of processes and services is performed to improve quality (Menkin 1999).

COORDINATION OF BENEFITS (COB)–A method of integrating benefits payable under more than one group health insurance plan so that the insured's benefits from all sources do not exceed 100 percent of his or her allowable medical expenses. Most insurers have a coordination of benefits department whose job it is to find duplicate coverage and coordinate benefits (NCHSR 1979).

COPAYMENT–A type of cost sharing whereby the insured or covered person pays a specified flat amount per unit of service or service of time (e.g., $2 per visit, $10 per prescription); the insurer pays the rest of the cost (U.S. House of Representatives 1976).

COST-BASED REIMBURSEMENT–Under this arrangement, a third party payer pays the hospital or other provider for the care received by covered patients at cost, not on the charges actually made for those services. The costs are often defined by the provider and are retrospective costs (Congressional Budget Office 1988).

COST EFFECTIVE–Relative term, implying that the net benefits and outcomes of an intervention are worth the cost required. Interventions need not be cost saving to be cost effective—many cost-effective interventions do not save money but are still judged to be worthwhile (University of Pittsburgh Medical Center 1995).

COST-EFFECTIVE ANALYSIS–Method of economic analysis that assesses both the cost and the effectiveness of an intervention, service, or program. Costs are measured in monetary units, such as dollars. Effectiveness is measured in units of outcomes experienced, such as number of years of improved survival, cases of disease prevented, or quality-adjusted life years (QALYs) gained (University of Pittsburgh Medical Center 1995).

COST OF ILLNESS–Estimation of the economic effect of a disease, including the costs of diagnosis and management and of the consequences of treated and untreated disease (University of Pittsburgh Medical Center 1995).

COST SAVING–The absolute reduction in costs and expenditures resulting from the substitution of one intervention for another (University of Pittsburgh Medical Center 1995).

COST SHARING–A health insurance policy provision that requires the insured party to pay a portion of the costs of covered services. Deductibles, coinsurance, copayment, and balance bills are the types of cost sharing (PPRC 1996B).

COST SHIFTING–When a third party reimburses at an inadequate rate to cover actual costs and the hospital attempts to recoup the difference by charging other payers higher rates (HCFA 1982).

COVERAGE DECISION–A decision by a health plan whether to pay for or provide a medical service or technology for particular clinical indications. Services are normally not considered for a coverage decision unless they have been approved by the U.S. Food and Drug Administration as being safe and effective. Experimental services are often considered for coverage decisions and may not be covered (PPRC 1996B).

CURRENT PROCEDURAL TERMINOLOGY (CPT)–The coding system for physicians' services developed by the CPT Editorial Panel of the American Medical Association, it is the basis of the Medicare coding system for physicians' services. See HCFA Common Procedures Coding System (HCPCS) (PPRC 1996B).

DAYS PER THOUSAND–A standard unit of hospital utilization measurement that refers to the annualized use (in days) of hospital or other institutional care for each 1,000 covered lives (Menkin 1999).

DEDUCTIBLE–The amount of covered expenses that must be incurred by the insured before benefits become payable by the insurer (NCHSR 1979).

DEFINED-BENEFIT COVERAGE–Coverage is an approach to providing medical benefits. With this coverage, the sponsor provides funding for a specific package of medical services and is responsible for paying for that package.

DEFINED-CONTRIBUTION COVERAGE–Coverage is another approach to providing medical benefits. With this coverage, the sponsor provides funding for a specific dollar contribution toward the cost of coverage and is responsible for paying only that contribution.

DIAGNOSIS RELATED GROUP (DRG)–A system of classifying patients on the basis of diagnoses for purposes of payment to hospitals. Each DRG represents a broad clinical category based on body system involvement and disease etiology, which are similar in use and resources. They are now used by Medicare, most state Medicaid programs, and many private insurance companies to make hospital payments on a prospectively determined, per case amount. See Prospective Payment System (PPS) (PPRC 1996B).

DIAGNOSTIC AND STATISTICAL MANUAL OF MENTAL DISORDERS, 3RD EDITION, REVISED (DSM III-R)–The manual used to provide a diagnostic coding system for mental and substance abuse disorders (Menkin 1999).

DIRECT GRADUATE MEDICAL EDUCATION COST (DME)–The cost recognized by Medicare as the direct education and training cost of medical residents in teaching hospitals. It includes resident salary and fringe benefits, faculty time, and overhead. Medicare reimburses teaching hospitals for a portion of these costs.

DISCHARGE–A formal release from a hospital or a skilled nursing facility. Discharges include people who died during their stay or were transferred to another facility.

DISENROLLMENT–The termination of an enrollee's coverage under a health plan, either voluntarily or involuntarily. Voluntary disenrollment occurs when a member quits because he or she does not wish to continue coverage under that plan. Involuntary disenrollment might occur if a member changes jobs, will not comply with recommended treatment plans, or commits offenses such as fraud, abuse, or nonpayment of premiums or copays (Menkin 1999).

DISPROPORTIONATE SHARE (DSH)–Urban hospitals with more than 100 beds that qualify for additional operating and capital disproportionate-share payments under the provision that 30 percent of total inpatient revenue comes from state and local governments.

DOWNSTREAM RISK–An arrangement where an entity (typically a provider group) accepts risk from another entity (typically, a licensed organization like an HMO) (PPRC 1997).

DRG WEIGHT–An index number that reflects the relative resource consumption associated with each DRG multiplied by the hospital-specific standard payment amount, which yields the amount paid for a specific case.

DRUG UTILIZATION REVIEW (DUR)–An evaluation of customer drug use patterns at all stages, including the prescribing and dispensing of the drug, to determine the effectiveness and appropriateness of prescribed drug therapy. DUR covers a range of activities including prospective, concurrent, and retrospective evaluation of pharmaceutical use and cost (Menkin 1999).

DUAL CHOICE–The practice of giving people a choice of more than one health insurance or health program to pay for or provide their health services. Characteristic of the Federal Employees Health Benefits Program. Required by the HMO Act. P.L. 93-222 of employers with respect to qualified HMOs (section 1310 of the PHS Act) (U.S. House of Representatives 1976).

DUALLY ELIGIBLE–A Medicare beneficiary who also receives the full range of Medicaid benefits offered in the beneficiary's state of residence (PPRC 1996B).

EFFECTIVENESS–The net health benefits provided by a medical service or technology for typical patients in community practice settings (PPRC 1996B).

EFFICACY–The net health benefits achievable under ideal conditions for carefully selected patients (PPRC 1996B).

ENCOUNTER–A record of a medically related service (or visit) rendered by a provider to a health plan enrollee, typically using a standard billing form or an HMO-specific encounter form. Encounters are tracked to monitor service utilization, even when providers are reimbursed under capitation or other arrangements not requiring direct billing for the service (Menkin 1999).

END-STAGE RENAL DISEASE (ESRD)–For purposes of enrollment under Medicare, individuals who have chronic kidney disease requiring renal dialysis or kidney transplant are considered to have end-stage renal disease. Eligibility for Medicare coverage usually begins with the third month after the month in which a course in renal dialysis begins (U.S. House of Representatives 1976).

ENROLL–To agree to participate in a contract for benefits from an insurance company or HMO. A person who enrolls is an enrollee or subscriber. The number of people (including dependents) enrolled with an insurance company or HMO is its enrollment (U.S. House of Representatives 1976).

ENROLLMENT PERIOD–Period during which individuals may enroll for insurance or HMO benefits. There are two kind of enrollment periods, for example, for supplementary medical insurance of Medicare: the initial enrollment period (the seven months beginning three months before and ending three months after the month a person first becomes eligible, usually by turning 65); and the general enrollment period (the first three months of each year) (U.S. House of Representatives 1976).

ENTITLEMENT AUTHORITY–In the federal budget, legislation that requires the payment of benefits or entitlement to any person or government meeting the requirements established by such law (U.S. House of Representatives 1976).

EQUITY MODEL–A form of for-profit healthcare delivery system in which the physicians or other providers are owners (Menkin 1999).

ERISA–The Employee Retirement Income Security Act of 1974. Landmark legislation that established federal standards of operation for qualified private employee benefit plans. ERISA preempts many state laws' governing benefits (EBRI 1991).

EVALUATION AND MANAGEMENT SERVICES–A nontechnical service, such as a visit or consultation, provided by most physicians to diagnose and treat diseases and counsel patients (PPRC 1996B).

EXPERIENCE RATING–A method of establishing premiums for health insurance in which the premium is based on the average cost of actual or anticipated healthcare used by various groups and subgroups of subscribers and thus varies with the health experience of groups and subgroups or with such variables as age, gender, or health status. It is the most common method of establishing premiums for health insurance in private programs (U.S. House of Representatives 1976).

EXPLANATION OF BENEFITS (EOB)–A statement mailed to a member or covered insured explaining how and why a claim was or was not paid (Menkin 1999).

FEDERAL EMPLOYEES HEALTH BENEFITS PROGRAM (FEHBP)–The group health insurance program for Federal employees; the largest employer-sponsored contributory health insurance program in the world. It is voluntary for the employees, about 80 percent of those eligible being covered (U.S. House of Representatives 1976).

FEDERALLY QUALIFIED HMO–An HMO that has satisfied certain federal qualifications pertaining to organizational structure, provider contracts, health services delivery information, utilization review as well as quality assurance, grievance procedures, financial status, and marketing information, as specified in Title XIII of the Public Health Services Act (PPRC 1996B).

FEEDBACK–Making available to providers and practitioners the data for or results of evaluative studies about themselves and their peers (Institute of Medicine 1994).

FEE-FOR-SERVICE–A method of paying healthcare providers for individual medical services rendered, as opposed to paying them salaries or capitation payments (PPRC 1996B). See Capitation.

FEE SCHEDULE–Schedule of insurance that specifies what the insurance plan will pay for a particular service or treatment (NCHSR 1979).

FIRST-DOLLAR COVERAGE–Insurance plans that have no deductible or coinsurance (NCHSR 1979).

FIXED COSTS–The costs that are incurred regardless of volume and thus independent of the volume of services provided. Fixed costs must be amortized over the resource's useful life. Capital equipment and real property are examples of fixed costs (University of Pittsburgh Medical Center 1995).

FLAT FEE–A single inclusive benefit for all charges incurred for a collection of services (e.g., pregnancy, childbirth, and complications arising therefrom). A limit (such as $1,000) may be applied per pregnancy or per year (U.S. House of Representatives 1976).

FORMULARY–The list of prescription medications that may be dispensed by participating pharmacies without health plan authorization. A drug is selected for the formulary on the basis of its effectiveness as well as its cost. The physician is requested or required to use only formulary drugs unless there is a valid medical reason to use a nonformulary drug. Formularies may be open or closed. Closed formularies are restricted by the number and type of drugs included in the list (Menkin 1999).

THE FOUNDATION FOR ACCOUNTABILITY (FACCT)–A not-for-profit organization that creates tools that help people understand and use quality information, develops consumer-focused quality measure, supports public education about healthcare quality. See www.facct.org.

FUNCTIONAL INDEPENDENCE MEASURE/FUNCTION-RELATED GROUPS–A patient classification system developed for classifying medical rehabilitation patients.

GAMING–Gaining advantage by using improper means to evade the letter or intent of a rule or system (PPRC 1996B).

GATEKEEPER–Term used to describe the coordination role of the primary care provider who manages various components of a member's medical treatment including all referrals for specialty care, ancillary services, durable medical equipment, and hospital services. The gatekeeper model is a popular cost-control component of many managed care plans because it requires patients to first see their primary care physicians and receive their approval before going to a specialist care physician about a given medical condition (except for emergencies) (Menkin 1999).

GENERALISTS–Physicians who are distinguished by their training as not limiting their practice by health condition or organ system, who provide comprehensive and continuous services, and who make decisions about treatment for patients presenting with undifferentiated symptoms. Typically include family practitioners, general internists, and general pediatricians (PPRC 1996B).

GRADUATE MEDICAL EDUCATION (GME)–The period of medical training that follows graduation from medical school, commonly referred to as internship, residency, and fellowship training (PPRC 1996B).

GRIEVANCE SYSTEM–A formal complaint (verbal or written) system required by state and federal law for HMO members and providers to voice complaints, seek remedies, or request a review of supplemental benefits. Grievances are submitted to the HMO's Membership Services Department, which is responsible for researching and working with the appropriate department to resolve the issue. A formal grievance hearing may be requested if the complaint has not been resolved to the satisfaction of the member or the provider (Menkin 1999).

GROSS DOMESTIC PRODUCT–The total current market value of all goods and services produced domestically during a given period; differs from the gross national product by excluding net income that residents earn abroad (PPRC 1996B).

GROUP INSURANCE–Any insurance plan by which a number of employees (and their dependents) of a given employer, or members of a similar homogeneous group, are insured under a single policy, issued to their employer or the group with individual certificates of insurance given to each insured individual or family (U.S. House of Representatives 1976).

GROUP MODEL HMO–An HMO that pays a medical group a negotiated, per capita rate, which the group distributes among its physicians, often under a salaried arrangement. See HMO, IPA, Network Model HMO, Staff Model HMO (PPRC 1996B).

HCFA Common Procedure Coding System (HCPCS)–Pronounced "hick picks," a Medicare coding system based on CPT, but supplemented with additional codes (PPRC 1996B). See Coding, Current Procedural Terminology.

Health Care Financing Administration (HCFA)–The federal agency responsible for administering Medicare and overseeing the administration of Medicaid by the states (United HealthCare Corporation 1994). See www.hcfa.gov.

Health Care Prepayment Plan (HCPP)–A health plan with a Medicare cost contract to provide only Medicare Part B benefits. Some administrative requirements for these plans are less stringent than those of risk contracts or other cost contracts (PPRC 1996B).

Health Economics–The application of the field of economics to healthcare. An assessment of the most efficient use of available resources, defined in terms of cost and outcome (University of Pittsburgh Medical Center 1995).

Health Maintenance Organization (HMO)–A health delivery system that offers plan enrollees comprehensive health coverage for hospital and physician services for a prepaid, fixed fee. HMOs contract with or directly employ participating healthcare providers (i.e., physicians, hospitals, and other health professionals) and HMO members are required to choose from among these providers for all healthcare services or pay out-of-pocket (AMCRA Foundation 1994).

There are five standard models of HMOs:

1. The **Independent Practice/Physician Association (IPA)** model HMO contracts with physicians in solo practice, and/or with independent practice/physician associations (**IPAs**) who, in turn, contract with their own member physicians. The majority of physicians in an IPA model HMO are in private practice and, in many cases, also have a significant number of patients who are not HMO members.
2. The **Group Model** HMO contracts with a single multispecialty medical group to provide care to the HMO's membership. The group practice may work exclusively with the HMO, or it may provide services to non-HMO patients as well. The HMO often pays the group on a prepaid capitation basis for some or all of the covered services.
3. The **Network Model** HMO contracts with more than one medical group to provide services to its members.
4. The **Staff Model** HMO employs physicians directly. The physicians are employees of the HMO and deal exclusively with HMO members.
5. The **Mixed Model** HMO is any combination of the model types described above (AMCRA Foundation 1994).

The prototype HMO is the Kaiser-Permanente system, a prepaid group practice that dominates markets on the West Coast. Rates of hospitalization and surgery are considerably less in HMOs than those occurring in the system outside such prepaid groups, although some feel that earlier care and providing fewer services may be better explanations (U.S. House of Representatives 1976).

HEALTH PLAN–An organization that acts as insurer for an enrolled population (PPRC 1996B). See Fee-for-Service, Managed Care, Medical Savings Account.

HEALTH PLAN EMPLOYEE DATA SET (HEDIS)–A standard data-reporting system developed in 1991 and is updated every few years to measure the quality and performance of health plans. A main goal of HEDIS is to standardize health plan performance measures for consumers and payers. HEDIS concentrates on four aspects of healthcare: 1) quality, 2) access and patient satisfaction, 3) membership and utilization, and 4) finance. The NCQA is responsible for coordinating and making changes each year (Menkin 1999).

HEALTH STATUS–Information typically from individuals themselves, on domains of health such as physical functioning, mental and emotional well-being, cognitive functioning, social and role functioning, and perceptions of one's health in the past, in the present, and for the future or compared with that of one's peers (also called health-related quality of life) (Institute of Medicine 1994).

HOME HEALTH AGENCY–A public agency or private organization that is primarily engaged in providing skilled nursing services and other therapeutic services in the patient's home, such as physical, occupational, or speech therapy, medical social services, and home health aid services (DHHS 1983).

HOSPITAL INPATIENT PROSPECTIVE PAYMENT SYSTEM–Medicare's method of paying acute-care hospitals for inpatient care. Prospective per-case payment rates are set at a level intended to cover operating and capital costs for treating a typical inpatient in a given DRG. Prospective payment systems are also being developed for Medicare payments for home health services, outpatient hospital services, skilled nursing facilities, and rehabilitation facilities.

HOSPITAL INSURANCE (HI) (also known as Part A)–An insurance program providing basic protection against the costs of hospital and related posthospital services for individuals covered by Medicare (DHHS 1983).

INCURRED BUT NOT REPORTED (IBNR)–Costs associated with a medical service that has been provided, but for which a claim has not yet been received by the carrier. IBNR reserves are recorded by the carrier to account for estimated liability based on studies of prior lags in claim submissions (United HealthCare Corporation 1994).

INDEMNITY–A benefit paid by a health insurance policy for an insured loss. Often used to refer to benefits paid in cash rather than in terms of services as provided by service-type plans. Also used to denote a benefit payment made without regard to the charges incurred (NCHSR 1979).

INDIVIDUAL (OR INDEPENDENT) PRACTICE ASSOCIATION (IPA)–An HMO composed of individual practices. Physicians are paid on a fee-for-service basis, and subject to quality assurance and utilization review (NCHSR 1979).

INPATIENT HOSPITAL DEDUCTIBLE–A fixed payment for hospital care that must be paid by the beneficiary before the Medicare program pays any additional costs. By law, the inpatient hospital deductible is adjusted each year to reflect the average cost of one day's hospital stay for all Medicare beneficiaries (EBRI 1991).

INSTRUMENTAL ACTIVITIES OF DAILY LIVING (IADL)–An index or scale that measures a patient's degree of independence in aspects of cognitive and social functioning including shopping, cooking, doing housework, managing money, and using the telephone.

INSURANCE–The contractual relationship that exists when one party, for a consideration, agrees to reimburse another for loss to person or thing caused by designated contingencies. The first party is the insurer; the second party, the insured; the contract, the insurance policy; the consideration, the premium; the person or thing, the risk; and the contingency, the hazard or peril. Generally, a formal social device for reducing the risk of losses for individuals by spreading the risk over groups. Insurance characteristically, but not necessarily, involves equitable contributions by the insured, pooling of risks, and the transfer of risk by contract. Insurance may be offered on either a profit or nonprofit basis to groups or individuals (U.S. House of Representatives 1976).

INTEGRATED DELIVERY SYSTEM (IDS)–A regional healthcare network providing a large range of services (i.e., a continuum of care) for patients within a set geographical area. The services may include wellness programs, preventive care, ambulatory clinics, emergency care, general hospital services, rehabilitation, long-term care, congregate living, psychiatric care, home health, and hospice care. An IDS usually establishes alliances and contractual relationships with other providers to offer services not provided directly by the IDS (Menkin 1999).

INTENSITY OF SERVICES–The number and complexity of resources used in producing a patient care service, such as a hospital admission or home health visit. Intensity of services reflects, for example, the amount of nursing care, diagnostic procedures, and supplies furnished.

INTERMEDIARY–A private or public organization with which HCFA enters into agreement to help administer benefits to institutional providers under the Hospital Insurance program. The intermediaries determine costs for Part A benefits and make payments to providers (DHHS 1983).

INTERNATIONAL CLASSIFICATION OF DISEASES (ICD-9-CM)–A diagnosis and procedure classification system designed to facilitate the collection of uniform and comparable health information. This system is used to group patients into DRGs.

LIFETIME RESERVE DAYS (LFD)–A beneficiary is entitled to 60 hospital lifetime reserve days for inpatient hospital care. At the time regular benefits are exhausted, the patient chooses whether or not to exercise the use of the reserve days (DHHS 1983).

LOSS RATIO–The ratio of benefits paid out to premiums collected for a particular type of insurance policy. Low loss ratios indicate that a small proportion of premium dollars was paid out in benefits, whereas high loss ratios indicate that a high percentage of the premium dollars was paid out in benefits (PPRC 1996B).

MALPRACTICE EXPENSE–The cost of professional liability insurance incurred by physicians or other providers (PPRC 1996B).

MANAGED CARE–Any system of health service payment or delivery arrangements wherein the health plan attempts to control or coordinate use of health services by its enrolled members. Arrangements often involve a defined delivery system of providers with some form of contractual arrangement with the plan. Formal utilization review and quality assurance systems are involved. Enrolled members face financial incentives to use the defined delivery system of providers (PPRC 1996B). See Health Maintenance Organization, Preferred-Provider Organization, and Point-of-Service Plan.

MANAGEMENT SERVICES ORGANIZATION (MSO)–An organization that provides a wide variety of administrative and practice management services to physicians. Some MSOs may limit their operations to selling physicians various administrative support services such as billing, group purchasing, and office administration. Other MSOs purchase the assets of physician practices outright, install office managers and other personnel, and hire physicians through professional services contracts (PPRC 1997).

MARGINAL COST–Additional cost incurred or savings accrued through the provision of an additional unit of service (University of Pittsburgh Medical Center 1995).

MASTER BENEFICIARY RECORD (MBR)–The basic social security master file of all retirement, survivor, disability, and health insurance beneficiaries (DHHS 1983).

MEDICAID–Title XIX of the Social Security Amendments of 1965; federal/state welfare program that provides medical care assistance to the indigent and medically indigent. Medicaid is a healthcare financing program for low-income people. There are federal guidelines for which services are covered. Enrollment guidelines are based on state and territorial government guidelines. The program is funded jointly by both state and federal contributions (EBRI 1991).

MEDICAL LOSS RATIO–The ratio between the cost to deliver medical care and the amount of money that a plan receives. Insurance companies often have a medical loss ratio of 92 percent or more; tightly managed HMOs may have medical loss ratios of 75 to 85 percent, although the overhead (or administrative cost ratio) is concomitantly higher (Menkin 1999).

MEDICAL SAVINGS ACCOUNT (MSA)–A health insurance option consisting of a high-deductible insurance policy and a tax-advantaged savings account. Individuals pay for their own healthcare up to the annual deductible by withdrawing from the savings account or paying out of pocket. A catastrophic insurance policy pays for most or all costs of covered services once the high deductible is met (PPRC 1996B).

MEDICAL SAVINGS ACCOUNT OPTION–Beginning in January 1999, up to 390,000 beneficiaries will have the choice (on a demonstration basis ending January 1, 2003) of enrolling in a Medical Savings Account (MSA) option. Under this option, beneficiaries would obtain high-deductible health policies that pay for at least all Medicare-covered items and services after an enrollee meets the annual deductible of up to $6,000. The difference between the premiums for such high-deductible policies and the applicable Medicare+Choice premium amount would be placed into an account for the beneficiary to use in meeting his or her deductible expenses (HCFA 1997B).

MEDICARE–Title XVIII of the Social Security Amendments of 1965; federal/Social Security insurance program that provides medical care assistance to elderly and disabled individuals (NCHSR 1979).

MEDICARE+CHOICE–Part C of Medicare. Medicare pays approved managed care plans to cover the services under Part A and Part B, usually combined with other supplemental services.

MEDICARE COST CONTRACT–is an agreement between an HMO and HCFA that provides health services to plan members based on reasonable cost. The plan receives an initial capitated amount and is audited at the end of the contract to determine the final rate that the plan should have been paid (AMCRA Foundation 1994).

MEDICARE CURRENT BENEFICIARY SURVEY (MCBS)–A longitudinal survey administered by HCFA that provides information on specific aspects of beneficiary access, utilization of services, expenditures, health insurance coverage, satisfaction with care, health status, physical functioning, and demographic information.

MEDICARE HEALTH CARE PREPAYMENT PLAN (HCPP)–Payment is received for Medicare Part B at a reasonable prepaid cost. HCPPs are distinguished from Medicare+Choice plans because HCPPs only partially cover Medicare benefits (AMCRA Foundation 1994).

MEDICARE MANAGED CARE–A method used to deliver health services and to pay hospitals and physicians caring for Medicare beneficiaries. This method attempts to control or coordinate the use of services to contain expenditures, improve quality, or both. It always involves beneficiaries making a choice to enroll in an alternative to traditional fee-for-service Medicare. The alternatives have a defined network of hospitals and physicians (NCHSR 1979), administrative systems for utilization management and quality assessment and improvement (HCFA 1982), and financial incentives for enrollees to use the network of hospitals and physicians (DHHS 1983).

MEDICARE RISK CONTRACT–An agreement between an HMO (or CMP) and HCFA requiring the plan to provide, at a minimum, all Medicare-covered services to eligible Medicare enrollees for a fixed monthly payment from the government, along with a monthly premium from the enrollee. The HMO is then liable for all covered services regardless of their extent or expense (AMCRA Foundation 1994).

MEDICARE SELECT–A type of Medigap policy in conjunction with a preferred-provider network. Enrollees using the preferred network have Medigap coverage. Enrollees using nonpreferred providers face Medicare cost sharing—that is, Medicare SELECT provides normal reimbursement for out-of-network usage (AMCRA Foundation 1994).

MEDICARE SUPPLEMENT–Sometimes called Medigap, these policies ensure that a health plan will pay a policyholder's coinsurance, deductible, and co-payments and will provide additional coverage for services not covered by Medicare, up to a preset amount. A supplemental health insurance policy designed to supplement Medicare. All insurers are required to offer only ten standard policies beginning with a basic policy that only pays for catastrophic expenses (AMCRA Foundation 1994).

MEDPAC (MEDICARE PAYMENT ADVISORY COMMISSION)–An independent federal body that advises the U.S. Congress on issues affecting the Medicare program (www.medpac.gov).

MEMBER MONTHS–The unit of volume measurement used by managed care plans to count the total number of months of coverage for each plan member. Each member month is the equivalent of one member for whom the managed care plan is paid for one month's premium income. Member months accumulate for year-to-date statistical purposes (Menkin 1999).

MORAL HAZARD–Occurs when the insured experiences higher health costs when there is insurance coverage than when it is absent.

MOST-FAVORED-NATION (MFN) CLAUSE–A contractual agreement between a provider and a payer stating that the provider will automatically provide the payer the best discount of any it provides anyone else (Menkin 1999).

NETWORK MODEL HMO–An HMO that contracts with several different medical groups, often at capitated rates. Groups may use different methods to pay their physicians (PPRC 1996B). See Group Model HMO, HMO, IPA, Staff Model HMO.

OPEN ENROLLMENT–A period when new subscribers may elect to enroll in a health insurance plan or prepaid group practice. In the Medicare+Choice program, a period of time each year that a Medicare beneficiary may join a Medicare managed care plan. In the Health Maintenance Organization Act of 1973 (P.L. 93–222), the term refers to periodic opportunities for the general public, on a first-come first-served basis, to join an HMO (U.S. House of Representatives 1976).

OPPORTUNITY COST–Estimate of foregone value that might otherwise have been achieved as a result of an alternative use of a resource (University of Pittsburgh Medical Center 1995).

OUTCOMES–What happens to a person as a result of healthcare. Outcomes include measures of the individual's health status and quality of life (or health-related quality of life), as well as numerous other measures such as presence or absence of disease, readmission to hospital, repeat surgery, and death (Institute of Medicine 1994).

OUTCOMES MEASUREMENT–The process of systematically tracking a patient's clinical treatment and responses to that treatment using generally accepted outcomes measures or quality indicators such as mortality, morbidity, disability, functional status, recovery, and patient satisfaction (Menkin 1999).

OUTCOMES RESEARCH–A specialized branch of research that attempts to identify and develop standards for severity-adjusted clinical outcomes of medical service for large groups of patients (Menkin 1999).

OUT-OF-AREA BENEFITS–Benefits, usually limited to emergency services, that an HMO provides to its members when they are outside the HMO's service area. Most managed care plans specify that out-of-area emergency care services will be provided and covered until the plan member can be returned to the HMO's service area for medical management of the case (Menkin 1999).

OUT-OF-NETWORK SERVICES–Healthcare services received by a plan member from a noncontracted provider. Reimbursement is usually lower when a member goes out of network (Menkin 1999).

PANEL SIZE–The number of patients served by a physician or physician group. If the panel is greater than 25,000 patients, then the physician group is not considered to be at substantial financial risk because the risk is spread over the large number of patients. Stop-loss and beneficiary surveys would not be required.

PART A OF MEDICARE (Hospital Insurance Program)–Pays providers directly and covers inpatient hospital care with a large deductible and further cost sharing over 60 days. Part A also covers skilled nursing facility care following a hospital stay, home health care, and hospice care.

PART B OF MEDICARE (Supplemental Medical Insurance Program)–Has a monthly beneficiary premium and pays providers directly. Part B covers physician and other medical services, outpatient hospital care, ambulatory surgical services, laboratory services, outpatient mental health services, and some preventive services with a deductible, and coinsurance of 20 percent for most services.

PART C OF MEDICARE (Medicare+Choice)–Pays approved managed care plans to cover the services under Part A and Part B, usually combined with other supplemental services.

PARTIAL CAPITATION–An insurance arrangement wherein the payment made by a health plan to a provider is a combination of a capitated (per-member-per-month) amount and payment is made on the basis of actual use of services; the proportion specified by contract for these components determine the insurance risk faced by the provider (PPRC 1996B).

PAYMENT RATE–The total amount paid for each unit of service rendered by a healthcare provider, including both the amount covered by the insurer and the consumer's cost sharing; sometimes referred to as payment level. Also used to refer to capitation payments to health plans (PPRC 1996B).

PEER REVIEW ORGANIZATION (PRO)–The name previously given to an organization contracting with HCFA to review the medical necessity and quality of care provided to Medicare beneficiaries. Now called Quality Improving Organization (PPRC 1996B).

PERFORMANCE MEASURE–A specific measure of how well a health plan does in providing health services to its enrolled population. Can be used as an indicator of quality. Examples include percentage of diabetics receiving annual referrals for eye care, screening mammography rate, and percentage of enrollees indicating satisfaction with care (PPRC 1996B).

PHARMACEUTICAL BENEFIT MANAGEMENT COMPANY (PBM)–Large pharmaceutical marketing enterprises that focus on purchasing pharmaceuticals at reduced prices from manufacturers and offering them at discounted prices to large employer health plans and hospitals (Menkin 1999).

PHARMACOECONOMICS–Application of health economics to pharmaceuticals. As with other health economic analyses, pharmacoeconomic analysis should assess all relevant costs and benefits, not merely acquisition or administration costs (University of Pittsburgh Medical Center 1995).

PHYSICIAN GROUP–A partnership, association, corporation, individual practice association (IPA), or other group that shares costs and distributes income from the practice among members.

PHYSICIAN-HOSPITAL ORGANIZATION (PHO)–A legal entity formed and owned by one or more hospitals and physician groups to obtain payer contracts and to further mutual interests. Physicians maintain ownership of their practices while agreeing to accept managed care patients under the terms of the PHO agreement. The PHO serves as a negotiating, contracting, and marketing unit (United HealthCare Corporation 1994).

PHYSICIAN INCENTIVE PLAN–Any compensation arrangement at any contracting level between a managed care organization (MCO) and a physician or physician group that may directly or indirectly have the effect of reducing or limiting services furnished to Medicare or Medicaid enrollees in the MCO.

PING-PONGING–The practice of passing a patient from one physician to another in a health program for unnecessary cursory examinations so that the program can charge the patient's third party for a physician visit to each physician. The practice and term originated and is most common in Medicaid mills (U.S. House of Representatives 1976).

POINT-OF-SERVICE (POS) OPTION–Offered by some traditional HMOs and PPOs to its enrollees to allow for out-of-network or "out-of-plan" coverage, but with economic incentives to enrollees to use network providers, such as lower copayments or coinsurance for their use. POS options are generally more expensive for purchasers (employers, etc.) of healthcare coverage (AMCRA Foundation 1994).

POINT-OF-SERVICE (POS) PLANS–Similar to PPOs in that they are characterized by a network of providers whose services are available to enrollees at a lower cost than the services of non-network providers. The difference is that whereas PPO enrollees are free to contact network specialists at their discretion, a POS participant must first receive authorization from a primary care physician (gatekeeper) to receive full benefits. Also, the out-of-network benefits of a POS plan are typically less than those of a PPO (AMCRA Foundation 1994).

PORTABILITY–The requirement that insurers waive any preexisting condition exclusion for someone who was previously covered through other insurance as recently as 30 to 90 days earlier (PPRC 1996B). See Preexisting Conditions.

PRACTICE GUIDELINES–Explicit statements about the benefits, risks, and costs of particular courses of medical action based on the medical literature and expert judgment. Intended to help practitioners, patients, and others make decisions about appropriate healthcare for specific clinical conditions (PPRC 1996B).

PREEXISTING CONDITION–A physical or mental condition that existed prior to the effective date of the person's insurance (NCHSR 1979).

PREEXISTING CONDITION EXCLUSION–A practice of some health insurers to deny coverage to individuals for a certain period, for example, six months, for health conditions that already exist when coverage is initiated (PPRC 1996B). See Portability.

PREFERRED PROVIDER ORGANIZATION (PPO)–A healthcare benefit arrangement designed to supply services at a reasonable cost by providing incentives to its enrollees to use designated healthcare providers (those that contract with the PPO at a discount), while also providing a lower level of coverage for services rendered by healthcare providers who are not part of the PPO network. Financial incentives for individuals to use preferred providers include lower copayments or coinsurance, and maximum limits on out-of-pocket costs for in-network use. Unlike with HMOs, out-of-network usage is allowed by PPOs, though at a higher cost to the enrollee.

Most PPOs involve an arrangement between a panel of providers (physicians, hospitals, and other healthcare professionals) and the purchasers of care, for example, employers or insurance companies. The panel of preferred providers agrees to a specified fee schedule in return for preferred status, and is required to comply with certain utilization review (UR) guidelines.

PPOs are not insurers. They generally do not assume any financial risk for arranging medical services. In many cases, the risk is assumed by self-insured employers or by another underwriter (AMCRA Foundation 1994).

PREMIUM–An amount paid periodically to purchase health insurance benefits (PPRC 1996B).

PREPAYMENT–Inconsistently used, sometimes synonymous with insurance, sometimes it refers to any payment ahead of time to a provider for anticipated services (such as an expectant mother paying in advance for maternity care). It is sometimes distinguished from insurance as referring to payment to organizations (such as HMOs), which, unlike an insurance company, take responsibility for arranging for and providing needed services as well as paying for them.

PRIMARY CARE CASE MANAGEMENT (PCCM)–A state-operated program wherein primary care providers contract directly with the state for the provision or coordination of medical services for Medicaid recipients. A key component of most programs is the payment of a case management fee to the primary care provider as compensation for coordination of care (Menkin 1999).

PRINCIPAL DIAGNOSIS–The condition established, after study, to be chiefly responsible for occasioning the admission of the patient to the hospital for care (DHHS 1983).

PRODUCTIVITY–The ratio of outputs (goods and services produced) to inputs (resources used in production). Increased productivity implies that an organization is producing more output with the same resources of the same output with fewer resources.

PROFESSIONAL ALL-INCLUSIVE CARE FOR THE ELDERLY (PACE)–A program administered by HCFA that uses managed care to serve frail elderly persons who have been assessed as eligible for nursing home placement and are, for the most part, dually eligible for Medicare and Medicaid. The program provides adult day care and case management in addition to Medicare and Medicaid benefits to help the program participant maintain independent living in the community, all for one combined Medicare-Medicaid payment.

PROFESSIONAL LIABILITY INSURANCE (PLI)–The insurance physicians purchase to help protect themselves from the financial risks associated with medical liability claims (PPRC 1996B).

PROFILING–Expressing a pattern of practice as a rate—some measure of utilization (costs or services) or outcome (functional status, morbidity, or mortality) aggregated over time for a defined population of patients—to compare with other practice patterns. May be done for physician practices, health plans, or geographic areas (PPRC 1996B).

PROSPECTIVE PAYMENT SYSTEM (PPS) OR REIMBURSEMENT–Any method of paying hospitals or other health programs in which amounts or rates of payment are established in advance for the coming year and the programs are paid these amounts regardless of the costs they actually incur (U.S. House of Representatives 1976).

PROSPECTIVE REVIEW–Review of necessity for hospitalization prior to admission to determine if it is medically necessary and if the hospital is the appropriate level of care.

PROVIDER SPONSORED ORGANIZATION (PSO)–A public or private entity established by healthcare providers, which provide a substantial proportion of healthcare items and services directly through affiliated providers who share, directly or indirectly, substantial financial risk (HCFA 1997B).

PRUDENT BUYER–The concept that Medicare should not reimburse a provider for a cost that is not a reasonable cost because it is in excess of the amount that a prudent and cost-conscious buyer would be expected to pay (U.S. House of Representatives 1976).

QUALITY-ADJUSTED LIFE YEAR (QALY)–A common method for estimating the value of alternative outcomes in terms of a common nonmonetary unit, derived from the expressed preferences of patients for alternative states of health. QALYs integrate the quality of life experienced with the outcome obtained as a result of an intervention. States associated with decreased functional status are weighted less than states with improved function (University of Pittsburgh Medical Center 1995).

QUALITY ASSESSMENT–Measurement of technical and interpersonal aspects of healthcare including access to and outcomes of that care (Institute of Medicine 1994).

QUALITY ASSURANCE–A formal, systematic process to improve quality of care that includes monitoring quality, identifying inadequacies in delivery of care, and correcting those inadequacies (PPRC 1997).

QUALITY IMPROVEMENT–Effort to improve the level of performance of a key process, which involves measuring the level of current performance, finding ways to improve that performance, and implementing new and better methods (Institute of Medicine 1994).

QUALITY-IMPROVING ORGANIZATION–Medicare contractors in each state that engage hospitals and other providers in projects that improve the quality of care for selected diseases or disorders affecting the Medicare population.

QUALITY OF LIFE–Assessment of patient functional status. A variety of methods may be used to estimate quantitatively such outcomes as cognitive, psychological, physical, role, social function, level of pain, and general well-being. Quality-of-life scales may be generic or disease specific (same measures used regardless of disease) (University of Pittsburgh Medical Center 1995).

REASONABLE COST–In processing claims for HI benefits, intermediaries use HCFA guidelines to determine the reasonable cost. The cost is based on the actual cost of providing such services and excludes any costs that are unnecessary in the efficient delivery of services covered by the health insurance program (DHHS 1983).

REFERRAL SERVICES–Any specialty, inpatient, outpatient, or laboratory services that are ordered or arranged, but not furnished directly.

REINSURANCE–The practice of one insurance company buying insurance from a second company for the purpose of protecting itself against part or all of the losses it might incur in the process of honoring the claims of its policyholders. The original company is called the ceding company; the second is called the assuming company or reinsurer (Menkin 1999).

RELIGIOUS FRATERNAL BENEFIT SOCIETY PLANS–As defined by the BBA of 1997 with regard to Medicare+Choice, plans that may restrict enrollment to members of the church, convention, or group with which the society is affiliated. Payments to such plans may be adjusted as appropriate to take into account the actuarial characteristics and experience of plan enrollees (HCFA 1997B).

RESERVES–Balance sheet accounts set up to report the liabilities faced by an insurance company under outstanding insurance policies. The company sets the amount of reserves in accordance with its own estimates, state laws, and recommendations of supervisory officials and national organizations. Reserves, while estimated, are all obligated amounts and have four principal components: (1) reserves for known liabilities not yet paid, (2) reserves for losses incurred but unreported, (3) reserves for future benefits, and (4) other reserves for various special purposes including contingency reserves for unforeseen circumstances (U.S. House of Representatives 1976).

RESOURCE-BASED RELATIVE-VALUE SCALE–A coded listing of physician or other professional services using units that indicate the relative value of the various services they perform: taking into account the time, skill, and overhead cost required for each service, but not usually considering the relative cost effectiveness of the services, the relative need, or demand for them, or their importance to people's health. Appropriate conversion factors are used to translate the abstract units in the scale to dollar fees for each service. Other relative-value scales have been based on historical charges.

RETROSPECTIVE REIMBURSEMENT–Payment to providers by a third-party carrier for costs or charges actually incurred by subscribers in a previous time period. This is the method of payment used under Medicare Part B (U.S. House of Representatives 1976).

RETROSPECTIVE REVIEW–Review of care for quality and appropriateness after it has been given.

RETURN ON INVESTMENT–Income for a period of time divided by total assets. This is frequently used to judge management and the feasibility of product or service lines (Menkin 1999).

RIDER–An amendment that modifies the terms of the group contract or certificates of insurance. It may increase or decrease benefits, waive a condition or coverage, or in any other way amend the original contract (NCHSR 1979).

RISK ADJUSTER–A measure used to adjust payment made to a health plan on behalf of a group of enrollees to compensate for spending that is expected to be lower or higher than average, based on the health status or demographic characteristics of the enrollees (PPRC 1996B).

RISK MANAGEMENT–An extensive program of activities to identify risks, evaluate them, and take corrective action against any that may lead to patient or employee injury, property loss, or damage with resulting financial loss or legal liability (Menkin 1999).

RISK POOL–A pool of funds set aside by a managed care plan involved in a risk-sharing arrangement with providers. This pool is created by withholding a portion of provider fees to create an incentive to control utilization and to cover any unexpected costs. Funds remaining in the pool after a set period of time are distributed to the providers (Menkin 1999).

RISK SELECTION–Any situation in which health plans differ in the health risk associated with their enrollees because of enrollment choices made by the plans or enrollees—that is, where one health plan's expected costs differ from another's due to underlying differences in their enrolled populations (PPRC 1996B).

SELF-INSURED HEALTH PLAN–Employer-provided health insurance in which the employer, rather than an insurer, is at risk for its employees' medical expenses (PPRC 1996B).

SENSITIVITY ANALYSIS–Method to assess the influence of changes in assumptions and estimates over the range of plausible values on results and conclusions. Because all data are characterized by some degree of uncertainty, sensitivity analysis is required of every economic analysis. Sensitivity analysis demonstrates the dependence or independence of the findings and conclusions on the uncertainty of the data estimates (i.e., whether or not the conclusions are altered as a result of which plausible variable or assumption value is used). Sensitivity analysis also identifies the critical variables that drive the analysis and for which the greatest precision is required and identifies those critical variables that are priorities for future research (University of Pittsburgh Medical Center 1995).

SERVICE BENEFITS–HMOs, federal employee plans, Blue Cross, and some Blue Shield Plans generally provide service benefits. A service benefit implies that regardless of how the cost or price of a service varies during the term or the contract, the service will still be provided with no additional charge (NCHSR 1979).

SOCIAL HEALTH MAINTENANCE ORGANIZATION (SHMO)–HCFA demonstration project that expands the Medicare benefit package to reduce or slow functional impairment of frail beneficiaries. Additional covered services include nursing home, homemaker, transportation, drugs, and case management services (PPRC 1997).

STAFF MODEL HMO–An HMO in which physicians practice solely as employees of the HMO and usually are paid a salary (PPRC 1996B). See Group Model HMO, Health Maintenance Organization.

STATE BUY-IN–Term given to the process by which a state may provide supplementary medical insurance (SMI) coverage for its needy, eligible persons through an agreement with the federal government under which the state pays their premiums (DHHS 1983).

STOP-LOSS REINSURANCE–Reinsurance purchased by primary insurers to protect against excessive claims losses. Under this arrangement, reinsurance is written on an aggregate basis and the reinsurer pays all or a percentage of the primary insurer's claims losses above a cumulative annual amount. The stop-loss may apply to an entire health plan or to any single component (Menkin 1999).

SUBROGATION–The contractual right of a health plan to recover payments made to a member for healthcare costs after that member has received such payment of damages in a legal action. Subrogation differs from coordination of benefits in that the liability is shared under COB between parties on a contractual or legal basis, whereas subrogation assigns the rights to another party (Menkin 1999).

SUBSTANTIAL FINANCIAL RISK–An incentive arrangement that places the physician or physician group at risk for amounts beyond the risk threshold if the risk is based on the use or costs of referral services. The risk threshold is 25 percent.

SUPPLEMENTAL MEDICAL INSURANCE (SMI)–SMI (also known as Part B) is a voluntary insurance program that provides benefits for physician and other medical services in accordance with the provisions of Title XVIII of the Social Security Act for aged, blind, and disabled individuals who fall below specified income and resource thresholds and who elect to enroll under such a program (DHHS 1983).

SUPPLEMENTAL SECURITY INCOME–A federal income support program for low-income disabled, aged, and blind persons. Eligibility for the monthly cash payments is based on the individual's current status without regard to previous work or contributions (PPRC 1996B).

SUPPLIER–A provider of healthcare services, other than a practitioner, that is permitted to bill under Medicare Part B. Suppliers include independent laboratories, durable medical equipment providers, ambulance services, orthotists, prosthetists, and portable x-ray providers (PPRC 1996B).

TAX DEFERRAL–Tax treatment granted to qualified retirement plans where taxes are not imposed when benefits are accrued (under a defined-benefit plan) or contributions are made (under a defined-contribution plan), but instead are imposed when benefits are paid to participants in cash (EBRI 1991).

TOTAL QUALITY MANAGEMENT–A philosophy and system for achieving constant performance improvement at every level. Key elements of TQM include companywide CQI efforts, self-directing work teams, employee involvement programs, flexible service delivery processes, quick changeover and adaptability, customer focus, supplier integration, and production cycle time reduction. Many healthcare organizations implement TQM programs as a competitive strategy (Menkin 1999).

TRIPLE OPTION PLAN–A type of managed care plan that allows members to choose any of three service options—HMO, PPO, or indemnity plan—each time they require medical care. A PCP manages accountability for care (Menkin 1999).

UB-92–Standard hospital discharge claims form used by Medicare and most other payers. Includes nine diagnosis fields and six procedure code fields to create the uniform bill (UB) 92.

UNBUNDLING–Separately packaging units that might otherwise be packaged together. For claims processing, that includes providers billing separately for healthcare services that should be combined according to industry standards or commonly accepted coding practices (United HealthCare Corporation 1994).

UNDERWRITING–In insurance, the process of selecting, classifying, evaluating, and assuming risks according to their insurability. Its fundamental purpose is to make sure that the group insured has the same probability of loss and probable amount of loss, within reasonable limits, as the universe on which premium rates were based (U.S. House of Representatives 1976).

U.S. PER-CAPITA COST–The national average cost per Medicare beneficiary, calculated annually by HCFA's Office of the Actuary (PPRC 1996B). See Adjusted per-Capita Cost, Medicare Risk Contract.

UTILIZATION REVIEW (UR) AND UTILIZATION MANAGEMENT (UM)–A formal assessment of the medical necessity, efficiency, or appropriateness of healthcare services and treatment plans on a prospective, concurrent, or retrospective basis (United HealthCare Corporation 1994).

UTILIZATION REVIEW ORGANIZATIONS (UROs)–are external reviewers who assess the medical appropriateness of a suggested course of treatment for a particular patient, thereby providing the patient and payer increased assurance of the appropriateness, value, and quality of healthcare services being provided. The most common form of UR, preadmission certification, is requested by the patient's physician for approval of any nonemergency admission to an inpatient facility. Other techniques include concurrent review, second surgical opinion, discharge planning, outpatient certification, and case management (AMCRA Foundation 1994).

VARIABLE COSTS–Costs that are incurred and whose consumption is volume-dependent. Labor and disposable supplies are examples of variable costs (University of Pittsburgh Medical Center 1995).

WITHHOLD–A percentage of payments or set dollar amounts that are deducted from the service fee, capitation, or salary payment, and that may or may not be returned, depending on specific predetermined factors like productivity and utilization (Menkin 1999).

WRAPAROUND COVERAGE–Method of integrating payment for health benefits provided by one policy with another policy without duplicating the primary coverage. The wraparound coverage policy normally pays for deductibles and coinsurance, as well as benefits not covered by the primary policy (PPRC 1996B).

COMMON ACRONYMS

AAHP	American Association of Health Plans
AAMC	Association of American Medical Colleges
AAPCC	Adjusted-Average Per-Capita Cost
AAPPO	American Association of Preferred Provider Organizations
AARP	American Association of Retired Persons
ACG	Ambulatory Care Groups
ACR	Adjusted Community Rate
ADA	Americans with Disabilities Act
ADL	Activities of Daily Living
AGPA	American Group Practice Association
AHA	American Hospital Association
AHCRQ	Agency for Health Care Research and Quality
AIDS	Acquired Immunodeficiency Syndrome
ALOS	Average Length of Stay
AMA	American Medical Association
ANSI	American National Standards Institute
APC	Ambulatory Patient Classifications
APG	Ambulatory Patient Groups
APR	Adjusted Payment Rate
ASC	Ambulatory Surgical Center
ASO	Administrative Services Only Contract
BBA	Balanced Budget Act of 1997 (See Legislation Section)
BC or BX	Blue Cross
BC/BS	Blue Cross/Blue Shield
BLS	Bureau of Labor Statistics
BMAD	Part B Medicare Annual Data Files
BS	Blue Shield
BSF	Benefits Stabilization Fund
CAHPS	Consumer Assessment of Health Plans Survey
CBO	Congressional Budget Office
CBS	Medicare Current Beneficiary Survey
CC	Complication and/or Comorbidity
CHAMPUS	Civilian Health and Medical Program of the Uniformed Services

CHIRI	Consumer Health Information Research Institute
CM	Case Manager
CMI	Case Mix Index
CMP	Competitive Medical Plan
CMSA	Consolidated Metropolitan Statistical Area
COB	Coordination of Benefits
COBRA	Consolidated Omnibus Reconciliation Act of 1985
COE	Center of Excellence
CPI	Consumer Price Index
CPI-U	Consumer Price Index—All Urban Consumers
CPS	Current Population Survey
CPT	Current Procedural Terminology
CQI	Continuous Quality Improvement
CRS	Congressional Research Service
DCG	Diagnostic Cost Groups
DEMPAQ	Developing and Evaluating Methods to Promote Quality
DHHS	U.S. Department of Health and Human Services
DI	Disability Insurance
DME	Durable Medical Equipment
DRG	Diagnosis Related Group
DSH	Disproportionate-Share Hospital
DUR	Drug Utilization Review
ECF	Extended Care Facility
ECI	Employment Cost Index
EKG	Electrocardiogram
EM	Evaluation and Management
EOB	Explanation of Benefits
EOC	Explanation of Coverage
EOMB	Explanation of Medicare Benefits ("This is not a bill")
ERISA	Employment Retirement Insurance Security Act of 1974
ESRD	End-Stage Renal Disease
FACCT	Foundation for Accountability
FAS	Financial Accounting Standard
FASB	Financial Accounting Standards Board
FDA	Food and Drug Administration
FEHBP	Federal Employees Health Benefits Program
FFS	Fee-for-Service
FQHC	Federally Qualified Health Center
FQHMO	Federally Qualified Health Maintenance Organization
FY	Fiscal Year
GAO	U.S. General Accounting Office
GDP	Gross Domestic Product
GHAA	Group Health Association of America (now called AAHP)
GME	Graduate Medical Education

HCFA	Health Care Financing Administration
HCPCS	HCFA Common Procedure Coding System
HCPP	Health Care Prepayment Plan
HEDIS	Health Plan Employer Data and Information Set
HHA	Home Health Agency
HI	Hospital Insurance (Part A of Medicare)
HIAA	Health Insurance Association of America
HIV	Human Immunodeficiency Virus
HMO	Health Maintenance Organization
IADL	Instrumental Activities of Daily Living
IBNR	Incurred But Not Reported
ICD-9-CM	International Classification of Diseases, ninth revision, clinical modifications (for use in the United States)
ICF	Intermediate Care Facility
ICU	Intensive Care Unit
IDS	Integrated Delivery System
IME	Indirect Medical Education
IMG	International Medical Graduate
IOM	Institute of Medicine
IPA	Independent Practice Association
IRS	Internal Revenue Service
JCAHO	Joint Commission on Accreditation of Health Care Organizations
MAC	Maximum Allowable Cost
MCBS	Medicare Current Beneficiary Survey
MCO	Managed Care Organization
MedPAC	Medicare Payment Advisory Commission
MEDTEP	Medical Treatment Effectiveness Program (of AHCRQ)
MHCA	Managed Health Care Association
MIG	Medicare Insured Group Demonstration
MIP	Managed Indemnity Plan
MIS	Management Information System
MMIS	Medicaid Management Information System
MPCC	Medicare Per-Capita Cost
MSA	Medical Savings Account
MSG	Multispecialty Group
MSO	Management Service Organization
NAHDO	National Association of Health Data Organizations
NAHMOR	National Association of HMO Regulators
NAIC	National Association of Insurance Commissioners
NAM	National Association of Manufacturers
NAMCS	National Ambulatory Medical Care Survey
NCHS	National Center for Health Statistics
NCQA	National Committee for Quality Assurance

NDC	National Drug Code
NGA	National Governors' Association
NHIS	National Health Interview Survey
NHSC	National Health Service Corps
NIH	National Institutes of Health, HHS
NLM	National Library of Medicine, HHS
NMES	National Medical Expenditure Survey
NMIHS	National Maternal and Infant Health Survey
NP	Nurse Practitioner
OACT	Office of the Actuary, HCFA, HHS
OBRA	Omnibus Budget Reconciliation Act of 1986
OIG	Office of the Inspector General, DHHS
OMB	Office of Management and Budget
OOP	Out-of-Pocket Payments
OPD	Outpatient Department
OPM	Office of Personnel Management
OTC	Over the Counter (drugs)
PA	Physician's Assistant
PACE	Program for All-Inclusive Care for the Elderly
PAR	Participating Physician and Supplier Program
PCCM	Primary Care Case Management
PCN	Primary Care Network
PCP	Primary Care Provider (or Physician)
PGP	Prepaid Group Practice
PHCO	Physician-Hospital-Community Organization
PHO	Physician-Hospital Organization
PMPM	Per Member Per Month (Capitation)
PORT	Patient Outcomes Research Team (in MEDTEP Program)
POS	Point-of-Service
PPO	Preferred Provider Organization
PPRC	Physician Payment Review Commission (now defunct; see MedPAC)
PPS	Prospective Payment System
PRO	Peer Review Organization
PSO	Provider Sponsored Organization
QA/QI	Quality Assurance/Quality Improvement
QIO	Quality Improving Organization
QISMC	Quality Improvement Standards for Managed Care
QMB	Qualified Medicare Beneficiary
RBRVS	Resource-Based Relative-Value Scale
RFP	Request for Proposals
RVS	Relative Value Scale
RVU	Relative Value Unit
SCP	Specialty Care Provider (or Physician)

SHMO	Social Health Maintenance Organization
SIPP	Survey of Income and Program Participation
SLMB	Specified Low-Income Medicare Beneficiary
SMI	Supplementary Medical Insurance (Part B of Medicare)
SMS	Socioeconomic Monitoring System, AMA
SNF	Skilled Nursing Facility
SSA	Social Security Administration
SSI	Supplemental Security Income
TEFRA	Tax Equity and Fiscal Responsibility Act of 1982
TPA	Third-Party Administrator
TQM	Total Quality Management
UB-92	Uniform Billing Form (1992)
UM	Utilization Management
UPIN	Universal Physician Identification Number
UR	Utilization Review
URAC	Utilization Review Accreditation Commission
URO	Utilization Review Organization
USPCC	United States Per-Capita Cost
VA	Department of Veterans Affairs
WEDI	Workgroup for Electronic Data Interchange

MEDICARE LEGISLATION

Balanced Budget Act of 1997—This legislation enacts the most significant changes to the Medicare and Medicaid Programs since their inception 30 years ago. Additionally, it expands the services provided by HCFA through the new Child Health Insurance Program (Title XXI). These changes:

- extended the life of the Medicare Trust Fund and reduced Medicare spending;
- increased healthcare options available to America's seniors;
- improved benefits for staying healthy;
- fought Medicare fraud and abuse; and
- looked at ways to help Medicare work well in the future.

Consolidated Omnibus Budget Reconciliation Act of 1985 (**COBRA**)—Created Medicare's Physician Payment Review Commission.

Deficit Reduction Act of 1984 (**DEFRA**)—Expanded Medicaid eligibility and made Medicare the secondary payer for covered health expenses of employees aged 65–69.

Employee Retirement Income Security Act of 1974—Established certain rules governing self-insured health plans whose employer meets certain requirements. Affected plans are exempt from state insurance regulation.

Health Insurance Portability and Accountability Act of 1996—This law improves access and portability of health insurance, grants broad new authority to the federal government to investigate and prosecute healthcare fraud and abuse, and provides for implementation of standards for the electronic transmission of healthcare information. *Health Care Portability and Accessibility*: individuals and families can have only one 12-month preexisting condition exclusion imposed on them with prohibition of pregnancy, newborns, and genetic testing as conditions for exclusion. *Medical Savings Accounts*: allowable for self-employed and individuals working at firms with two to 50 employees who purchase a high-deductible health plan. This is a four-year trial that is limited to 750,000 enrollees. *Self-Employed Insurance Deduction*: gradually increases the tax deduction for health insurance expenses from 30 to 80 percent by 2002 for the self-employed. *Long-Term Care Insurance*:

employer contributions to long-term care plans are nontaxable. *Preventing Health Care Fraud and Abuse*: the law establishes three programs—Fraud and Abuse Control Program, Medicare Integrity Program, and Beneficiary Incentive Program. These programs are aimed at reining-in fraud and abuse. *Administrative Simplification*: encourages standards for electronic transmission of health information to improve efficiency and effectiveness of the Medicare and Medicaid programs, as well as standards for security and privacy of information.

Health Maintenance Organization Act Amendment of 1988—Relaxed some requirements of the 1973 HMO Act by making it easier for employers to negotiate rates and coverage. Repealed the requirement that an employer that offers health insurance and has more than 25 employees must offer the dual option of enrollment in a federally qualified HMO at the request of such an HMO.

Health Maintenance Organization Act of 1973—P.L. 93-222, enacted during the Nixon administration to establish new federal standards for health plans, called Health Maintenance Organizations (HMOs) with federal oversight.

Medicare Catastrophic Coverage Act of 1988—Increased Medicare benefits to provide catastrophic health coverage and prescription drug benefits; expanded Medicaid benefits for pregnant women, children, and in-community spouses of elderly in nursing homes. (Medicare provisions were repealed in 1989.)

Medicare+Choice—This legislation enables HCFA to contract with more types of managed care and fee-for-service plans (e.g., coordinated-care plans like HMOs, PPOs, and PSOs; private fee-for-service; religious fraternal benefit society plans; and medical savings account options (MSAs). These different types of contractors are called Medicare+Choice or "Medicare Part C." (Note that the following may be different for MSAs.)

No participating plan may discriminate and all must accept any beneficiary on a first-come first-served basis. All marketing materials must be reviewed by HCFA. All services currently covered by Medicare must be covered by the Choice providers (except for hospice care). Plans must also keep the beneficiary informed with information on benefits, exclusions, access, providers, preauthorization, grievance, appeals, and costs, among others. Medicare+Choice plans must also establish a quality assurance program, establish grievance, appeals, and coverage determination procedures; ensure patient confidentiality; and maintain advance directives.

Medicare+Choice plans will be reimbursed by the government under capitated PMPM rates based on a blend of the area-specific rate and the national rate (90/10 in 1998 to 50/50 in 2003). Premiums among enrollees must be uniform, and the maximum out-of-pocket expenses cannot exceed those under Medicare fee-for-service. Plans must be state licensed as a risk-bearing entity that can offer health insurance and must assume the full financial risk for Medicare coverage of their enrollees. A minimum of 5,000 urban enrollees or 1,500 rural enrollees must be maintained. See bill for more information (HCFA 1997).

Omnibus Budget Reconciliation Act of 1986 (**OBRA '86**)—Made changes to Medicare reimbursement to physicians and hospitals.

Omnibus Budget Reconciliation Act of 1989 (**OBRA '89**)—Created the RBRVS fee schedule for physician payment under Medicare.

Omnibus Budget Reconciliation Act of 1990 (**OBRA '90**)—Required that states pay Medicare premiums and cost sharing for QMBs, Medicare beneficiaries with incomes below 100 percent of the federal poverty level; all states must pay Part B premiums (not Part A or cost sharing) for beneficiaries with incomes below 110 percent of the poverty level in 1993 and below 120 percent in 1995 (Committee on Ways and Means 1994).

Omnibus Budget Reconciliation Act of 1990 (**OBRA '90**) (**Budget Agreement**)—Established Medicare SELECT for allowing PPOs to enter the Medicare market. Required the National Association of Insurance Commissioners to develop rules for Medigap insurance that would permit only ten standard policies to be sold. HCFA required to regulate the states and their oversight of the Medigap market.

Retirement Benefits Bankruptcy Protection Act of 1988—Required companies that file for reorganization under Chapter 11 of the bankruptcy code to continue paying life and health insurance benefits to retirees. Such companies are prevented from modifying their plans unless they can prove it is necessary to do so to avoid liquidation.

Social Security Amendments of 1965—Enacted Medicare and Medicaid. Permitted half of expenses paid for medical insurance, not in excess of $150, to be deducted from taxable income.

Tax Equity and Fiscal Responsibility Act of 1982 (**TEFRA**)—Eliminated the separate $150 deduction for half of health insurance premiums and included health insurance premiums as medical expenses that may be deducted subject to the adjusted gross income floor. Limited deductions for medical expenses to amounts in excess of 5 percent of adjusted gross income.

Tax Reform Act of 1986—Established new nondiscrimination rules for health and welfare plans under Internal Revenue Code section 89 (subsequently repealed by Congress in 1989). Limited deductions for medical expenses to amounts in excess of 7.5 percent of adjusted gross income. Allowed a deduction for 25 percent of the amount paid for health insurance for self-employed individuals, spouses, and dependents.

INDEX

ABOUT THE AUTHOR

Louis F. Rossiter, Ph.D., wrote this book while he was professor of health economics for the graduate program in the Department of Health Administration at Virginia Commonwealth University, Medical College of Virginia (MCV) Campus, Richmond, Virginia.

In addition to his years of teaching and sponsored research at Virginia Commonwealth University, Dr. Rossiter was the first director of the Williamson Institute for Health Studies on the MCV Campus. He took a leave of absence (1989–1992) to serve as senior policy advisor to the Administrator of the Health Care Financing Administration, where he lead the policy development in the agency, especially related to managed care for Medicare and Medicaid.

Believing that the best economic research is a practical demonstration, Dr. Rossiter has been involved in evaluating or creating managed care initiatives for Medicare since 1983. Besides serving on the original expert panel to select the very first Medicare managed care plans in the Reagan administration, he was the coprincipal investigator of the national evaluations of the Medicare managed care experience in the 1980s and early 1990s. In both $3.2 million evaluations, conducted by the Williamson Institute with Mathematica Policy Research, he oversaw the study design of health outcomes for the elderly enrolled in Medicare HMOs. With other members of the study team, he has published numerous papers on the costs, quality, and impact of Medicare managed care on beneficiaries and health plans. In recognition of his knowledge as a health economist and evaluator of healthcare delivery systems, Dr. Rossiter was appointed by (then) Secretary Louis Sullivan, M.D., to the National Advisory Council for the Agency for Health Care Policy and Research, D.H.H.S. (1991–96).

Dr. Rossiter currently serves on the National Advisory Committee for the Robert Wood Johnson Foundation's Changes in Health Care Financing and Organization (HCFO) initiative. Combined with his over-fifty publications and numerous edited books, he brings a unique perspective of the economist who has studied and helped to manage Medicare managed care.

He is currently deputy secretary for Health and Human Resources, Commonwealth of Virginia.